In Search of Meaning

Thierry C. Pauchant and Associates

In Search of Meaning

Managing for the Health of Our Organizations, Our Communities, and the Natural World

Jossey-Bass Publishers • San Francisco

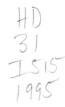

Substantial discounts on bulk quantities of Jossey-Bass books
are available to corporations, professional associations, and other
organizations. For details and discount information, contact the
special sales department at Jossey-Bass Inc., Publishers.
(415) 433-1740; Fax (415) 433-0499.

For sales outside the United States, please contact your local
Paramount Publishing International office.

Manufactured in the United States of America. Nearly all Jossey-Bass
books and jackets are printed on recycled paper that contains at least
50 percent recycled waste, including 10 percent postconsumer waste.
Many of our materials are also printed with vegetable-based inks;
during the printing process these inks emit fewer volatile organic
compounds (VOCs) than petroleum-based inks. VOCs contribute to
the formation of smog.

Excerpts on p. 132 from Shakespeare's *King Henry V* and *The Life and
Death of King Richard II* are reprinted by permission of Oxford University
Press.

Library of Congress Cataloging-in-Publication Data

In search of meaning : managing for the health of our organizations,
   our communities, and the natural world / Thierry C. Pauchant and
   associates. — 1st ed.
      p.   cm. — (The Jossey-Bass management series)
   Includes bibliographical references and index.
   ISBN 0-7879-0031-1
   1. Management.   2. Organizational behavior.   I. Pauchant, Thierry
C.   II. Series.
HD31.I515   1995
658—dc20   94-31010
                                                                 CIP

FIRST EDITION
HB Printing   10 9 8 7 6 5 4 3 2 1   *Code 94112*

The Jossey-Bass
Management Series

Consulting Editors
Organizations and Management

Warren Bennis
University of Southern California

Richard O. Mason
Southern Methodist University

Ian I. Mitroff
University of Southern California

Contents

Contents

Preface

The field of management is in crisis. The signs of this crisis are many: a lack of organizational performance, chronic unemployment, industrial disasters and pollution, and the overall difficulties encountered in change. Many managers and employees are also disillusioned by the premise that modern management principles can guarantee prosperity and peace. Further, many managers complain that academics do not produce the knowledge and tools necessary for addressing this crisis. While business schools currently struggle to modify their curricula, many so-called gurus flood the business community with what they believe to be magical solutions. Some call for a management revolution and top management's vision of excellence; others insist that management consists of one-minute actions or try to sell "portable" MBAs; still others urge their audience to adopt a "big bang" view of organizations; and managers struggle at work with "total quality" or "re-engineering," which, they are told, should bring back total competitiveness and total prosperity.

We do not propose gimmicky solutions in this book. Rather, we ponder deeply the causes of the crisis in management today. We believe that this crisis is not only economic but also existential; it is rooted in our most basic fears and hopes and goes far beyond considerations of competitiveness or productivity alone. The authors of *In Search of Meaning* share a common faith: the faith that courageously facing the crisis will help the men and women working in organizations discover potential solutions. As we argue in this book, a crisis need not be only negative. While the rush for magical solutions in a turbulent time is understandable, courageous human beings know better than to attempt to deny the very reality of this turbulence. A crisis can also be positive. Its painful experience can lead individuals to reflect on its nature and determine different actions on the basis of individual, collective, and organizational learning.

In this book, we attempt to respond to a comment being made in many organizations around the globe: "It just doesn't make sense anymore!" It is important to recognize that this statement does not merely imply that one can no longer make sense of one's work and one's organization. This lack of intellectual understanding is one of the subjects most talked about in current management books and also in organizations; it emphasizes notions such as complexity, paradox, turbulence, and uncertainty or—even more voguishly—the notion of chaos. However, to "make sense" also implies something more subjective and personal: it also means that one cannot any longer find meaning in one's activities. The desire to make sense poses not only the problem of *lack of understanding* but also the problem of *loss of meaning*.

Whether from Canada, France, Germany, or the United States, the authors of this book are all very conscious of the reality of this search for meaning in many organizations. Echoing Friedrich Nietzsche's warning in the nineteenth century of the rise of absurdity or Edmund Husserl's alarm in the 1930s of the coming crisis of Occidental humanity, today's cries of despair are audible in any number of organizations, if one is courageous enough to listen to them.

Perhaps what is new today is that one must literally plug one's ears not to hear this despair. Moreover, such cries are not only evident from the forgotten, the powerless, the poor, the unemployed, and the dying, which is tragic enough; they are also perceptible from employees and managers commonly defined as successful. And today nature itself is echoing the pain of human beings; that is, environmental pollution is echoing the pollution of the soul.

One of the commonalities of the authors of this book is their courageous acknowledgment of these pollutions. Another is their discontent with current managerial theory and practice that propose gimmick after gimmick in attempting to deny the cries of despair. From traditional organizational behavior to conventional strategic management, most proposed solutions are only more of the same: more analyses; more empowerment; more speed; more markets; more control; more innovation, consumption, competition, seduction, vision, production, precision, rationalization, perfection.

Another commonality among the authors of this book is their relativizing of the utilitarian and economic functions of both organizations and work. For them, organizations are not only means for providing goods and services to a market or only means for producing an economic added value; organizations are also places where individuals work, dream, suffer, and live and where they should be able to grow, learn, and actualize themselves. As readers will see in this book, we have perhaps arrived at a point in history where the added value generated through production has become inferior to the destruction it engenders, both for humans and for the natural world of which human beings are inherently a part. Thus, between the lines, many authors hint that the dream of industrialization and production as currently defined (that is, of promising to bring lasting prosperity and security) has been shattered. It seems that today many individuals are more conscious of such threatening issues as world hunger, ecological pollution, unemployment, international instability, and blatant inequality, among others, leading to an often painful requestioning of both personal and organizational meaning.

Finally, a key aspect of this book is the existential point of view taken by the authors. They all emphasize that the deep issues confronting many managers and other employees today must be addressed in terms of the existential tradition.

We invite the readers of *In Search of Meaning* to accompany us on a voyage through which they will gain a deeper understanding of the sources of the loss of meaning, of destruction, and of the crushing cries of despair, a voyage through which we hope they will discover concrete avenues for seriously addressing these issues.

Overview of the Contents

The Introduction provides a number of definitions to help read- ers become familiar with the existential concepts referred to in this book and describes each chapter in relation to the others. The first two chapters clarify additional issues in existentialism and discuss the pitfalls associated with erroneous attempts to fulfill existential needs. The authors of these chapters discuss how the current notion of business effectiveness leads to a loss of subjective meaning (Chapter One) and how "existential ad- dictions" trigger alarming medical and physiological problems (Chapter Two).

The following three chapters present the problems associ- ated with the search for excellence, perfection, and total qual- ity in organizations. In these chapters, the authors discuss the tortuous existential ground of this search and its negative effects on the subjective and natural worlds (Chapter Three); the prob- lematic distribution of status, power, and benefits in organiza- tions (Chapter Four); and the dangers of cultural "existential creations" (Chapter Five).

In the next four chapters, the authors attempt to address existential issues through the acknowledgment and management of paradoxes (Chapter Six), the building of a community through genuine dialogue with others (Chapter Seven), the necessary task of acknowledging and managing the dark side of organi- zational life (Chapter Eight), and the necessity of deriving ex- istential meaning from one's cultural and religious backgrounds (Chapter Nine).

In the final two chapters, the authors explore the posi- tive and negative impacts of existential issues in two organiza- tions: an attempt to rediscover meaning through the process of remythologization in a religious organization (Chapter Ten) and the disastrous effects of a lack of existential responsibility in a financial institution (Chapter Eleven).

The Conclusion proposes a definition of existential health, suggests several avenues for further research, and emphasizes that existential issues affect not only the subjective and social lives of individuals but their physiology and the natural world as well.

Audience

This book is first for those managers, executives, professionals, and other employees who wish to rediscover or enhance a sense of personal and collective meaning in their organizations. In particular, the book will be most useful for people in key leadership positions, human resources, and organizational development. Second, this book will be especially useful for management educators, consultants, change agents, and teachers and students in the organizational field. It can be used as a supplementary text in courses or training programs in organizational behavior, theory, development, and change, or it can be used as a stand-alone text. One contributor is already using the book for a graduate course on meaning at work. Finally, this book is also addressed to management theorists and researchers. We hope that it will legitimize the use of an existential perspective in management and encourage others to conduct additional and much needed research in this domain.

Montreal, Quebec   THIERRY C. PAUCHANT
September 1994

Acknowledgments

My first insight for *In Search of Meaning* came to me while I was writing my Ph.D. dissertation at the University of Southern California in 1986. My subject of study and the methodology I used were both existential. Following Ian Mitroff's path, I wrote my dissertation on the field of crisis management, realizing in the process that existentialists such as Rollo May define the object of existential psychotherapy as the *study of individuals in crisis.* Under Warren Bennis's tutorship, I also used in this dissertation a methodology derived from Heinz Kohut's approach in self-psychology, discovering that Kohut's work, too, has been compared to that of a number of existentialists, such as Søren Kierkegaard. When interviewing managers in organizations about their experience during a crisis, I further realized that many echoed the issues discussed by existentialists such as Barrett, Becker, Camus, Miller, or Weil. However, I could not find in the management literature much help for expressing this echo, and I envisioned a book that would make explicit the links between the wealth of experience discussed by existentialists and the experiences and behaviors I found in organizations.

This book is a first step in that direction. As will become evident, its contributors do not use only the traditional perspectives of management; in addition, they rely on many great authors of existential works who honor the human spirit, including Ernest Becker, Albert Camus, Victor Frankl, Otto Rank, William Shakespeare, or Paul Tillich. These authors offer a fresh and necessary perspective on the experiences and behaviors of the men and women working in organizations. Thus my warm thanks to Ian Mitroff and Warren Bennis at USC, as well as to Burt Nanus, Jim O'Toole, Omar El Sawy, and Warren Schmidt.

My thanks, too, to Will McWhinney, Fred Massarik, and Bob Tannenbaum for our exchanges during my studies at the University of California, Los Angeles, and later on. I am particularly grateful to the members of the group we recently formed at the École des Hautes Études Commerciales (HEC), the Group for Education and Research on Management and the Ecology (GERME), for our discussions on the relationships between the subjective, social, and natural worlds: Omar Aktouf, Isabelle Deschamps, Taïeb Hafsi, Paul Lanoie, Michel Provost, and Jean-Philippe Waaub. Thanks also to my colleagues Gaétan Ayotte, Alain Chanlat, Jean-François Chanlat, Richard Déry, Allain Joly, Veronika Kisfalvy, Laurent Lapierre, Danny Miller, Gérard Ouimet, Suzanne Rivard, and Francine Séguin for their interest in this book.

In addition, I would like to thank the following people for our exchanges on existentialism and organizations during the past few years: James Hurley in Australia; Robert Cobbaut and Didier Van Den Hove in Belgium; Iran Machado in Brazil; Nicole Aubert, Christophe Dejours, and Eugène Enriquez in France; Burkard Sievers in Germany; Craig Lundberg, Howard Schwartz, Paul Shrivastava, and Bill Wolf in the United States; and Gordon Lawrence and Dennis Smith in the United Kingdom.

I would like also to thank the managers, professionals, and employees from many organizations and the students in management who have helped me during the past years in better understanding the reality of existential issues in management; Dorinda Cavanaugh, Patrice Goyette, Céline Legrand, Lucie Pagé, and Muriel Richard for their help in editing; André Cyr, who has translated from the French the chapters by Omar Aktouf, Nicole Aubert, and Estelle Morin; HEC's graphic design department for their assistance; Cedric Crocker and Bill Hicks at Jossey-Bass, who kept faith in this project and helped me along the way; and the Conseil de Recherches en Sciences Humaines du Canada (CRSH), the Fonds pour la Formation de Chercheurs et l'Aide à la Recherche (FCAR), and the HEC research department for their financial assistance.

Finally, I wish to reiterate my thanks to all the contributors to this book, which is obviously the result of our collective effort. I have learned much from our exchanges on the paramount reality of existential issues in organizations and on the difficulty of managing them. Today I have an even better understanding of the tremendous work still in front of us to make this existential reality more directly usable by the men and women working in organizations. I have an especially warm *merci* for Estelle Morin, both a contributor in this book and the prime contributor in my life; as a colleague and my wife, she has encouraged and helped me a great deal in my task of editor and in much, much more.

T.C.P.

The Authors

Thierry C. Pauchant is associate professor of management at the École des Hautes Études Commerciales, the University of Montreal's business school, and associate director of the Group for Education and Research on Management and Ecology. He received his Ph.D. degree (1987) from the University of Southern California in strategic and crisis management. Pauchant has published more than sixty scientific articles and two books on strategic and crisis management, the existential ground of managerial actions, and the social and ecological responsibilities of managers and employees. Through the years he has been a manager, a consultant, and a scientific researcher for organizations such as AT&T, Corning, Desjardins, Holiday Inn, Laventhol and Horwath, the French Ministry of Tourism, the University of Montreal, and Environment Canada. He is currently studying for a diploma in environmental sciences at McGill University.

Omar Aktouf received his Ph.D. degree (1983) from the École des Hautes Études Commerciales, University of Montreal, in management. He is professor of management at the École des Hautes Études Commerciales, Montreal, and guest teacher at the École Supérieure de Commerce de Paris and École Supérieure de Commerce de Marseille. He is a member of the advisory board and scientific committee of the Standing Conference on Organizational Symbolism. Aktouf's work has been published in major English and French academic journals, and his books and textbooks incorporate his main methodological approach to management and corporate studies: ethnomethodology, symbolics, and radical humanism.

Nicole Aubert is professor of organizational behavior at the École Supérieure de Commerce de Paris. She received her Ph.D. degree (1982) from the University of Paris IX in organizational science. Her research interests include the human aspects of management, the psychopathology of work, and the human consequences of the search for organizational effectiveness. Aubert has written several books, including *Le stress professionnel* [Professional Stress] (1989), *Le coût de l'excellence* [The Cost of Excellence] (1991, with V. de Gaulejac), and *Management, aspects humains et organisationnels* [Human and Organizational Aspects of Management] (1991, with others).

Paul E. Bracke is a psychologist in private practice in Oakland and Palo Alto, California. He received his Ph.D. degree (1985) from Stanford University in counseling psychology. As a consultant to the Meyer Friedman Institute in San Francisco, Bracke trains group leaders and conducts group programs designed to change Type-A behavior. He has conducted research on the long-term effectiveness of reducing Type-A behavior in individuals who have suffered heart attacks and on the role of the family in the development of Type-A behavior. He is a coauthor of articles on the treatment of Type-A behavior and on the future of existential-humanistic psychotherapy.

James F. T. Bugental is emeritus professor, Saybrook Institute, San Francisco; and emeritus clinical faculty member, Stanford University Medical School. He received his Ph.D. degree (1948) from Ohio State University in psychology. He is the author of *The Search for Existential Identity* (1976), *Psychotherapy and Process* (1978), and *The Art of the Psychotherapist* (1987). Past president of the Association for Humanistic Psychology and of the California Psychological Association, Bugental has taught or lectured at over two hundred universities, hospitals, professional schools, and professional societies in the United States, Canada, Mexico, England, and Germany.

Frederick I. Herzberg is known as the father of job enrichment, a strategy to increase human creativity and happiness at work, and for the motivation-hygiene theory, based on one of the most replicated studies in the history of industrial psychology, *Motivation to Work* (1959). He extended his theory to existential levels in *Work and the Nature of Man* (1966). Author of five books and over two hundred articles, Herzberg has consulted in thirty-five countries, is a contributing editor to *Industry Week* magazine, and is currently distinguished professor of management at the University of Utah. He received his Ph.D. degree (1950) from the University of Pittsburgh in psychology.

Robert Kramer lectures on research methods and statistics at the School of Business and Public Management, George Washington University. He is editor of *Otto Rank: Selected American Lectures* (forthcoming). Since 1975 Kramer has served as a research analyst at the U.S. Bureau of Labor Statistics, where he now also serves as facilitator for the union-management Quality of Worklife steering committee. Kramer is a doctoral candidate at the School of Business and Public Management, George Washington University, in organization and management.

Estelle M. Morin is associate professor at the École des Hautes Études Commerciales in Montreal and a psychologist in private practice. She teaches psychology and organizational behavior at the undergraduate and graduate levels, with an existential and Jungian orientation. Her research interests center primarily on the meaning of work, personality theory, and crises and effectiveness. She received her Ph.D. degree (1990) from the University of Montreal in psychology. Morin is a coauthor of *L'efficacité des organisations* [The Effectiveness of Organizations] (1994, with A. Savoie and G. Beaudin).

Narayan Pant is assistant professor of policy and strategy at the University of Alberta, Canada. He received his Ph.D. degree (1992) from the Leonard N. Stern School of Business, New York University, in business policy and strategy. In addition to teaching, he conducts research and writes on issues ranging from how to strategize given limited forecasting ability (and how to fit strategies to unknown futures) to how to anticipate pathological outcomes in organizations.

Howard S. Schwartz is professor of organizational behavior at the School of Business Administration at Oakland University in Rochester, Michigan. He studied philosophy at Antioch College, the University of Pittsburgh, and the University of California, San Diego. He received his Ph.D. degree (1980) from Cornell University in organizational behavior. Schwartz's main interest has been unconscious processes in organizations. He is the author of *Narcissistic Process and Corporate Decay: The Theory of the Organization Ideal* (1990), and his most recent work has been on the psychodynamics of political correctness.

Burkard Sievers is professor of organization development at Bergische Universität, Wuppertal, Germany. He received his Ph.D. degree (1972) from the University of Bielefeld, Germany, in organizational sociology. As demonstrated in his most recent book, *Work, Death, and Life Itself* (1994), he is interested in the traditional myths of management and organization as they relate to human mortality.

Kenwyn K. Smith is associate professor of organizational behavior at the University of Pennsylvania and director of its Center for Workplace Studies. His research focuses on the impact of organizational dynamics on the physical and emotional health of employees. Professor Smith teaches at Penn's School of Social Work and at the Wharton School. He received his Ph.D. degree (1974) from Yale University in organizational behavior and is a specialist in organizational change, group dynamics, and the management of conflict. He has written extensively on these topics.

In Search of Meaning

Introduction: Toward a Field of Organizational Existentialism

Thierry C. Pauchant

Simone Weil, in "A propos de la condition humaine," wrote: "If the objective is to escape from oneself, it is simpler to play or to drink. And it is even simpler to die. All entertainments (of this type) . . . are a disguised form of suicide . . . because an existence which has as its object to escape from life leads in the final analysis to a search for death. Death is the only refuge against life" ([1933] 1988a, pp. 318–319).

This introduction echoes Weil's remark; describes the history and overall direction of the existential tradition, and suggests reasons for addressing existential issues in organizations. It also reviews the existing research in management and introduces each of the chapters included in this book.

What Is Existentialism?

The first line of Scott Peck's best-seller *The Road Less Traveled* begins with the affirmation that "life is difficult" (1978, p. 15). As of 1994, this book had been on the *New York Times* best-seller list each and every week for ten years! Existentialists would agree with Peck's contention. As a whole, they recognize both the

1

beauty and the tragedy of life and posit that what they call the authentic individual fully recognizes this duality of life.

Existentialists' recognition of a dark side of life has often led people to conclude that this tradition is overly morbid or pessimistic. However, this is a great misconception for three reasons. First, to recognize that life consists not only of the search for immediate pleasure but also of difficulties and tragedies that lead irreversibly to death is a sign of courage and maturity because tragedies do indeed happen. Moreover, the denial of these realities leads to mental and physical illness for both the human and natural worlds. Second, existentialists do not focus only on the dark side of life; they also recognize the many moments of triumph, peak experience, joy, and transcendence. Third, existentialists realize that the bright and dark sides of life are not only opposites. From an existential and dialectical point of view, life and death are opposites, but they are also complementary; each needs the other to define itself. Further, for existentialists, these two sides of life are the result of every creative action, essentially linked to each other, and built into the structure of life itself, into the so-called human condition and into nature.

For me, the term *existentialism* means primarily and simply a courageous and full embracing of life, an embracing of life's tragic and magical sides, and a willingness to look both life and death in the eye. Globally, existentialists are concerned with the concrete human experience of the human condition; typical of the subjects they address are life, death, responsibility, meaning, loneliness, despair, tragedy, anxiety, joy, love, transcendence, and spirituality. Notice that these topics are not often discussed in the corporate boardroom or the classroom. In general, the quest to embrace life fully seems to have vanished from many organizations and work in general. Today many managers and other employees prefer to speak of career planning, marketable innovations, pension plans, or the need for developing strategic advantages or aspiring to financial rewards, success, security, power, status, and fame.

Because the existential tradition springs from a deep recognition of both life and death, its use can lead to two important contributions in management. The first is to make another sense of organizational reality. As we will see in this book, the use of the existential perspective allows a different understanding of the purpose of work activities and helps one make sense of the complexity and turbulence much talked about today in organizations. The second contribution is to identify diverse ways of addressing significant concerns rarely discussed or even acknowledged in organizations.

It should be emphasized that existentialists never propose to resolve, once and for all, the basic issues of the human condition; rather, they show that these issues are built into the human condition and need to be recognized and worked through *during the entire span of life.* Despite the fact that existentialists refuse to entertain the myth of final or magical solutions, they do propose a number of very concrete actions that "authentic" individuals can implement in an attempt to rediscover a sense of personal meaning. These actions are often very different from those advocated in the traditional managerial literature, with its emphasis on so-called excellence, constant innovations, competitive advantages, turnaround strategies, vision/empowerment, total quality, or re-engineering.

As used in this book, the term *organizational existentialism* is not meant to imply that an organization can have a sense of experience. Organizations do not experience anything; people do. The field of organizational existentialism is thus concerned with better understanding the subjective experiences and the actions of the *people* who work in organizations or interact with them, and it proposes different ways of addressing the basic issues of the human condition, such as the loss of personal meaning.

A Managerial Definition of Existentialism

Existential philosophers have insisted that it is probably impossible to define precisely what existentialism is. For example, Walter Kaufmann (1956, p. 11) has declared that "existentialism is not a philosophy but a label for several widely different revolts against traditional philosophy" and that it "is not a school of thought nor reducible to any set of tenets." Similarly, Maurice

Friedman (1964, p. 3) has proposed that "existentialism is not
a philosophy but a mood embracing a number of disparate
philosophies." To complicate the matter further, many existentialists, such as Camus and Heidegger, have explicitly refused
to be identified with this tradition.

Although I have not been trained as a philosopher, I offer
here my own version of the overall direction embraced by the
existential tradition, with an eye toward its application in management. *For me, the existential tradition points first of all to the personal realization that one is living concretely as part of the entire world.*
At first glance, this realization may seem very conceptual or
even rather trivial, especially in relation to the daily tasks of
an employee or a manager in an organization. However, as this
book will show, it is a very concrete and important realization
for guiding one's work, whether at the CEO or employee level,
because it involves a host of consequences. I will indicate a number of general consequences here and provide a more structured
framework for grouping them later.

This existential realization brings with it, for example,
a biological view of oneself and the universe, thus leading one
to realize more fully the necessity of *death* as well as the fragility
of the planet as an ecosystem. At a time when many actions
taken in organizations can be seen as a denial of death, this realization seems particularly important. Also, at a time when the
negative impact of industrial activities on the ecology becomes
more and more problematic, it seems that this insight into the
desirability of reuniting in one single whole the social and natural
worlds is badly needed.

Another consequence of the personal realization posited
is a potential awareness of one's culture, both societal and organizational, and an understanding that a specific cultural system, or a particular religion, represents only *one possibility* for
viewing and acting in the world. This view leads in turn to the
realization that one cannot help but be *responsible* for one's own
choices. At a time when organizations are employing members
of more and more ethnic, cultural, and religious groups, it also
seems that this realization becomes paramount. It could, for
example, allow more respect for others' cultures and a greater

understanding of the consequences of one's cultural heritage grounded in a specific time period. As another example, it seems that an enhanced understanding of one's ultimate responsibility is very necessary considering the current proliferation of nonethical behaviors in business and the fact that the cultural ethos of our societies is becoming more and more amoral, technological, and utilitarian.

The personal realization that one concretely exists as part of the larger world also brings the insight that, in spite of this embeddedness, one is paradoxically and in the final analysis alone and irremediably isolated from others. Existentialists do emphasize that the self-realization of an individual proceeds from the encounter with another through a genuine dialogue (Bohm, 1990; Friedman, 1994). For example, as stressed by Martin Buber, Heinz Kohut, Gabriel Marcel, Carl Rogers, and Paul Tillich, the "I" needs a "you" to become an "I," thus putting the quality of the relationship at a central place. However, they also emphasize the inescapable *loneliness* of the individual, the ultimate gap between the self and the other, the self and the world. At a time when organizations are advocating the myth of team spirit for achieving greater effectiveness, the realization of loneliness is paramount because it allows one to understand that social belonging can become an escape from one's individuality.

Finally, the realization that one is part of the entire world but unavoidably cut off from it, that one is fundamentally responsible for one's choices and doings despite uncertainty, and that life leads to death brings with it the fundamental question of the personal sense of *meaning*. As we will see in the following chapters, existentialists emphasize the need for a dialectical view of life rather than the much more common linear logic based on strict either/or categories. Thus, for example, death is not seen by existentialists as the ultimate enemy to fight or deny but as inextricably linked to life itself; the realization of death allows one to be more truly alive. Again, at a time when we speak at length about corporate identity, change, complexity, turbulence, crisis, chaos, and survival, it seems that the ability to shift from a linear understanding—say, from turbulence to survival, disorder to order, or flux to stability—to a dialectical view could help managers and other employees make more sense of their situation and actions. This different logic could, for example, assist people in more fully recognizing the condition in which they are placed, acknowledging at last that life is difficult, the observation that launched this introduction. In turn, this different logic could lead individuals to attempt to address the foregoing issues courageously rather than avoid them through the use of diverse surrogates, defense mechanisms, and other gimmicks.

We will return to these consequences of using an existential perspective throughout this book. Meanwhile, we turn briefly to the historical origin of the existential tradition. While this discussion may seem overly philosophical to some readers, I believe that it will help them better understand the overall thrust of this tradition and thus better realize its usefulness in management.

Historical Origin of the Existential Tradition

Many people who have been exposed to some existential concepts are under the impression that this tradition emerged on Paris's Left Bank under the leadership of Jean-Paul Sartre. Although I admire Sartre's genius and insights, especially in his literary works, it is also obvious that his fame has turned many people away from the existential tradition as a whole. Usually these people have had the tendency to infer — erroneously — from Sartre's work that existentialism is overly dark, rhetorical, intellectual, and difficult to understand; that it uses extravagant mumbo jumbo, considers the individual's action as the center of the world, and is drastically opposed to spirituality. Given Sartre's relative influence, it is important to state very clearly that *existentialism is not Sartrianism.* To put the matter another way, to view organizations and work from an existential perspective does not of necessity lead one to see the world through Sartre's lenses. As William Barrett, one of the key philosophers to introduce the existential tradition in North America, emphasizes (1958, p. 11): "Jean-Paul Sartre is not Existentialism — it still seems necessary to make this point for American readers;

he does not even represent . . . the deepest impulse of this philosophy. . . . French existentialism as a popular movement . . .
is a small branch of a very much larger tree. And the roots of
this larger tree reach down into the remotest depths of the
Western tradition."

Echoing Barrett, many existential philosophers, with exceptions such as Kaufmann (1956) and Foulquié (1989), have
proposed that the father of existential philosophy was a pre-
Socratic philosopher who lived around 500 B.C.: *Heraclitus of
Ephesus.* The philosophical origin of this tradition is therefore
closely identified with the birth of Western philosophy and Western science, themselves traditionally attributed to Thales of
Miletus at about 600 B.C. Heraclitus's work has influenced many
key existential authors. He was, for example, one of Paul Tillich's
favorite philosophers (Pauck and Pauck, 1989, p. 97); Martin
Buber turned extensively to Heraclitus in his work (Friedman,
1964, p. 17); Martin Heidegger and Friedrich Nietzsche extensively studied the pre-Socratics and drew in particular from Heraclitus (Heidegger and Fink, 1993); and students of Nietzsche's
work even argue that Nietzsche saw Heraclitus in his Zarathustra
(Lowith, [1935] 1991). In the same vein, Friedman (1964, pp.
22–23) places some of Heraclitus's works first in his reader on
existentialism.

This incursion into the historical origin of the existential
tradition might at first seem out of place in a book on management. However, setting the birth date of the existential tradition during the pre-Socratic period, some twenty-five hundred
years ago, has many implications for its use in management.
For example, this historical perspective de-emphasizes the importance of the Sartrian branch of existentialism and the influence of World War II; that is, it shows that existentialism
did not spring merely from a dark period or as a specific mood
of a particular time and place. Putting the existential tradition
in a much larger and older perspective allows one to understand
that existential issues have concerned human beings for thousands of years. Moreover, recognizing that the tradition springs
from the pre-Socratic period helps one better understand why
many existentialists ground themselves in the concrete world

as these early philosophers were much concerned about discovering the proper ways for humans to live as part of the entire cosmos.

I would like to close this brief discussion of the historical origin of the existential tradition with a quotation from William Barrett. In it Barrett argues that both Kierkegaard and Nietzsche — two great men in nineteenth-century existentialism who were influenced by Heraclitus — attempted to recapture the original pre-Socratic spirit and thereby influenced two giants of twentieth-century existential philosophy, Martin Heidegger and Karl Jaspers. I leave to the reader the task of comparing this philosophy of life to the current infatuation in management with narrow specializations or very elaborated models that are presented as universal and absolute truth.

> In ancient Greece . . . instead of a specialized theoretical discipline philosophy there was a concrete way of life, a total vision of man and the cosmos in the light of which the individual's whole life was to be lived. . . . The motive of philosophy [was] very different from the [current] cool pursuit of the savant engaged in research. . . . The modern university is as much an expression of the specialization of the age as is the modern factory. . . . [However] neither Kierkegaard nor Nietzsche was an academic philosopher. . . . Neither developed a system; both in fact gibed at systematizers and even the possibility of a philosophic system. . . . Ideas [were] not even the real subject matter of these philosophers. . . . More than thinkers, Kierkegaard and Nietzsche were witnesses who suffered for their time what the time itself would not acknowledge as its own secret wound. No concept or system of concepts [lay] at the center of either of their philosophies, but rather the individual human personality itself struggling for self-realization. No wonder both are among the greatest of intuitive psychologists [Barrett, 1958, pp. 5, 6, 12, and 13].

When Philosophy Meets Psychology and Literature

All existentialists are not philosophers. Many of them are psychologists, psychoanalysts, or psychiatrists; others are theologians or mythologists; still others are novelists, playwrights, or poets. Indeed, one of the strengths of the existential tradition is that it allows inquiries other than the sole but paramount indepth inquiry of basic assumptions. As will become evident, one of the greatest contributions of existentialism is not only to ask "how" questions, that is, questions about means, such as how to achieve success. Through the philosophical method, existentialists also ask deeper "why" questions, questions that challenge the motivation behind an action, such as Why should one achieve success as currently defined? In addition, the existential tradition leads to a better understanding of the subjective experience of individuals through the use of psychology. Here one is no longer only analyzing the soundness of arguments or perspectives but is also concerned with understanding the deep and subjective motivations behind these perspectives, as hinted at by Barrett at the end of the foregoing quotation. Moreover, existentialists move beyond philosophical and psychological methods for conducting their inquiries by also using drama, novels, and poetry to express, in a different and more poignant way, the experiences of the human condition and their consequences. In the modern exposition of existentialism, which utilizes these different approaches, we can see the mark of the pre-Socratics, including Heraclitus, who blended the philosophical-scientific method with psychology, theology, literature, and the arts, drawing from what today are called the social and natural sciences. The pre-Socratics did not have to contend with today's schisms between the sciences themselves and between the sciences and the arts, and many existentialists have remembered the earlier *transdisciplinary* tradition.

The following table provides some idea of the wealth and range of the existential tradition. This table includes the names of famous authors who are recognized as existentialists or who have borrowed extensively from existential tradition in their work. It should be stressed that, with the very rare exceptions of R. D. Laing and Carl Rogers, none of these authors has yet been seriously considered in modern management thought and practice. This table is based on the references used in major texts on existentialism (such as Barrett, 1958; Becker, 1973; Foulquié, 1989; Friedman, 1964; May, 1950; and Yalom, 1980a). The placement of a particular author in one or another column should not be seen as definitive because many authors, such as Sartre, have made contributions in more than one area.

Philosophy Theology Mythology	Psychology Psychiatry Psychoanalysis	Poetry Novels Plays
Hannah Arendt	Silvano Arieti	Samuel Beckett
William Barrett	Ernest Becker	William Blake
Simone de Beauvoir	Menard Boss	Miguel de Cervantes
Jacob Boehme	Norman O. Brown	Dante
Martin Buber	James Bugental	Fyodor Dostoevsky
Joseph Campbell	Leslie Farber	T. S. Eliot
Albert Camus	Paul Feyerabend	Jean Genet
Meister Eckhart	Victor Frankl	Jean Giono
José Ortega y Gasset	Erich Fromm	Goethe
Martin Heidegger	Karen Horney	Nikolai Gogol
Karl Jaspers	Walter Kaufmann	Ernest Hemingway
Søren Kierkegaard	Heinz Kohut	Hermann Hesse
Arthur Koestler	Elisabeth Kübler-Ross	Franz Kafka
Gabriel Marcel	R. D. Laing	André Malraux
Maurice Merleau-Ponty	Rollo May	Thomas Mann
Thomas Merton	Alice Miller	Herman Melville
Friedrich Nietzsche	Clark Moustakas	Arthur Miller
Blaise Pascal	Otto Rank	Henry Miller
Jean-Paul Sartre	Carl Rogers	George Orwell
Friedrich Schelling	Erwin Strauss	Rainer Maria Rilke
Paul Tillich	Harry Stack Sullivan	William Shakespeare
	Irwin Yalom	Leo Tolstoy

As if this list were not long enough, one could, as indicated by Barrett (1958) or Yalom (1980a), include additional major authors who have used existential concepts in their work: John Dewey, Sigmund Freud, Stanislav Grof, Edmund Husserl, William James, Carl Jung, Karl Marx, Abraham Maslow, Simone Weil, and Alfred North Whitehead.

Echoing existential philosophers, authors in existential psychology and literature also emphasize a number of basic issues that articulate the human condition. Irwin Yalom (1980a), for example, has proposed that the field of existential psychotherapy attempts to address four interdependent existential subjects that human beings experience: *death, responsibility, loneliness,* and *meaning.* I will only briefly comment on each of them here because I have already touched on them, and each chapter in this book will discuss them in detail.

The realization of the inescapability of *death* is, according to Yalom (1980a, p. 8), the "most easily apprehended ultimate concern," but it is also often experienced as a terrible truth. This realization frequently results in an existential tension for individuals who wish to persist or in a fuller appreciation of life itself if death can be assimilated (Kübler-Ross, 1969). The issue of *responsibility* springs from the insight that one is living as a part of a larger world, whose rules and structures are often experienced as uncertain. From this insight, one is frequently confronted with the tension that exists between the wish for order and certainty and the experience of disorder and uncertainty — but with the realization that one is responsible for one's actions despite uncertainty. The experience of *loneliness* springs from the fundamental realization of one's isolation from others and the world. This insight often causes one to experience conflicts between the wish for belonging and the experience of isolation. Finally, the issue of *meaning* emerges from the realization that death is inescapable, that one must assume the weight of one's responsibility, and that one is ultimately alone. An existential conflict frequently arises from these realizations as one is confronted with the necessity of creating one's meaning and yet wishes to be given a sense of meaning by an outside force.

Current Existential Issues in Organizations

As we near the end of this millennium, the need to address existential issues in organizations seems particularly important. I have already discussed in another publication (Pauchant, 1993) some of the signs of existential suffering visible in society at large and in organizations in particular. In that work, I present a number of studies and indicators suggesting that the extent of existential problems is presently important. For example, studies indicate that most people in America obsessively focus on the self, that the number of suicides in the younger generation has dramatically increased in most Western nations, that drugs furnishing an illusion of one's being truly alive have become dangerously popular, and that many therapists have pointed out that most of their clients are suffering today from boredom or neurotic anxiety. These signs are also visible in organizations, including an increase in drug and alcohol addictions, dramatic behaviors, and workaholism; additional signs are many managers' inability to delay gratification, their lack of empathy, the rise of charismatic and grandiose leaders, and the current popularity of the "search for excellence," expressed, for example, in "total quality management," "re-engineering," and striving for an idealized perfection.

As noted in the preface, it would be a mistake to believe that the issues of boredom, anxiety, alienation, loss of meaning, and despair are experienced only by people who lack financial rewards, power, status, and "success" or who have lost their jobs. This notion seems particularly prevalent today as many advocate the development in organizations of more so-called participative management and empowerment, greater responsibility, and an enhanced sense of accomplishment. However, a number of studies clearly indicate that managers with a wide range of prestige, money, power, responsibilities, status, and accomplishment can also suffer from the same symptoms, thus relativizing the claim made for the benefits of greater participation, at least from an existential view. To cite only one study, after interviewing more than four thousand "successful" senior executives, managers, and professionals in the United States, Jan Halper (1988, p. 9) concluded that many are "disillusioned by the fruits of their success, for it has often resulted in emptiness and confusion."

It is enlightening to realize that the existential sufferings experienced in organizations and in the process of working are the very ones that existentialists have described for centuries.

For example, Becker (1973, p. 6) argues that "the crisis of modern society is precisely that the youth no longer feel heroic in the plan for action that their culture has set up"; Bugental (1976, p. 2), in a commentary that he develops further in Chapter Two of this book, proposes that "each of us is invisibly crippled"; Heidegger (1963) emphasizes the dangers of the experience of "self-estrangement"; Nietzsche (1972) proposes that the disease of contemporary human beings is that their "soul has gone stale"; and Sartre (1966) advances the concept of "bad faith," in which individuals attempt to escape despair by embracing a set of roles and tasks through which they—in an illusory manner—"define" themselves. In the same vein, Maslow (1971, p. 44) describes the "sickness of the soul" when self-actualization cannot be achieved.

While the current extent of existential suffering in and out of organizations has multiple origins, many of which are discussed in this book, it seems that the realization that our times have radically changed, as compared to the recent past, has had a strong impact on this condition. Edgar Morin (1990), for example, suggests that we have already left the twentieth century and entered what he calls the Damoclean Era. He identifies four major trends that are affecting people's sense of security and also increasing the visibility of death, the first crucial existential concern identified by Yalom (1980a). First, Morin points to current ecological problems, such as depletion of the ozone layer and the threat of global warming, which lead to a questioning of the viability of life on earth as we know it. Second, he emphasizes that the international security of the world will likely worsen in the future; while the superpowers are in the process of reducing their strategic weapons, smaller nations governed by deranged leaders have access to such weapons, and terrorism and nationalism are increasing. Third, Morin cites the new AIDS threat that has recently appeared from sexual relations and concerns all the populations of the globe. Fourth, he notes that our psyche is attacked by drugs, media propaganda, and the current importance of bureaucratic, technocratic and utilitarian rationalities.

In terms of the organizational world, we could add three

more trends that seem to fit the Damoclean view expressed by Morin: (1) the increase in industrial and environmental accidents and crises, leading to a painful requestioning of the safety of advanced and complex technologies; (2) the recent increase in global competition as new countries enter markets and win over older, Western nations in several of those markets, leading to such consequences as bankruptcies and government deficits; and (3) the slow but growing realization that the promises offered by managerialism and industrialism for increased prosperity, security, peace, and employment have not been realized, leading to a questioning of past societal choices and personal and organizational meaning.

Although the foregoing views may be overly pessimistic, the diversity and actuality of these issues suggest the strength of character and political courage that will be needed to face them squarely and not succumb, as Kierkegaard warned, to dread. Perhaps Rollo May (1969, p. 13) has summarized the potential consequences for many individuals of the realization of such a Damoclean view:

> Our [age] is an era of radical transition. The old myths and symbols by which we oriented ourselves are gone, anxiety is rampant; we cling to each other and try to persuade ourselves that what we feel is love; we do not will because we are afraid that if we choose one thing or one person we'll lose the other, and we are too insecure to take that chance. . . . The individual is forced to turn inward; he becomes obsessed with the new form of the problem of identity, namely, Even-if-I-know-who-I-am, I-have-no-significance. . . . The next step is apathy. And the step following that is violence. For no human being can stand the perpetually numbing experience of his own powerlessness.

Views of Senior Authors in Management

As previously indicated, the management literature has mostly shied away from the recognition of existential issues in organi-

zations. Such authors as Camus, Dostoevsky, Heidegger, Tillich, and Tolstoy are rarely acknowledged in that literature or
introduced in MBA courses or organizational training. Perhaps
the belief is that, by magic, managers, other employees, and
students in business do not experience such issues or need to
address them! It is more likely, however, that the anxiety associated with the acknowledgment of existential issues raises
some powerful defense mechanisms that hinder the addressing
of such issues and the works of these authors.

Nevertheless, a number of senior and/or influential authors in such management areas as organizational behavior, organization development, crisis management, organization theory,
and strategic management have recently begun to recognize
some of these issues. Among these authors are Warren Bennis,
Michel Crozier, Frederick Herzberg, James March, Ian Mitroff,
Henry Mintzberg, and Gareth Morgan, who could help legitimize the relevance of addressing existential issues in organizations. However, in spite of these initiatives, to date, only a few
works have specifically addressed the existential dimension in
management.

For example, Warren Bennis has argued that existential
meaning for individuals living in a society, in and out of organizations, springs from individual and collective dreams. Central
for Bennis is the paramount function of leaders to articulate these
dreams in society, to make a distinction between higher aspirations and mere ambitions. According to Bennis (1989, p. 39),
our "founding fathers . . . were dreamers, and dreamers on a
grand scale. Today, we do not dream but merely fantasize about
money and things. As a dreamless sleep is death, a dreamless
society is meaningless. As individuals, we need dreams in the
way we need air, and as a society, we need true leaders—
uncommon men and women who, having invented themselves,
can reinvent America and restore the collective dream by expressing for and to us that irreverent, insouciant, peculiarly
American spirit." Similarly, Michel Crozier has emphasized the
necessity of studying people in organizations from both a cognitive and conceptual perspective and a more subjective and existential one. As he (1992, p. 49) succinctly states, "the organizational problems are both conceptual and existential."

In an interview echoing Rollo May's remark quoted earlier, Frederick Herzberg has proposed that the previous "mystery systems" used by people in Occidental nations for transcending physical reality have recently broken down, a theme upon which he expands in Chapter Nine of this book. Drawing from the existential tradition, he observes that "we pushed quantity of products and experiences so that people could forget their own loss of meaning." Further, he calls for the necessity of assisting managers and employees alike in their search for their own character: "I can't find very much significance any more in our institutions . . . pep talks and company statements won't carry any meaning: people will rely on their own search for meaning and significance in developing character and ethics . . . [but] if we don't have enough humanities education, people will hear nothing when they talk with themselves" (quoted in Pascarella, 1980, pp. 47, 48–49).

Emphasizing the existential motivation behind many debates and arguments over management theory and practice, James March (quoted in Schein, 1987, p. 15) has observed that "arguments are the arenas in which educated men establish their right to imagine themselves alive." Also, echoing the remark made previously by Herzberg on the need for the humanities in business education and practice, March is presently teaching a course at Stanford's business school on organizational leadership, using as required texts Cervantes's *Don Quixote,* Shakespeare's *Othello,* and Tolstoy's *War and Peace.*

In a study on crisis management, Ian Mitroff has similarly emphasized the need for better understanding and addressing the existential dimension, however hindered by conditions in "bounded emotionality." As I wrote with him (Pauchant and Mitroff, 1992, p. 5): "The fundamental difference between a crisis-prone organization and a crisis-prepared one lies in the concept of responsibility, in the existential sense of the term. Individuals who manage crisis-prepared organizations are more able to confront the anxiety triggered by crises and to act decisively. Being less "bounded emotionally," they are more able to be ethically, emotionally, and cognitively responsible toward themselves, their employees, their business partners, and their surrounding environment."

Similarly, Henry Mintzberg (1987, pp. 6, 8) has emphasized the existential function of business strategies, a factor very rarely explicitly addressed in the field of business policy and strategic management: "Strategy does not only focus employees' attention . . . it also provides to everybody [employees and public] a sense to their existence. . . . Strategy is a cure against anxiety created by complexity, uncertainty and fragmented knowledge. . . . The primary role of strategies in organizations [is to] provide answers to the big questions."

Finally, in a book that has achieved some popularity in business schools, Gareth Morgan (1986, pp. 212–214, 233–235, 365) briefly presents Ernest Becker's work on the denial of death and the quest for immortality, succinctly introduces Heraclitus's philosophy and explains how it can contribute to a different view of organizations, and notes the potential value of works by Beckett, Camus, Melville, Sartre, and Shakespeare to help one understand organizations' subjective and ideologic dimensions.

Explicit Existential Studies in Management: A Brief Review

Despite the importance of the existential dimension for organization theory, education, research, and practice, currently only a very small number of authors in management have published specific research studies drawn explicitly from the existential tradition. Reviewing the literature at the end of the 1970s, Burrell and Morgan (1979) had difficulty finding examples of studies that relied on what they called a "radical humanist approach" in management. While they mentioned a dozen general works that address society at large more than organizations in particular, they only refer to three studies specifically conducted at the organizational level; however, even these studies drew primarily from the works of Marx and Habermas, who can only partially be considered as existentialists (Burrell and Morgan, 1979, pp. 320–321). Years later, Morgan (1986) again reviewed the literature and mentioned only three of the studies described below.

Thus far in my own research, I have only identified about thirty management scholars (in addition to the few mentioned above) who have explicitly used some tenets of the existential tradition in their work. These authors are cited in alphabetical order to provide the interested reader with a reference list of works already conducted in the existential domain and to suggest the variety of subjects that can be addressed from this perspective.

Aktouf (1990b) has documented in a case study the existence of a different and more "enlightened" kind of leadership in one organization. Aubert and Pagès (1989) and Aubert and de Gaulejac (1991) have indicated the tremendous stress and despair experienced in France by employees of so-called excellent companies that require them to be constant "warriors" and "winners." Boland and Hoffman (1983) have described how employees in a machine shop use humor as a way of preserving their personal well-being. Bouchard (Chanlat, 1990, pp. 589–611) has similarly proposed that the expression of symbolism in organizations springs from an existential wish to create. Denhardt (1987) argues that the superior-subordinate relationship is based on the imagery of the master-slave relationship that sprang from a quest for immortality. In another work, Denhardt (1981) explores the way in which the world of organizations affects employees' and managers' sense of meaning, action, and sense of continuity. Enriquez (1989) argues that employees of "excellent companies" in France have a tendency to become "prisoners," losing their own "body, thinking and psyche."

Guillet de Monthoux (1983) challenges the traditional views of decision-making and bureaucracy theory through anarchism and existential philosophies. Kramer (1989) assesses Denhardt's (1981) "theology" and proposes that this religious orientation needs to be included in organization theory. Massarik (1984) advises managers to come back to the basic raw material of daily experience to enhance their managerial knowledge, and Massarik (1985) describes the process of deep sharing for communicating and developing a sense of personal meaning. McWhinney (1991), drawing in particular from Otto Rank, explores some of the roots of evil in organizations. Mitroff and Pauchant (1990) describe twenty-four dangerous games — that is, games that can lead to organizational or industrial disaster —

presently being played in organizations in an attempt to diminish managers' existential anxiety. Reporting on an early study conducted in a so-called excellent company in France, Pagès, Bonetti, de Gaulejac, and Descendre (1979) propose that such companies have a tendency to become "religious systems," incarnating the wish for immortality. Using the notion of *mitsein* developed by Heidegger, Pagès (1984) suggests that the glue holding a healthy group together is each member's paradoxical realization of his or her ontological loneliness.

Pauchant and Mitroff (1992) develop the concept of *bounded emotionality,* which is articulated from the existential tradition and goes beyond the more restrictive concept of *bounded rationality,* to explain the current lack of interest in many organizations in preventive crisis management. Pauchant and Morin (1994) insist on the political and existential courage needed in an organization in order to develop a crisis management strategy. Pauchant (1991) proposes a typology of the charismatic leadership subjective experience derived from Heinz Kohut's self-psychology model, and Pauchant (1993) discusses some of the signs of existential despair in organizations. Peter Reason (1993) proposes that to embrace an existential outlook leads to a sacred experience in management practice and research. Rice (1960) discusses some of the implications of the existential perspective for the businessperson. Schwartz, in a series of articles (1983, 1985, 1987a), emphasizes that Maslow's concept of self-actualization was originally based on a realization of the dark side, discusses the implications of the denial of death on organizational change efforts, and argues that antisocial actions of organizationally committed individuals are motivated by a quest for self-identity and meaning. Schwartz (1987b) also proposes that the idea of a perfect organization leads to totalitarianism, with disastrous effects such as slavishness, shamefulness, cynicism, loneliness, and alienation, and in a later book (1990a), he develops his theory of the organization ideal.

In yet another series of articles, Sievers (1986a, 1986b) argues that a number of concepts in management, such as participation and motivation, are "scientific inventions" being taken as surrogates for existential meaning. In later works (1990a–1990d) he suggests that the issue of death in organization theory and practice must be seen as part of the normal course of life and not be "diabolized" and (1992, 1994) that organizations can be seen as theaters where individuals can transcend their existential suffering. Drawing in particular from the work of Rollo May and Paul Tillich, Smith and Berg (1988) discuss some of the paradoxes evident in the functioning of groups. Finally, drawing in part from Elisabeth Kübler-Ross's work, Tannenbaum and Hanna (1985) propose a model for better understanding and assisting the change process in organizations.

Choice of Contributors, Style, and Structure

The chapters included in this book have been written by some of the authors cited in the preceding section. In 1991, I sent a letter to thirty or so authors, explaining the purpose of this book and attaching an article I had written on the necessity of developing an existential perspective in management (Pauchant, 1993). About twenty of them responded that they would be willing to contribute a chapter to the book. I then asked each of them to send me a short chapter outline so that I could be sure that the chapters would not overlap and that they would cover the field of management broadly. Over a period of two years, fourteen of these authors sent me an actual chapter. Although three of the chapters were either too theoretical or not sufficiently grounded in the existential tradition, the remaining eleven chapters, together with a chapter of my own, constitute the content of this book. This volume therefore brings together some of the very few management scholars around the world who are knowledgeable about the existential tradition and have used it in their own work.

In an attempt to remain true to the existential tradition, I asked each contributor to avoid mumbo jumbo, to write in a personal and active style, not to be afraid to use the first person, and to address concrete problems by translating the existential perspective into pragmatic managerial diagnosis and suggested action. In the chapters, the reader will find traditional and conceptual academic formats, dialogues between two people, discussions of the results of empirical studies conducted by the authors, in-depth case analyses and case vignettes, and discussions that borrow from works of art, rely on an historical perspective, and tell a story. Although these differences in style will be evident to the reader, they honor the existential tradition and address a variety of existential issues. In addition, each chapter includes key references in existentialism to assist the reader who wishes to turn to additional sources.

An Overview of the Chapters

The contributors to this book address in various ways many of the topics traditionally discussed in the general field of management, including organizational change, behavior, theory, development, crisis, research, strategy, and effectiveness; they address issues of supervision, motivation, hierarchy, power, communication, culture, and organizational learning; and they provide fresh views on the search for excellence, the function of leadership, and the purpose of work and organizations in general.

To help the reader, the early chapters of the book are the most explicit. They provide many definitions of existential concepts, whereas the later chapters tend to take an understanding of these notions for granted and proceed from there. There has also been an attempt to group the chapters according to common themes, although none of the contributors have strictly separated the four major themes addressed in existentialism: death, responsibility, loneliness, and meaning. Rather, they integrated these themes while focusing on a few in particular.

Chapters One and Two define a number of existentialist terms and describe some of the negative effects of existential suffering at the subjective and physical levels. In Chapter One, Estelle Morin, drawing from an empirical study, discusses the narrowness of criteria used for measuring organizational effectiveness. Concerned primarily with the work of existential psychiatrists Victor Frankl and Irvin Yalom, she defines the concept of meaning at work and shows why the current notion of organizational effectiveness leads to a general lack of meaning and neurosis in organizations. Morin also proposes several avenues for helping individuals discover meaning in their lives in general and at work in particular.

In Chapter Two, Paul Bracke and James Bugental remind us that the consequences of what they call existential addiction are not only mental and social but physiological and medical as well and lead to chronic fatigue, heart disease, viral infections, and cerebral hemorrhages. Bracke and Bugental note that *karoshi,* or death from overwork, is presently the second leading cause of death for working men in Japan and that more than 50 percent of individuals in the United States exhibit Type-A behavior. These authors present four individual case analyses and discuss a number of potential therapeutic interventions.

The next three chapters address some of the negative effects of the now in vogue search for excellence, perfection, total quality, and re-engineering. In Chapter Three, Thierry Pauchant argues that the excellence trend springs from a denial of death and life. The analysis of Peters and Waterman's bestseller *In Search of Excellence,* seen as the origin of this trend, shows that these two authors specifically base their argument on the work of existentialist Ernest Becker but that they denature that work. By examining Becker's original work, Pauchant shows how the excellence trend, which claims to lead to prosperity and a sense of immortality, has instead increased a number of subjective and physical injuries to both humans and nature and suggests ten ways of addressing this issue.

In Chapter Four, Omar Aktouf examines the power relationships in organizations. Drawing from an analysis of the history of British royalty by some of Shakespeare's characters and current examples in organizations, he shows that today's corporate executives have inherited an illusive glory that is leading to the deification of top managers and the depersonalization of employees. Commenting on the dangers of totalitarianism, Aktouf concludes by suggesting the necessity for "republicanizing" organizations by rehumanizing top managers and repersonalizing employees to achieve a dual sharing of power and profit.

In Chapter Five, Nicole Aubert proposes that the Sartrian view of the realization of oneself through one's action is seen today as primarily attainable in organizations. Commenting on the individualistic basis of this view and on the decrease in political and religious ideals, she shows that this quest leads instead to a loss of personal meaning. Based on interviews conducted in what have been characterized as "excellent companies," Aubert argues that the managerial system has been replaced by an "imaginary system" in an attempt to control not only the body but also the heart and dreams of the individual. She concludes the chapter by describing the challenge of restoring personal meaning at work while remaining competitive.

The following four chapters return to some of the issues discussed in earlier chapters and present general directions for potential change. In Chapter Six, Kenwyn Smith discusses some of the managerial implications of taking responsibility and using one's existential courage in the midst of change. Presented as a dialogue between a manufacturing firm's CEO and a wise old man, this chapter highlights some of the vicious circles, dialectical processes, and self-defeating strategies that are often present in today's organizations. Stressing the need to courageously acknowledge one's subjective experience of powerlessness, doubt, and confusion, Smith offers a number of practical managerial actions based on an existential and dialectical understanding of leadership, organizations, and work.

In Chapter Seven, Robert Kramer develops further the notion of dialogue and shows that Carl Rogers's approach has been greatly influenced by Otto Rank's existentialism. From this perspective, the development of a relationship is not only a means for achieving greater productivity but also one of the only ways available for making bearable the never-ending dual anxiety of the fear of life and the fear of death. Kramer notes the challenges that this realization brings to a more traditional view of manager-employee supervision and describes three core competencies for developing such relationships: congruence, unconditional positive regard, and empathic understanding.

In Chapter Eight, Howard Schwartz proposes that we look beneath seemingly carefree behaviors to understand the tragic side of life in organizations. Using several examples and individual case analyses, he proposes that the denial of the dark side,

such as the experience of loneliness, leads individuals to construct the fantasy of an organizational ideal, which culminates
in a denial of reality, self-estrangement, projection of evil onto
others, and totalitarianism. Schwartz emphasizes the need to
acknowledge this dark side and reminds us that this need is emphasized in Maslow's concept of self-actualization.

In Chapter Nine, Frederick Herzberg expands upon his
motivation-hygiene theory by discussing four existential questions: Why me? Whom do I turn to? What should I do? Who
am I? Comparing what he calls the mystery systems of the West
(Hellenism, Judaism, Christianity, and Islam) to those of the
East (Taoism, Hinduism, and Buddhism), Herzberg shows that
these diverse systems offer different answers to the four questions posed. He then advises managers in the West to ground
themselves in their own mystery system, acknowledging their
weaknesses, be they scientific, shamanic, or religious.

The final two chapters present case analyses involving two
very different organizations and propose that the management
of existential issues can have a radical effect on the health of
these organizations, their employees, and the environment. In
Chapter Ten, Burkard Sievers looks at the suffering experienced
in organizations, which are viewed as arenas for the experience
of both eros and death. Sievers's case analysis of a religious
organization allows him to study the paradoxes that exist in
organizations explicitly based on a spiritual ideal. On the basis
of his analysis of the myths, values, beliefs, and symbols developed in this one particular organization, he proposes that the
management of equality among members is often the main
source of discontent and suffering. Sievers then suggests the need
for a remythologizing of this organization derived potentially
from the rediscovery of its patron saint and, finally, expands
his conclusions for other organizations.

In Chapter Eleven, Narayan Pant tells the story of the
collapse of a bank. Referring to Camus's novel *The Plague,* he
shows that this crisis springs from the ordinary behaviors of ordinary people in an ordinary community. In Pant's tale, no one
really exercises the courage to be, and this lack of responsibility is the real plague that affects each individual in the commu-

nity and leads to a crisis. However, Pant is careful to emphasize that assuming responsibility would not have led to traditional bravery or heroism but to a sense of common decency and the courage to face one's system of meaning.

In the conclusion, I define conditions of existential health in organizations, propose several avenues for further research, and remind the reader that existential issues affect not only the subjective and social lives of individuals but their physiology and the natural world as well, thus calling for the need of managerial science and practice to draw from both the social and natural sciences.

Part One

The Challenge of Finding Meaning in Work

1

Organizational Effectiveness and the Meaning of Work

Estelle M. Morin

The concept of organizational effectiveness holds a central position in the management of private and public organizations and in the field of organizational research. Over the last decade, concerns for efficiency, productivity, excellence, and total quality have become increasingly widespread in Western organizations. These concerns are often motivated by the perception of threats to the survival of the organization. They also seem to be justified by the ever greater international competition for markets and resources. In this chapter, I shall review a number of phenomena that have been explored by several contributors to this book, particularly Aubert, Pauchant, Schwartz, and Sievers. In different ways, these authors claim that the employees of organizations in which the cult of performance is paramount gradually lose the meaning of work, an observation also made by Le Mouël (1991). In this chapter, I hypothesize that the loss of meaning in contemporary organizations is partly due to the current representations of effectiveness, and I propose concrete ways to rediscover the meaning of work.

In this discussion of the phenomena related to the meaning of work and existence, I draw largely on the work of two existential psychiatrists, Victor E. Frankl and Irvin D. Yalom. Frankl was one of the first psychiatrists to apply existentialist thinking, particularly the notion of meaning, to psychotherapy. In addition, Frankl (1963) developed the concept of *logotherapy* to

29

describe a form of helping relationship that orients analysands' comprehension efforts toward the future while focusing their attention on the tasks that they must accomplish for themselves and on the meaning that they must give to their own future. Frankl's own experience in the concentration camp at Auschwitz helped him immensely in better understanding the central importance of meaning in the life of the individual. One of the major lessons that he drew from this tragic experience is that it is ultimately futile to look for *the* meaning of life because an answer is probably impossible to find; the question should rather be phrased as, What does life expect from the individual, now, today, and tomorrow? According to Frankl (1963, pp. 123–124): "These tasks, and therefore the meaning of life, differ from man to man, and from moment to moment. Thus it is impossible to define the meaning of life in a general way. Questions about the meaning of life can never be answered by sweeping statements. 'Life' does not mean something vague, but something very real and concrete."

Also according to Frankl (1963), meaning is a vital necessity for human beings for two major reasons: (1) Because of civilization and socialization, individuals are no longer able to grasp the behavior patterns that are dictated by their instincts; they must ascribe a meaning to their behavior that is acceptable for them and for the society in which they live. (2) Until recently, tradition prescribed rules of behavior and moral obligations that provided human beings with a certain form of security. With the waning of tradition, individuals are now deprived of an important source of meaning. Since they can no longer follow their instincts or the prescriptions of tradition, they must be able to discover meaning on their own. As Frankl (1967, pp. 33–34) states, "At present, instincts do not tell man what he has to do, nor do traditions direct him toward what he ought to do; soon he will not even know what he really wants to do and will be led by what other people want him to do, thus completely succumbing to conformism."

Several psychiatrists and psychologists, including Irvin D. Yalom, Edith Weisskopf-Joelson, and Robert W. Hanna, have followed Frankl, and some of their contributions are described in this chapter. I have chosen to devote special attention to the works of Yalom because he has become very popular not only because of his scientific publications, such as *Theory and Practice of Group Psychotherapy* (1970) and *Existential Psychotherapy* (1980a), but also because of his novels, such as *When Nietzsche Wept* (1992) and *Love's Executioner and Other Tales of Psychotherapy* (1989).

This chapter is divided into five parts. The first part describes the findings of an empirical study on the representations of organizational effectiveness that I carried out with André Savoie and Yvan Bordeleau at the University of Montreal. The results of this study have led me to identify three tendencies that may contribute to the loss of meaning in modern organizations. The second part describes the consequences on the work experience of the logic of effectiveness that derives from such representations. The third explores the notions of meaning and the meaning of work and of existence, primarily on the basis of the works of Frankl and Yalom. The fourth part outlines the consequences of the loss or absence of meaning on mental health. In that section, I also present a clinical description of existential neurosis and explain its etiology and symptomatology. The fifth and final part concludes with an outline of the various means that could be used to achieve more humane management practices based on the lessons of existential psychotherapy.

Representations of Organizational Effectiveness

There are few empirical studies in the literature on the evaluation of organizational effectiveness. According to Bedeian (1987), the only experimental results are presented in a study directed by Quinn (Quinn, 1988; Quinn and Rohrbaugh, 1983). In addition, the contributions of Seashore and Yutchman (1967) and Friedlander and Pickle (1968) should be mentioned. However, these empirical studies contain an important bias: their definition of the components of organizational effectiveness was formulated according to the *researchers' own representations* of the organization, of effectiveness, and of its evaluation. To avoid this type of bias, we have selected a method that draws on the expertise of the evaluators themselves, that is, on experts who specialize in the evaluation of organizational performance and who have an in-depth knowledge of this field.

In our research, we used the Delphi technique (Van de Ven and Delbecq, 1974) to draw on the expertise of eighteen senior executives from thirteen private and five public organizations (Morin, 1989). At the end of the study, the participants had selected forty-six performance indicators that were then used to describe four components of organizational effectiveness. The first component is related to employees and refers to the *quality of human resources,* with particular emphasis on employee development. The second component covers the technical and economic efficiency of the organization, particularly in the areas of profitability and productivity. The third component represents the organization's stability and growth, which have been secured through the protection of financial resources and through the quality of goods and services. Finally, the fourth component describes the position of the organization in its market, based on the evaluation of external groups such as investors and consumers or in comparison with the positions of its competitors.

Table 1.1 presents the criteria and indicators that were used and approved by the majority of participants. These are classified according to the components of organizational effectiveness to which they belong.

This study is interesting in that it captures a narrow definition of the concept of organizational effectiveness *provided by the managers themselves.* What may be even more interesting is the fact that this study offers empirical documentation on the prevailing orthodoxy of the current generation of senior managers with regard to the notion and evaluation of organizational effectiveness on the eve of the twenty-first century. The importance that managers place on the criteria of classic economic theory is particularly striking. To ensure the survival of the organization, managers must obviously pay a great deal of attention to performance criteria such as economic and technical efficiency, productivity, the stability and growth of the organization, the support of external groups, and competitiveness. This being said, however, common sense dictates that while these criteria are

Table 1.1. Components Criteria and Indicators
of Organizational Effectiveness.

Quality of Human Resources	*Technical and Economic Efficiency*
Employee mobilization (Knowledge of organizational objectives, rate of employee turnover, remuneration, employee commitment, incentives for employee initiative)	Resource economy (Rate of inventory turnover, percentage of error reduction, of rejects and waste, comparison of profitability with that of competitors)
Employee morale (Rate of employee turnover, work climate)	Productivity (Comparison of production costs with those of competitors and those of previous years, comparison of actual versus forecast expenses, ratio of the volume or quantity of production to the number of man hours)
Employee productivity (Knowledge of expected production results, control over quality of work, employee performance, knowledge of organizational objectives, remuneration)	
Employee development (Employee mobility)	

Support of External Groups	*Stability and Growth of the Organization*
Shareholder satisfaction (Profit per share)	Product quality (Improvement in the quality of the product, number of returns, number of complaints from customers, mechanisms to detect signals from the environment)
Customer satisfaction (Quality control, delivery time, quality of customer service, customer loyalty, number of complaints from customers)	
Organizational competitiveness (Comparison of production costs with those of competitors, comparison of profitability with that of competitors, product competitiveness, mechanisms to detect signals from the environment)	Financial performance (Increase of annual turnover and profitability in comparison with the results of past years)

all essential, *they are not sufficient in themselves.* In addition, it is highly significant to note that a large number of the dominant concerns and values of Western societies since the end of the Second World War are not even represented in Table 1.1. For instance, note the absence of criteria related to multiculturalism, the integration of minorities, business or industrial ethics, environmental and ecological issues, and so on. Our managers were apparently not interested in these issues even though they have been at the center of the public, political, and academic discussions of the last decades.

We shall see later in this chapter how this concept of organizational effectiveness can explain some of the loss of meaning that afflicts a growing number of managers and employees. For the time being, however, I shall limit the discussion to the identification of three tendencies that are derived from the representations of effectiveness presented in Table 1.1.

First Tendency: Attention to Three Economic Actors

The managers in our sample still adhere to the tenets of classic economic theory best exemplified in the work of Friedman (1962), who argues that the organization must absolutely satisfy the interests of three groups of actors *only:* shareholders, employees, and customers. According to classic economic theory, other groups, such as governments, suppliers, communities, and society in general, are at best peripheral to the continued prosperity of the organization. The fact that managers tend to devote excessive attention to these three interest groups generates a form of discrimination that leads to the neglect, if not the outright denial, of the interests of the other groups that may be affected by the activities of the organization.

Second Tendency: The Primacy of Economic Success

The central place of economic success is obvious in the managers' representations of organizational effectiveness in the late 1980s. The analysis of the data generated by this study shows that a majority of indicators (76 percent) are related to the economic component and that they occupy a dominant position in the structure of their relationship with other indicators (Morin, Savoie, and Beaudin, 1994). One of the direct consequences of the primacy of economic success is the *exclusive recognition of those factors that contribute to the financial performance of the firm.* Moreover, the importance of economic success is such that it results in the lack, if not the loss, of social, moral, spiritual, and environmental values in the management of organizations. Referring to Buber (1963), I would submit that the overvaluation of economic success, organizational growth, and competition is ultimately detrimental to the notion of effectiveness, which then becomes a mere matter of meeting a set of preestablished objectives. In addition, this approach distorts the nature of the work experience and generates a loss of meaning.

Third Tendency: The Depersonalization of Social Partners

The depersonalization of social partners is the third tendency derived from the denial of all but three interest groups and from the exclusive valorization of the economic results of the organization. From this perspective, customers are regarded as economic agents whose sole function is to purchase the goods or services offered by the organization. Similarly, the people who work for the organization are labeled "employees" or even worse "human resources," which implies that virtually their only importance is their capacity to devote their talents to the economic success of the organization. The inherent danger in this type of vision is that it leads directly to the denial of the actors' humanity, to the adoption of so-called objective and impersonal attitudes toward these people (Weisskopf-Joelson, 1967), and to the rejection of their psychological, sociological, cultural, and spiritual complexity.

A Critique of the Current Representations of Organizational Effectiveness

Once again, I wish to stress that I am not attempting to downplay the importance of the economic perspective in organizational effectiveness or to supplant it with another one, because economic efficiency is most certainly a necessity in business. In fact, my criticism is directed at the *priority* that managers now place on the economic perspective in the evaluation of organizational performance. This precedence distorts the meaning of effectiveness and simultaneously affects the meaning of human work and human existence.

To better understand such tendencies, we must bear in mind that the choice of the components of organizational effectiveness is based on social *representations* (Doise, 1985; Morin, 1989; Morin, Savoie, and Beaudin, 1994). These components have therefore been selected from a number of different possibilities. As representations, they reflect a value system as well as a set of beliefs and practices. Thus, they lead to the adoption of specific positions (such as attitudes and judgments) and to the organization of a number of actions (such as behaviors and strategies). Needless to say, the operationalization of organizational effectiveness along criteria such as customer satisfaction, increased productivity, or other similar criteria indicated in Table 1.1 leads to consequent actions and strategies (Chanlat and Séguin, 1987). In general terms, *organizational effectiveness may be defined as a judgment made by an individual or a group upon the organization and, more specifically, on its expected activities, products, results, or effects* (Morin, 1989, p. 202).

This being said, it is indeed surprising that the current representations of organizational effectiveness are still totally similar to what they were at the beginning of the century! The results of our field study with experts in the evaluation of organizational performance are very similar to the concepts presented by several authors, such as Bass (1952), Campbell (1977), England (1967), Friedlander and Pickle (1968), Friedman (1962), Likert (1958), Mayo (1933), Quinn and Rohrbaugh (1981), Scott (1987), Seashore and Yutchman (1967), Simon (1947), Steers (1977), and Taylor (1911). These results can be seen as a positive sign of the stability of the representations of organizational effectiveness over time, but they can also be indicative of their fossilization during the past eight decades. The major social movements of the twentieth century, such as the women's liberation movement, the recognition of human rights and freedom, the development of ecological awareness, the advent of multiculturalism, and the introduction of preventive measures in the area of occupational health and safety, have apparently not modified top managers' view of the organization. Moreover, these major events in contemporary history seem to have had no impact on the efforts aimed at the improvement of organizational performance, in spite of the attempts to humanize organizations (such as employee assistance programs, affirmative action programs, job access programs, and so on). I would submit that this *cleavage* between the social and cultural reality and the administrative reality is partly responsible for the problems that managers face in mobilizing employees and for the difficulty that individuals have in making work a meaningful experience. The current dominance of organizational values over social values in general (Bellah and others, 1985; Pagès, Bonetti, de Gaulejac, and Descendre, 1979) and the rigidity of the notion of organizational effectiveness in managers' representation systems are two phenomena that seem to hamper the quest for meaning in the workplace. They also tend to reinforce administrative orthodoxy through the learning mechanisms that they generate and stimulate the current popularity of managerial fads such as total quality or the search for excellence. Before discussing these proposals, I would like to go back to the original meaning of the word *effectiveness* in order to illustrate its impact on the meaning of work and to demonstrate the semantic restriction that it has undergone in modern organizations.

Rediscovering the Notion of Effectiveness

According to Martin Buber (1958, p. 8), "The overvaluation of productivity that is afflicting our age has so thrived and its par-technical glance has set up a senseless exclusiveness of its own that even genuinely creative men allow their organic skills to degenerate into an autonomous growth to satisfy the demand of the day."

Echoing Buber's remark, the word *effectiveness* comes from the Latin *efficacitas,* which is made up of two elements, ex — "out of" and *facere* — "to do," meaning the making or the accomplishment of something that is intended or desired. It implies the ability to do something, the power to act upon objects. For the human being, to be able to do something means to make it visible that "I," as the subject, am active in the world, that "I" exist. According to Jankélévitch (1980, p. 94), "We might even say that existence consists only and exclusively in 'making to exist,' that existence is absolutely nothing beyond this function or this power."

If we adopt a wider perspective rooted in the etymology of the word, being effective means acting in the world, expressing ourselves in the world; it involves the capacity of leaving the world (through death) and of bequeathing evidence of our existence. Moreover, according to Fromm (1975, p. 235), the notion of effectiveness is also linked to our power, our will, and our existence; it provides tangible evidence that we are alive and human:

> Man's awareness of himself as being in a strange and overpowering world, and his consequent sense of impotence could easily overwhelm him. If he experienced himself as entirely passive, a mere object, he would lack a sense of his own will, of his identity. To compensate for this he must acquire a sense of being able to do something, to move somebody, to "make a dent," or, to use the most adequate English word, to be "effective." We use the word today in reference to an "effective" speaker or salesman, meaning one who succeeds in getting results. But this is a deterioration of the original meaning of "to effect."

Fromm's concept is echoed in several studies on the meaning of work. In the Western world, individuals are essentially motivated to demonstrate their abilities; to prove their mettle; to exercise and develop their talents; to express themselves through work; in sum, to be effective (see Gini and Sullivan, 1987; Locke and Latham, 1990; Schumacher, 1979). More specifically, the need for effectiveness is associated with the following tendencies: self-accomplishment and personal competence (White, 1959), self-coherence (Antonovsky, 1987), and self-efficacy (Bandura, 1977).

In sum, effectiveness is a major concern for the human being. It corresponds to the motivation to demonstrate one's existence, to transcend one's own death by leaving traces of one's existence (Becker, 1973; Camus, 1951). From an existentialist perspective, the notion of organizational effectiveness recovers its original meaning, that is, the capacity of a social organization to do something that will demonstrate the value of its individual members. From this perspective, we are collectively effective when we manufacture objects or deliver services that reflect our values and our beliefs, while being useful to society and to nature. The ethical dimension is central to this perspective: What image of ourselves do we intend to leave as a social organization? The ethical question refers to representations of organizational effectiveness that are radically different from the current dominant representations that were described in the preceding section. *It rests not only on economic values but also on social, moral, and even spiritual values.*

Restricting the concept of organizational effectiveness to the pursuit of economic success at all costs — which leads to the constant growth of organizations and legitimizes worldwide competition — actually generates disastrous consequences for the meaning of work and human existence (Aubert and de Gaulejac, 1991; Fromm, 1947; Le Mouël, 1991; Pauchant, 1993; Ruffin, 1984; Sievers, 1994; Weisskopf-Joelson, 1967). As we shall see in the next section, the first consequence of the overvaluation of success, growth, and competition is the development of a logic of perfection, which consolidates the ego of individuals and drives them to senseless narcissistic development. The second consequence is the weakening, if not the outright destruction, of social, moral, spiritual, and ecological values in our society, along with the impoverishment of the meaning of work and existence. After discussing these consequences, I shall elaborate on the notion of meaning, of meaning of work, and of meaning of existence; this will allow for a better understanding of the function of meaning with regard to mental health and individuation.

The Loss of Meaning in Modern Organizations

The prevailing logic of effectiveness in modern organizations exhorts people not to make mistakes in their activities, to produce (make) perfect objects or services. This is the implicit requirement of zero-defect and just-in-time programs, in which the good or the service must correspond perfectly to the quality standards of the designers and the demands of consumers. Moreover, it seems that individuals willingly commit themselves to this type of work because perfection is something that the human being regards as an ideal to be pursued (Patch, 1984). However, we must bear in mind that *the finitude of the human being, as a limited, imperfect, mortal being, is an inherent condition of existence, and the acceptance of this condition is necessary for mental health and for the potential progress of human society.* Conversely, the denial of this finitude leads to mental illness (Frankl, 1967).

The logic of perfection that flows from our current representations of organizational effectiveness generates at least two types of nonsense; the first is caused by the downfall of heroes and outstanding organizations, and the second by the impossible quest for human perfection. These types of nonsense are explained in the following paragraphs.

The *quest for excellence,* or the "total quality" game, sets the individual, the subject in the phenomenological sense, on an existential quest for perfection in which he can never be successful. This leads to the first type of nonsense. Since the subject may be aware of his perfectibility, he may therefore also be aware of his imperfection and of its corollary, that he cannot be perfect. When "being effective" is experienced as "being perfect" and when the subject realizes the impossibility of attaining "perfection," of reaching an "ideal," it becomes literally impossible for him to achieve something meaningful. This quest for perfection inexorably leads the individual to the nonsense of work because work then provides him with concrete evidence of his own impotence; he becomes a pure living object, devoid of identity and self (Cushman, 1990; Fromm, 1973).

To paraphrase the proposals made elsewhere in this book by Aubert and Pauchant, managers organize rituals aimed at publicly rewarding those who respect the *diktats* of the famous total quality model. This leads others to believe in the credibility of the model while providing them with figures with whom they can identify. For instance, many of the so-called success stories published in professional journals or in works such as *In Search of Excellence* (Peters and Waterman, 1982) reinforce the application of such rules in the management of organizations and in the execution of daily activities. However, we are now aware of the ephemeral nature of these "successes"; sooner or later, the heroes or the outstanding organizations run into new problems — and these often prove to be fatal (Le Mouël, 1991; Morin, 1993; Vedder, 1992; Pauchant and Mitroff, 1992; Pauchant and Morin, 1994). This is where the second type nonsense of this logic of perfection comes into play. When people who have internalized these ideals of perfection as real objects are forced to realize that their heroes have feet of clay, they are pervaded with a sense of disillusion and a loss of meaning that result from the cleavage in their own history (Hanna, 1985).

The finitude of the human being and the fallibility of the identification models are two realities with which the individual is confronted, and they remind him of the necessity of finding meaning not only in his work but also in his life. The individual needs a system of values and beliefs and a sense of history that will allow him to understand and interpret, if not all, at least many of the aspects of his life and to find meaning in them. This sense of history was previously provided by systems of religious, spiritual, or metaphysical beliefs (Frankl, 1967; Yalom, 1980a; Weisskopf-Joelson, 1967) that have now largely disappeared. With the weakening of moral, religious, and spiritual values in our so-called modern (or postmodern) society, the individual is confronted with the problem of the meaning of his existence and, in the case of organizational life, of the meaning of work. At the same time, he is also deprived of the support that was previously provided by such systems. The solution of this existential problem is therefore simultaneously more difficult and more imperative than ever.

The loss of the sacred nature of work that accompanies the intensification of existential problems has been noted by several researchers, including Schwartz and Sievers, who are contributors to this book, Hanna (1985), Mitroff (1983), Pascale and Athos (1981), and Weisskopf-Joelson (1967). Drawing on Yalom (1980a, 1980b), I would argue that the weakening of moral and spiritual values is a direct consequence of the reinforcement of amoral and material values. I believe it is important to specify that for me, as well as for Frankl (1967) and for Pascale and Athos (1981), spirituality does not necessarily involve a reference to a deity. Frankl, Yalom, Weisskopf-Joelson, Jung, and several others have often stated that the human being is a spiritual being that differentiates himself from animals through his quest for meaning, for *logos*. Hence, I use the words *spiritual* and *spirituality* in reference to the nonmaterial dimensions of humankind.

I have tried to demonstrate how the current representations of organizational effectiveness may affect the meaning of work and of human existence. It is important to develop a better understanding of the phenomena associated with the notion of meaning in order to restore meaning to the work and lives of individuals. However, it is also important to be aware of the limits of what can be accomplished. We shall see in the next section that meaning is the result of a subjective experience. The individual involved is the only person who may make sense out of his work or out of his life; nobody else can do it for him. Incidentally, the individual nature of meaning is one of the major criticisms that Sievers (1994) levels at the motivation theories derived from the field of organizational behavior. It is therefore futile to look for ways of making work meaningful, but it is possible to draw on the principles of existential psychotherapy presented by Frankl, Yalom, and others to help managers and workers restore meaning to their daily activities.

The Meaning of Work and of Human Existence

According to several authors, including Brief and Nord (1990), Deleuze (1969), Hanna (1985), and Jung (1981), meaning is an effect and a product of human activity. I would add that meaning is also an effective structure that consists of three components: *significance, orientation,* and *coherence.* In this section, I first elaborate on the notion of meaning in general and then explore the meaning of work through these three components.

The definitions of these components are based on the work of several authors, including Brief and Nord (1990), Csikszentmihalyi (1990), Frankl (1966, 1967), Legrand (1986), Merleau-Ponty (1942), Weisskopf-Joelson (1967), and Yalom (1980a).

The first component, *significance,* implies a specific manner of approaching and understanding the phenomenological experience, as well as the value or importance that is conferred upon this experience. The second, *orientation,* presupposes a project, a plan, or an intent that orients the subject's actions, an inclination toward an object in the most general sense of the word. The third component, *coherence,* refers to the integration of the data from the subject's consciousness, regardless of their contradictions, which the subject achieves by striking a balance between his inner life and social life.

To discover the meaning of an object, we must therefore first discover the manner in which the subject conceives the object. This will also highlight the subject's underlying values. In addition, we must discover the subject's orientation toward the object and the object's degree of coherence with his phenomenological experience. These three components have been described and discussed by the authors noted below.

Brief and Nord (1990) explain the meaning of work through the two definitions of the word *meaning* provided in *Webster's International Dictionary.* They explain that the first meaning of the word — "sense" — refers to the understanding or knowledge of an object, in this case, work. The second meaning of the word — "the purpose" or "the intent" — refers to what goes on in the subject's thinking process with respect to the reasons for which he works and to what he intends to accomplish or realize through his work. These researchers highlight the prospective and retrospective characteristics of meaning in general and of the meaning of work in particular. They use the word *meaning* in reference to the beliefs, values, and attitudes generated by the different processes that have been studied by a large variety of disciplines, such as anthropology, economics, history, philosophy, psychiatry, political science, and sociology.

The word *sense* also has two definitions. The first comes from the Latin *sensus,* meaning "the act of feeling," and refers to the capacity to perceive, judge, and discover the intelligibility of beings, actions, and things. The meaning that derives from this root generally refers to the original significance of something. The second definition comes from the Germanic root *sin,* meaning "direction," and here the word *sense* refers to the concept of a position in reference to an object, to the order of a series of events, and to the orientation of the subject's behavior. The word *sense* is therefore linked to a finality (of the action or of the object). In the same vein, Merleau-Ponty (1942, p. 173, our translation) submits that "the concept of significance is related to the final cause in the same manner that the relationship between a function and a variable is related to the effective cause." Thus, the duality of the word *sense* justifies the association of the meaning of a project with the observed activity. According to Legrand (1986, p. 309, our translation), "The current state of the epistemological, not to say 'philosophical,' research on the meaning of the operation of knowledge clearly carries this connotation: it is an attempt to know simultaneously the *significance* and the *project* ["the purpose," "the intent"] involved in the operation."

Csikzentmihalyi (1990) adds a third connotation to the word *meaning,* namely, that of harmony and balance in the structure of the experience and in the integration of the various actions in a continuous unified flow of experience. For the subject, feelings, thoughts, and actions are congruent; this inner congruence allows the subject to develop a state of psychological security and serenity that helps him deal with the difficult moments in his life. According to Frankl (1963, p. 121), this is what Nietzsche meant when he claimed that "he who has a *why* to live for can bear with almost any *how.*" Similarly, Dilthey (1962, p. 107) highlights the integrating character of meaning; according to him, meaning develops through the relationship that the subject establishes with the object, through the dialectic relationship between the self and the exterior world: "The concept of meaning arises, first of all, in relation to the process of understanding. It contains the relation of something outward, something given to the senses, to something inward of which it is the expression."

Yalom (1980a) also confirms the necessity of coherence as the third component of the word *meaning.* In fact, he defines meaning in reference to coherence and to the intent expressed by something. For him, the quest for meaning is in fact a quest for coherence. In addition, this psychiatrist also refers to the two first components of meaning, significance and orientation. Although he uses the terms *meaning* and *significance* interchangeably, he reminds us that the notion of significance is more specific than that of meaning because in English, it also carries the notion of importance or consequence. Hence, the notion of significance, which is included in the idea of meaning, highlights the underlying values as well as the representations of the object. Yalom also discusses the notion of purpose, which is often used in reference to the meaning of an object. As already suggested, this idea of purpose refers to the intent, the objective, or the function involved.

As an effect of coherence, meaning is discovered through the acts of commitment that are oriented by a transcendental finality. Frankl (1967, p. 31) supports this point of view: "We do not just attach and attribute meanings to things, but we rather find them; we do not invent them, we detect them."

Meaning is therefore the consequence of a highly subjective experience, although it includes a certain degree of objectivity that allows one to recognize it from a pattern of experience. In addition, the discovery of meaning is not based on rational mechanisms because it is rooted in existence (Frankl, 1967). For meaning to provide a coherent effect, one must commit oneself in a responsible manner to an objective or a cause that goes beyond one and forces one to transcend one's interests and abilities. According to Frankl, meaning is revealed as an illumination, which causes the coherent effect, and through acts of commitment that originate in the center of one's personality. Frankl goes so far as to claim that these acts proceed from the basic "trust in Being" and adds that meaning, or better yet *logos,* is not only the emergence of existence itself but also something that confronts existence: "In a word, each man is questioned by life; and he can only answer to life by *answering for* his own life; to life he can only respond by being responsible" (1963, p. 172).

The works of Frankl (1967) and Yalom (1980a) lead us to believe that the individual can achieve coherence between his or her inner life and social life through *acts of commitment.*

Moreover, for these acts to produce meaning, they must be oriented toward a finality that transcends the individual.

Having defined meaning through these three components, we can now use this structure to describe the current state of research on the meaning of work. If we agree that work is an object of meaning, we can describe (1) the *significance of work* for the individual as both a definition and a value, (2) the *orientation of the individual toward work* as defined as the personal objective or purpose of work in his life, and (3) the *coherence of the work experience* as resulting from acts of commitment toward an objective or a cause that allow the individual to transcend himself.

The Significance of Work

Significance, the first component of meaning, refers to the manner of defining an object and to the value that is conferred upon it. Thus studying the significance of work implies identifying what it represents for the individual as well as its importance in his life. These questions have generated a great deal of research over the past several years. Presented below is a brief summary of the current state of knowledge regarding the centrality of work (that is, its importance or value in people's lives) and the definition of work.

The Centrality of Work. Evaluating the centrality of work supposes evaluating its importance or its value in the life of the individual. According to the empirical research on the subject, work constitutes a significant activity for the human being because of its relationship to life. Anthony (1980, p. 419) explains this situation as follows: "As work has been the lot of man from time immemorial, man has invested work with something of the significance which he believes inheres in life. It is not so much that man makes his life through his work as that his life largely coincides with his work."

Morse and Weiss (1955) report that 80 percent of the subjects they surveyed indicated that they would continue to work even if they could afford to live comfortably without a job. According to these researchers, work is important because it gives the individual the feeling of belonging to a larger society, of having something to do, and of having a goal in life. Other studies, including those of MOW International Research Team (1987), Maurer (1968), Orzack (1959), Tausky (1969), and Vecchio (1980), have yielded similar findings. Although the percentages vary from one sample to the next, all of these studies indicate that a vast majority of individuals regard work as an important value in their life. Moreover, in their survey of the literature on the centrality of work, England and Whiteley (1990) report that work is important and significant for a majority of people, based on the following considerations:

> The time that individuals devote to work in their lives
> The numerous functions that work accomplishes for people
> The fact that work is closely linked with other important aspects of daily life, such as family, leisure, religion, and community life

The Definition of Work. The definition of work and the identification of the differences between working and holding a job have generated a substantial research effort. The Meaning of Work (MOW) project is the most far-reaching research project on this topic. (This project is led by an international research team made up of fourteen researchers, including George W. England, Itzak Harpaz, S. Antonio Ruiz Quintanilla, and William Whiteley. The team has conducted its surveys in eight countries: Belgium, England, Germany, Israel, Japan, the Netherlands, the United States, and the former Yugoslavia. The total sample of 14,700 subjects completed their interview questionnaires between 1977 and 1984.) To discover how individuals define work, the MOW International Research Team (1987) developed fourteen possible descriptors, which are listed here in the clusters that the team found:

> *Concrete work definition*
> Something that you have to do
> Compensated by a salary

In a working place
At a certain time
Is unpleasant

Social work definition
Something that contributes to society
Provides the feeling of belonging
Generates a profit for somebody else

Duty work definition
Something you have to account for
Belongs to your tasks

Burden work definition
Something physically strenuous
Mentally strenuous

Other, unclassified, work definition
Something that adds value to something
What someone tells you to do

In another study, England and Whiteley (1990) report six patterns of definition on the basis of these fourteen descriptors.
     Brief and Nord (1990) submit that the only element that
integrates the various definitions of the term *work* is "a purposeful
activity." This notion generally refers to expending energy
through a set of coordinated activities aimed at producing something useful (Firth, 1948; Fryer and Payne, 1984; Shepherdson, 1984). Work may be pleasant or unpleasant, and it may
or may not be associated with monetary exchanges. Moreover,
it does not necessarily have to be accomplished in the context
of a job. According to the interviews carried out by Fryer and
Payne (1984), work is a useful activity that is determined by
a predefined objective that goes beyond the pleasure derived from
its accomplishment. The word *job* refers to the occupation of
the individual, which corresponds to his or her remunerated activities in an organized economic system. According to Fryer
and Payne (1984), jobs always involve relationships of institu-

tionalized exchanges. The concept of job is also associated with remuneration in the form of wages or salary. It often involves the consent of the individual to let somebody else dictate the nature of his or her work and the manner of its accomplishment.

The Impact of the Current Representations of Effectiveness. Work cannot be reduced to the limited concept of job because of its importance in people's lives (Anthony, 1980) and the usefulness that it confers upon human existence (Sievers, 1994). According to Brief and Nord (1990), restricting the meaning of work to an activity that the individual accomplishes in order to earn a salary generates negative personal and institutional consequences. This type of restriction generates or reinforces contractual relationships between the individual and his or her employer and confers more importance on remuneration than on the spirit of service and community. It also devalues non-remunerated activities such as volunteer work and housework, which because they are no longer considered as work are no longer recognized or valued. At the institutional level, this use of the notion of work also creates a situation in which negotiators devote more attention to salary than to dealing with human relations within the organization or to the psychological treatment of the people who work there.

Orientation to Work

To know an individual's orientation toward work, the second component of work's meaning, researchers have analyzed the goals or objectives that people pursue through their work, as well as the functions of work.

The Purposes of Work. The MOW International Research Team (1987) has identified eleven objectives that individuals may pursue through their work:

An interest in the work
A good match between job requirements, abilities, and experience (the use of personal skills)

Variety
Autonomy (freedom to decide how to do the work)
A good salary
Opportunities for upgrading or social advancement
Job security
Good physical working conditions
A convenient work schedule
Good relations with superiors and colleagues
The opportunity to learn new things

Once an individual's personal objectives in work have been identified, it is only a short step to discover the purposes of work. By means of a factorial data analysis, the MOW International Research Team (1987) has identified two main purposes of work: (1) its economic or utilitarian function (salary and job security) and (2) its expressive function (interesting work, autonomy, and matching competences).

The MOW International Research Team's (1987) findings confirm those of Kaplan and Tausky (1974). These authors have reported six significances of work, which they have grouped according to instrumental function (work as means of realizing external projects) and expressive function (work as an activity that allows individuals to express themselves and to be satisfied with their performance). With respect to its instrumental function, work is seen as (1) an economic activity, or a way to earn a living, and (2) a programmed, routine activity, or a way to keep busy. With respect to its expressive function, work is seen as (1) an intrinsically satisfying activity, (2) a source of status and social prestige, (3) morally acceptable, and (4) a source of satisfying experiences in human relations.

Work has served different purposes throughout history. It has been regarded as a way to secure a living, to atone for original sin, to save one's soul, to contribute to the progress of human society, and to improve the quality of one's life. According to Borrero and Rivera (1980), work still serves several purposes in modern societies. It provides rhythm for daily activities and allows individuals to earn a living, to develop friendly relations, to increase their personal value, to accomplish something useful, to express themselves, to increase their knowledge, to learn, and to serve others. According to Anthony (1980), work is much more than a way of acquiring social status, obtaining rewards, or demonstrating personal talents; it is also an activity that allows for the formation of human relationships and the development of moral and spiritual responsibilities within individuals.

The Impact of the Current Representations of Effectiveness. As we have just seen, work generally serves two purposes: a utilitarian purpose (for instance, earning a living, keeping busy) and an expressive purpose (for example, serving others, exercising personal creativity). However, Yalom (1980a) points to the fact that work has lost its intrinsic utility and service purposes in many modern organizations. In addition, current administrative practices tend to fragment work to such an extent that it becomes impossible for individuals to do something in their own image, to use their creativity, to make a part of themselves exist (Yalom, 1980a). Although such practices may contribute to making work more productive, that is, to increase its added value, they also generate feelings of noneffectiveness, nonexistence, and loss of meaning for the workers involved (Aktouf, 1986; Braverman, 1974; Marx, 1976).

The Coherence of Work

The third component of the meaning of work, coherence, refers to the harmony that individuals derive from their work through acts of commitment accomplished for a cause that transcends them. Unfortunately, there is very little information regarding this component in the literature on the meaning of work. However, a certain number of proposals may be formulated on the basis of the writings of Becker, Frankl, Maslow, and Yalom.

Commitment at Work. The notions of responsibility and commitment hold an important position in existential psychotherapy. As Frankl (1967, p. 27) suggests, "Man is responsible for the fulfillment of the specific meaning of his personal life. But he is also responsible before *something*, or to *something*, be it society, humanity, or mankind, or his own conscience. However, there is a significant number of people who interpret their own existence not just in terms of being responsible to something, but rather to *someone*, namely, to God."

According to Becker (1975), Frankl (1967), and Yalom (1980a), individuals must accept their responsibility to humankind and to the world in which they live by choosing, for better or for worse, the monuments of their own existence, of their passage on earth. For Becker (1975), as for Frankl (1967), the desire to bequeath something to posterity, regardless of its nature (material or immaterial), is a way of transcending death. Yalom (1980a) goes so far as to defend the idea that the imminence of death makes the quest for meaning even more important for individuals. Death leads to the awareness of the fragility of existence and of the responsibility of individuals to themselves as well as to others.

The Impact of the Current Representations of Effectiveness. According to the etymology of the term, being *effective* is first and foremost an *existential experience* in which individuals act in the world, express their identity and creativity, and bequeath to the world something that will remind others of their existence. However, Western cultures do not encourage this type of behavior. The lack of commitment that characterizes the prevailing attitudes of our society does not help individuals find meaning at work or in life (Yalom, 1980a).

Moreover, current practices in the areas of mobilization and organizational development emphasize commitment to the organization, more specifically, to its assigned objectives. If these objectives are unrelated to the individual, they do not really call for the individual to surpass or transcend himself or herself, although they may represent a challenge. Organizational objectives would only acquire this type of value if they could converge toward transcendent values, such as the courage of being, rebellion against oppression, human solidarity, love, and virtue (Yalom, 1980a). In the same vein, management practices lead the individual to believe that self-accomplishment is the objective to be achieved. However, Frankl (1963, 1967) and Maslow (1970) have clearly demonstrated that, *for the human being, the need for transcendence corresponds to the necessity of surpassing oneself, not in the restricted sense of self-accomplishment but in the wider sense of accomplishing something that forces one to step out of one's inner boundaries, to distance oneself from one's egocentric interests in order to concentrate one's efforts on an authentic mode of existence with others in the world.* Self-accomplishment, according to Frankl, is not an objective but rather a consequence of this necessity to surpass oneself. Frankl (1967) and Maslow (1970) have also observed a frequent undesired consequence of the search for self-accomplishment for purely selfish purposes: narcissism.

Existential Vacuity: Etiology and Symptomatology

Individuals who do not succeed in finding meaning in their actions, relationships, or lives are condemned to a state of boredom, discontent, and impotence, which Frankl (1967) labels *existential frustration* or *existential vacuity.* According to this psychiatrist, these individuals tend to assuage the discomfort of existential vacuity by increasing their activities aimed at satisfying their need for pleasure or power. First, such individuals tend to seek pleasure mainly in erotic activities. Second, they attempt to increase their influence on their environment through the pursuit of wealth, social prestige, or professional success. Other compensatory mechanisms also exist, such as alcoholism, drug abuse, social deviance, and other means of escape, such as workaholism, gambling mania, gossip mania, and so forth. Frankl also argues that individuals who do not fulfill their destiny, who do not find meaning in their lives, tend to withdraw to their own inner worlds, to be concerned only with themselves. Weisskopf-Joelson (1967) makes the same observations in reporting on her clinical studies and highlights the current importance of narcissistic considerations in modern Western societies.

The lack or loss of meaning therefore produces a state of existential frustration for human beings. If this frustration lasts, it may lead to a nervous disorder that Frankl (1967) calls *noogenic neurosis.* This disorder is mainly characterized by a loss of interest, a lack of initiative, and a feeling of vacuity that is often expressed as the lack of an objective and the loss of meaning in one's life. Maddi (1967) also observed the same type of disorder, which he terms *existential neurosis*. Apart from the lack of meaning, its main symptom is the chronic incapacity to believe in the plausibility, the importance, the usefulness, or the interest of virtually any type of personal commitment. Frankl (1967) detected this type of discomfort primarily in the United States but also in a majority of other industrialized countries, such as Germany, Switzerland, and Austria.

According to Yalom (1980a) and Frankl (1967), existential, or noogenic, neurosis differs from other nervous disorders because of its etiology. Its symptomatic elements are signs of a thwarted will, and its behavior patterns are indicative of a nonsense crisis. Yalom (1980a) adds that the onset of existential neurosis may be triggered by the increase of free time and the reinforcement of noncommitment or nonresponsibility attitudes. According to Yalom (1980a, pp. 447–448), "A citizen of today's urbanized, industrialized secular world must face life [without] a religiously based cosmic meaning-system and wrenched from articulation with the natural world and the elemental chain of life. We have time, too much time to ask disturbing questions; as the four- and three-day work weeks loom ahead, we must brace ourselves for increasingly frequent crises of meaning. 'Free' time is problematic because it thrusts freedom upon us."

Frankl (1967) presents four symptoms of noogenic neurosis, which, as we have seen, is a crisis of nonsense. First, the individual adopts an attitude of ephemerality toward life. He lives one day at a time, provisionally, without expecting anything from tomorrow. Second, the individual nurtures a fatalistic attitude toward life. He adopts a nihilistic point of view: life doesn't make sense and doesn't serve a purpose. Third, the individual's thoughts and behavior are in total conformity with collective requirements, to such an extent that he becomes an anonymous being who commingles easily with the crowd. The state of estrangement that then pervades the individual often leads to a cleavage between his inner life and the outside world. According to Weisskopf-Joelson (1967), there are two possible

reactions to this: the individual either escapes into his inner world
by adopting a schizoid attitude or stagnates in a socially valued
lifestyle by adopting a character—a *persona* in Jungian terms,
or a *marketing character* in Fromm's (1978) words. The fourth
symptom described by Frankl develops as a result of this cleavage; the individual is perfectly prepared to become a fanatic,
to deny his differences with others in order to better deny his
own personality. Yalom (1980a) observes the same development
among individuals who suffer from this disorder. He notes two
types of reactions to this crisis of existential values: (1) conformism (doing what others do) and (2) submission to totalitarianism (doing what others wish). Both symptoms mask the fear
of and the flight from freedom (which paradoxically entails the
obligation of making choices), as well as the avoidance of personal responsibility for one's existence.

Maddi (1967, 1970; Kobasa and Maddi, 1979) has confirmed these observations in his research on existential neurosis. He presents three similar clinical pictures, which he labels
crusadism, nihilism, and *vegetativeness.* First, crusadism is characterized by a strong desire to devote oneself to an important and
dangerous cause regardless of its objective. This attitude allows
one to commit oneself compulsively to a social movement that
will alleviate one's anxiety. Yalom (1980a) and Weisskopf-
Joelson (1967) noted this type of attitude among their patients.
One plunges body and soul into these activities with such frenetic
energy that one succeeds in eliminating the tension caused by
the nonsense of one's own existence. This reaction is often picked
up by organizations dedicated to the pursuit of "excellence," which
channel it toward the improvement of their economic performance. The second reaction, nihilism, is characterized by the
perverse pleasure of destroying and by an active and pervad-
ing propensity to discredit the efforts of others as they are trying to accomplish meaningful things. This attitude is a consequence of despair. In an organization, it may emerge as the
resolute will to "beat" competitors, to denigrate the value of their
goods and services. Finally, vegetativeness is an extreme form
of disarray that results from the absence of meaning that is
characterized by a severe state of disorientation and apathy. Its

main components are the chronic incapacity of believing in the purpose or the value of life, a jaded and taunting disposition interspersed with depressive episodes, and finally a low level of activity. It offers striking similarities to professional burnout. This attitude has also been described by Kets de Vries and Miller (1985) in reference to the "apathetic" type, in whom cynicism and depression appear jointly.

The Lessons of Existential Therapy for Management

The proposals put forward in the conclusion of this chapter are divided into two categories: (1) helping individuals rediscover the meaning of their work and (2) preventing further discomfort by widening the definition of organizational effectiveness.

Rediscovering the Meaning of Work

In this chapter, I have tried to demonstrate that meaning is an extremely important need for human beings. In Western societies and modern organizations, the question of the meaning of work and existence becomes inevitable as a result of the weakening of religious and spiritual systems. I wish to reiterate that the finitude of human beings and the fallibility of identification models are two problems that remind the individual of the necessity of meaning. It behooves managers *to help* their employees and to help one another when they are confronted with this type of problem (Rondeau and Boulard, 1992). The loss or the absence of meaning is a major problem that affects attitudes, behavior, and mental health. In regard to the observations made in this chapter, I wish to advance the proposals outlined below, which are based on the application of existentialist psychotherapy as described by Frankl and Yalom to work situations.

Valorizing the Expressive Functions of Work. As we have seen, work serves two purposes in life: a utilitarian purpose and an expressive purpose. Nowadays, managers and employees alike are primarily interested in the first purpose, and this contributes to the devaluation of the second. However, we must acknowledge the importance of the expressive functions of work on people's attitudes, behavior, and mental health. Just as the body needs food, the human mind also needs "food." Individuals need to express their creativity and to transcend themselves in order to achieve self-accomplishment. Managers must revalorize the expressive functions of work by encouraging and equitably rewarding creativity, service, and personal commitment efforts.

The overvalorization of the utilitarian nature of work is one of the consequences of the overvalorization of economic success and the mindless consumption it engenders. Because of the importance that is placed on the production of goods and services, managers seek to increase productivity through all kinds of means. This ultimately leads to robotized production aimed at diminishing salary costs and therefore contributes to high unemployment rates. In many industrial nations, around 15 percent of the work force is now unemployed. The people who have lost their jobs are not only deprived of their income but also of work itself and its expressive and individuation functions. The idea that I wish to defend here is that workers warrant at least as much attention as do goods and services. Work must not be considered as only another production factor but also as an instrument of individual and social development.

Once again, individuals must be able to ascribe meaning to their actions, relationships, and lives in order to preserve their mental health. They need to commit themselves to a cause that they deem valuable. This search for meaning implies a human need for transcendence, a need to surpass oneself that is not aimed at self-accomplishment but that constitutes a form of personal commitment to a cause that forces one to look beyond egocentric interests and concentrate one's efforts on an authentic mode of existence with one's neighbors. According to Frankl (1967, p. 29), "Life can be made meaningful in a threefold way: first, through *what we give* to life (in terms of our creative work); second by *what we take* from the world (in terms of our experiencing values); and third, through *the stand we take* toward a fate we no longer can change (an incurable disease, an inoperable cancer, or the like)."

It is surprising that such ideas have had so little impact in the organizational environment in view of the fact that they were advanced by one of the most famous pioneers of modern management, Chester I. Barnard, who first presented them at a conference at the Newark Exchange Club on June 14, 1932 (as cited by Wolf, 1974, p. 48):

> For some time now, we have let ourselves become indoctrinated with the belief that the important things are to get money, to impress one's neighbors by possessions, to acquire shallow power, to secure notoriety, to place pleasure above character, to make oneself the center of the Universe. It seems to me high time to teach the truth and preach the faith. Man cannot live by prosperity alone. Sweat and brain are but the tools of a process that must be guided to a goal that is beyond self, not within self. The cooperation that is essential to our mere survival must come from the spirit; it cannot come from a brute selfishness that measures success in power to destroy; that mistakes cunning for intelligence; that confuses daring speculations for courage; that calls leadership that which only leads astray; that mistakes manners for culture and clothes for character.

Rekindling Individual Commitment. Yalom (1980a) places particular emphasis on the therapist's duty to help analysands fully assume their responsibilities toward themselves and others because he believes that *commitment* is a powerful antidote to nonsense. He explains that the quest for meaning is just as paradoxical as the quest for pleasure because the more one looks for it, the less one finds it. Conversely, one becomes able to find the meaning of one's life by making a free and sincere commitment to life. Yalom also claims that all individuals have an inner disposition to commit themselves. Thus, the main task of the analyst is to help individuals sever the links that hamper their commitment and to encourage them to assume fully their responsibilities. Similarly, organizations should not foster individual commitment within the context of growth for growth's sake but within projects that have an intrinsic value, that will stimulate individuals' creativity and their capacity to serve. This concept of work was central in the thinking of the conceptual fathers of modern management, but it has apparently been lost over the years. For instance, Barnard (1968, p. 146) suggested that managers should attempt to satisfy personal ideals in order to foster individual commitment: "Ideal benefactions as inducements to cooperation are among the most powerful and the most neglected. By ideal benefaction, I mean the capacity of organizations to satisfy personal ideals usually relating to non-material, future, or altruistic relations. They include pride of workmanship, sense of adequacy, altruistic service for family or others, loyalty to organization in patriotism, etc., aesthetic and religious feeling. They also include the opportunities for the satisfaction of the motives of hate and revenge, often the controlling factor in adherence to and intensity of effort in some organizations."

Fostering the Individuation of Employees. Yalom (1980a) also suggests that the therapist must support individuals' efforts to find meaning in the series of events that constitute their personal histories. Similarly, managers are in a position to foster and support their employees' efforts to discover personal and collective meanings (Hanna, 1985). In particular, managers can help their employees establish objectives that are meaningful for them and that are congruent with the priorities of their work unit. For instance, it seems that individuals are concerned about the social not to say humanitarian usefulness of what they are doing. If this is the case, work in the organization could be given a social or humanitarian orientation. Managers should also be able to open up a future in which the need for self-transcendence is more respected. Career management systems constitute a unique opportunity to do so insofar as they avoid the pitfalls of trivialization and of succumbing to collective pressures. To foster individuation, one must support the individual's efforts toward his or her own development, which of necessity is a unique process. Finally, the standards and the expectations of managers can have inhibiting effects on individual development. In their relations with their employees, managers must therefore be particularly careful to encourage them to develop their inner abilities to the fullest extent (Lesage and Rice, 1978).

Investing Energies in Meaningful Activities. Yalom (1980a) demonstrates the necessity of actually knowing the person who suffers from a lack of meaning in order to valorize whatever makes sense in his life. He submits that in order to help the individual discover the meaning of his existence, one must first *draw his attention away from his problems and then focus it on those aspects of his personality or activities that are still meaningful for him,* on the task that he must accomplish in order to restore meaning to his life, or on significant people. Because of this principle, Yalom's technique, which he calls *dereflection,* goes in the opposite direction of Freudian psychoanalysis, which focuses the analysand's attention on his problems in an attempt to solve them. Dereflection aims at developing the individual's curiosity for those things that provide meaning, while simultaneously nurturing his interest in others. To use this technique, however, one must delve into the activities and relations that are significant for the individual: What are his beliefs and values; wishes, interests, and goals; preferred activities? What does this person believe to be important in his life, and what gives this person the will to live? The use of this technique in relationships with subordinates who have lost the meaning of their work implies that the manager is truly interested in knowing these individuals and in helping them find ways to stimulate their commitment by focusing their attention on activities or objectives that are meaningful for them.

Widening the Notion of Organizational Effectiveness

In this chapter, I have also tried to demonstrate how human beings' pursuit of effectiveness is intrinsically linked to the search for the meaning of existence. The study of the current representations of organizational effectiveness has allowed us to understand their consequences on social life, ethics, morality, and ecology, as well as on people's mental health. Moreover, I have attempted to demonstrate how the predominantly economic nature of the concept of effectiveness leads to a logic of perfection aimed at the pursuit of excellence, which ultimately results in nonsense at work and, hence, in existential vacuity. To avoid such problems in the future, we must rediscover the root meaning of the notion of effectiveness, which necessarily implies widening its definition. As we have seen in this chapter, the notion of organizational effectiveness must imply not only economic values but also social, moral, spiritual, and ecological ones. In concrete terms, this means, for instance, that organizations should no longer be evaluated solely on the basis of their economic results, as per the criteria indicated in Table 1.1, but also according to their social, moral, and ecological performance. Moreover, these changes in the evaluation of organizational effectiveness must go beyond token gestures of corporate good citizenship and correspond to an authentic will on the part of managers to restore reciprocity and balance in their organization's exchanges with society in general and with individuals in particular. Obviously, defining effectiveness within an existentialist framework forces us to consider a much larger number of actors or interest groups. While managers must continue to pay attention to the satisfaction of the interests of shareholders, customers, and employees, as indicated in Table 1.1, they must also pay attention to other groups of stakeholders, such as minorities, citizens, governments, and of course, nature.

The existentialist perspective on organizational effectiveness concurs with several major administrative currents, such as social issues in management (Vogel, 1986), corporate social performance (Carroll, 1979; Drucker, 1984; Gilmore, 1986; Lewin and Minton, 1986; Lydenberg, Tepper Marlin, O'Brien Strub, and Council on Economic Priorities, 1986; Preston, 1978; Zahra and Latour, 1987), and business ethics (Corson and others, 1989; Ellmen, 1987; Gore, 1993; Meeker-Lowry, 1988). Some of the criteria developed by researchers cited here illustrate the array of the results that managers could take into consideration in the evaluation of organizational effectiveness.

Social and Moral Responsibilities of the Organization. In my analysis of the current representations of organizational effectiveness, I indicated the lack of criteria referring to the social and moral responsibilities of the organization. In the United States, the Council on Economic Priorities has proposed eleven criteria for evaluating the performance of 138 companies that distribute their goods and services in the U.S. market. The council has also published a guidebook called *Shopping for a Better World* (Corson and others, 1989), which explains how the consumer can perform a quick analysis of the moral and social responsibilities of a given company and shop accordingly. Following are the council's suggested criteria:

Amount of charity donations
Number of women in management positions
Number of visible minorities in management positions
Degree of involvement with the military
Testing of products on animals
Degree of openness about policies and social programs
Participation in community services (for instance, education, volunteer work, housing)
Degree of involvement with nuclear energy
Commitment to the protection of the environment
Degree of development of fringe benefits related to family matters (for instance, maternity leave, day-care centers, job sharing)

Ellmen (1987) has initiated the same type of research in Canada, although his five suggested criteria for evaluating company performance are less specific:

Location of head office
Quality of administrative practices regarding employees
Racial equality
Peaceful (that is, nonmilitary) nature of activities
Noninvolvement in nuclear energy

The Ecological Responsibility of the Organization. The current notion of organizational effectiveness completely ignores the value of ecology, although it would be easy for managers to evaluate their companies' efforts toward the protection and the valorization of the environment. This is what the Coalition of Environmentally Responsible Economics (Karrh, 1990) is attempting to do through its ten decision guidelines on environmental issues. These guidelines are called the *Valdez* principles, after the *Exxon-Valdez* disaster in Alaska:

Protection of the biosphere
Durable use of natural resources
Reduction and disposal of waste
Intelligent use of energy
Risk reduction
Marketing of safe goods and services
Compensation for damage inflicted
Openness about potential dangers and incidents
Appointment of directors and managers to board directors
Annual evaluation and audit

Two Guiding Principles

The evaluation of organizational effectiveness has been and will certainly remain a challenge for managers. The recommendations of a number of well-known researchers in this field provide an indication of the breadth of the conceptual and methodological problems involved in the evaluation of organizational performance.

In view of the complexity of the concept of effectiveness, Cameron and Whetten (1983) suggest two guiding principles. First, the definition of the construct must reflect the complex and paradoxical nature of effectiveness. In other words, it must be able to accommodate a larger variety of behaviors, preferences, and performance standards. Second, the evaluation criteria must be appropriate to the organization being evaluated. Van de Ven (1980) adds that these criteria must be concrete observable measures of the organization. They must also be able to generate enough variance to discriminate among the different degrees of performance. He rightly suggests that one should be parsimonious in the selection of criteria and recommends opting for criteria that are both easy and cheap to measure while remaining valid and reliable.

The difficulty involved in the evaluation of organizational effectiveness is such that Goodman, Atkin, and Schoorman (1983) have proposed a moratorium on research in this field. I am fully aware that I am making the manager's job more difficult by suggesting a widening of the concept of effectiveness. Moreover, the criteria that have been presented in this chapter are far from generating a consensus among researchers. This being said, however, we must also consider that the criteria provided by this type of research as well as the methodologies to which they lead are likely not only to improve the quality of life in our society and the protection of nature but also to allow for the restoration of meaning in the workplace.

2

Existential Addiction:
A Model for Treating
Type-A Behavior
and Workaholism

Paul E. Bracke and James F. T. Bugental

While all times seem troubled to those living them, ours repeatedly confronts us with the pervasive destructive force of addictions to work and compulsive activity. For far too long, our culture has explicitly and implicitly rewarded the workaholic, the superachiever, and the worker who scorns the nine-to-five work day and views relaxation and entertainment as indications of moral weakness. Ironically, the Type-A individual, who is at greater risk than others for premature coronary heart disease, is often awarded a "purple heart" for leading a driven and destructive vocational life.

Beyond the fact that heart disease continues to be the leading cause of death for both men and women, our generation's addictions to work and compulsive action have spawned exotic diseases of pervasive fatigue and sudden death (Sutherland, Pershy, and Brody, 1990; American Heart Association, 1991). The chronic stress of Type-A behavior and workaholism appears to suppress the immunological system, which then becomes vulnerable to viral infections, including chronic fatigue syndrome. Although the causes of chronic fatigue remain unclear, recent research has revealed striking similarities between the physical effects of chronic fatigue and cocaine abuse. This suggests that chronic fatigue may result from addictive lifestyles, such as those involving Type-A behavior and workaholism (Leherer and Hover, 1989).

The Japanese Ministry of Health reports that *karoshi,* or death from overwork, is the second leading cause of death for Japanese working men, accounting for 10 percent of all deaths in that population (Yates, 1988). This type of death usually occurs among men between the ages of forty and fifty who compulsively work twelve- to sixteen-hour days, without vacations, for months or even years. Most striking is the finding that two-thirds of these karoshi deaths are due to cerebral hemorrhages, that is, strokes.

Epidemiological research indicates that between 50 percent and 75 percent of individuals in both urban and rural settings exhibit significant Type-A characteristics (Rosenman and others, 1966; Multiple Risk Factor Intervention Trial Group, 1979; Moss and Dielman, 1986). Thus, Type-A behavior is pervasive despite its having been established as an independent risk factor for premature heart disease (Miller and others, 1991; Booth-Kewley and Friedman, 1987).

The staggering incidence and destructiveness of such syndromes as Type-A behavior and workaholism suggest a need for extending our understanding of these disorders in order to offer improved treatment and hope for prevention. Conceptualizing these contemporary compulsions as existential addictions will help explain the fundamental motivations that seduce so many people in our culture to give up their lives — symbolically and literally — to work and to desperate, continual activity.

We contend that the preponderance of Type-A and workaholic individuals seek their deadening immersion in work as a means of avoiding the basic existential issues of being human. Further, we hope that the addition of existential addiction to our diagnostic schema will bring greater clarity and increased attention to a pervasive but culturally denied source of physical destruction, social alienation, productivity erosion, and spiritual decline. Existential addiction, like any other addiction, exerts a wasteful drain on human effort, creativity, and well-being.

Contemporary Addictions

While the Type-A behavior pattern and workaholism are existential addictions that share many common features, distinguishing between them is essential to extending our understanding, treatment, and prevention of these destructive syndromes. Moreover, examining the relationships between existential anxiety and these pervasive conditions can help explain the high incidence of both Type-A behavior and workaholism.

Type-A Behavior Pattern

The Type-A behavior pattern (TAB) was identified in the late 1950s as a complex clinical syndrome believed to be related to premature coronary heart disease (CHD) (Friedman and Rosenman, 1959). Essentially, TAB involves a chronic struggle against time, events, and other people—a struggle that increases the risk of CHD due to chronic overstimulation of sympathetic nervous system pathways, which results in elevated cholesterol level, blood pressure, and heart rate among other physiological processes that promote atherosclerosis.

A series of studies have established that men and women assessed as Type A have higher cholesterol levels than other men and women, even in the absence of any dietary changes and higher levels of stress hormones believed to be related to CHD. (For a fuller description of these studies see Friedman and Ulmer, 1984.) More important, TAB has been shown to be an independent risk factor for CHD in healthy individuals (Rosenman, Brand, Scholtz, and Friedman, 1976).

Type A is a pattern involving behavioral dispositions (for example, aggressiveness), specific behaviors (for example, rapid and emphatic speech), and emotional responses (for example, anger and hostility) (Thoresen and Bracke, 1993). Beneath an outward facade of competence and control, Type-A people are believed to suffer from an internal sense of insecurity and inadequate self-esteem. Thus, Type-A behavior has been conceptualized as an attempt to eliminate personal insecurity and boost self-esteem through an excessive drivenness to accomplish a set of ambitious but often poorly defined goals, such as receiving recognition and advancement (Rosenman, Swan, and Carmelli, 1988). Type-A individuals are addicted to productivity, perfection, and control.

Unfortunately, the role of anxiety over life's basic conditions, or existential factors, in promoting TAB has been virtually unexamined (Bracke, 1992). Only recently has the possible role of social and cultural factors in promoting TAB been examined (Bugental and Bracke, 1992; Van Egeren, 1991). There has also been speculation that Type-A behavior is an addiction to the mood-elevating stress hormones (for example, norepinephrine) and to a high-pressure lifestyle.

Workaholism

Like Type-A behavior, workaholism is rampant and pervasively destructive. This is not surprising since even a brief examination of addiction to work clearly indicates that it has much in common with Type-A behavior. Consider the following characteristics of people addicted to work: (a) difficulty in relaxing due to the need to do more and more in order to feel good about themselves; (b) excessive responsiveness to the expectations of others and rare awareness of their own personal needs; (c) self-esteem based largely on how others evaluate their work performance; (d) a tendency to operate in a crisis mode, usually because of severely overscheduling themselves; (e) a pervasive and growing compulsiveness and an obsessive driven quality that is also exhibited in areas other than work; (f) a tendency to become socially isolated; (g) an intense drive to control time, events, and other people; and (h) perfectionism broadly applied (Fassel, 1990; Schaef and Fassel, 1988).

It would appear, then, that addiction to work may be a progressively degenerative form of the Type-A behavior pattern or at the very least share many of its destructive qualities. There is, for instance, some speculation that, like people exhibiting Type-A behavior, work addicts are addicted to the "high" of stress hormones as well as to the actual process of working

(Fassel, 1990). In addition, workaholism is essentially an addiction to action that may be manifested as impatience, as anger at colleagues who are viewed as obstacles, or as an internal racing mind.

Like other addictions, workaholism is believed to be primarily caused by inadequate self-esteem. The workaholic's self-esteem issue is the fear that there may be "no one inside worth knowing" or, worse, that there may be "no one at all there" (Fassel, 1990). It has also been proposed that workaholics are perfectionists, obsessively attempting to protect themselves from confronting anxious inner issues.

Most important to the concept of existential addiction is the recognition that the individual's tendency to work addiction often joins with the addictive pull of the organization to insulate the worker from the painful dilemmas and realities of modern life (Fassel, 1990). In short, the addictive process takes one out of touch and prevents any awareness and exploration of life's deeper questions. Thus, the workaholic, like the Type-A individual, colludes with the professional organization and other cultural institutions to avoid confronting life's fundamental dilemmas.

Existential Addiction

An existential addiction is a way of being in the world in which an activity, usually work, evolves into the central or singular focus of a person's life. Increasingly, an existential addiction supplants all other aspects of life. This type of addiction is distinguished not by its behavioral characteristics but rather by the underlying forces and motivations that promote and perpetuate it. An existential addiction may therefore be manifested as Type-A behavior or addiction to work. Such an addiction is accurately viewed as an existential one when it develops from a desperate need to avoid existential anxiety and not from inadequate self-esteem, personal insecurity, or avoidance of personal issues. Further, it is an existential addiction in that it displaces as a source of meaning all other values or purposes in a person's life. It becomes the sole justification for being.

Individuals experiencing an existential addiction are avoiding painful confrontations with the fundamental conditions of being human. While a comprehensive discussion of existential anxiety (see Bugental, 1965, 1976; May, 1983; Yalom, 1980a) is beyond the scope of this chapter and is discussed by other authors in this book, the following concepts are essential for understanding and identifying the existential addiction.

Through awareness, we implicitly experience the basic conditions of living, each of which confronts us with a particular challenge or dilemma that gives rise to existential anxiety. If this anxiety is integrated into one's life, it becomes a strong and healthy motivation to live life fully and in accord with one's needs and values, that is, to be authentic (Bugental, 1965). If one finds life's basic issues too devastating, however, one may develop an existential addiction as a means of avoiding existential anxiety. The existential addiction limits awareness and choices as it deadens and constricts one's life — often through a compulsive immersion in one's work. At the core of an existential addiction is a dread-inspired obsessiveness that promotes total immersion in work and an addiction to sheer compulsive "doing."

In essence, an existential addiction is an "existential anxiety avoidance disorder" employed to reduce or attempt to avoid the anxieties inevitable in confronting life's fundamental conditions of change, death and contingency, responsibility, relinquishment, and "a-partness." Each of these conditions is described below.

Because we are physically embodied, continual change is inevitable. Life itself is a dynamic process. Because we are aware of our physical being, we are subject to anxiety of pain, illness, or destruction.

Confronted with finiteness, we naturally experience anxiety arising from awareness of death and fate (Tillich, 1952; Bugental, 1965; Yalom, 1980a). Because we are limited, we are confronted by the infiniteness of potential and by the limited ability we have to control outcomes in life (that is, powerlessness). Contingency means that the number and possibilities of all the influences that together determine what will happen in the next instant or hour or in a lifetime are beyond our knowing and control (Bugental, 1965). Contingency does not deny our power to have some effect; it obliterates the illusion of certainty.

Because we have the capacity to choose and act on our choices, we are inevitably confronted with responsibility for what we choose and do and for what we have not chosen and not done. Thus guilt, sadness, and regret are inevitable aspects of life.

Because we are free to choose, we are inevitably confronted with relinquishing what might have been. Relinquishment is also the act of choosing to let go rather than being forced to give up something. Through choice and relinquishment, we can create personal meaning. When we surrender choosing — through conformity, for example — we experience meaninglessness or emptiness.

We are always in relation to others and yet always separate. We are thus confronted with our a-partness, an anxiety-producing paradox (Bugental, 1965). Finding ourselves separate yet related, we experience existential anxiety generated by the threat of isolation and loneliness or, conversely, by the threat of engulfment.

When Type-A behavior is an existential addiction (Bracke, 1992), the Type-A drive to accomplish an escalating number of tasks in less and less time serves to eliminate self-awareness. Moreover, the excessive need for control that characterizes Type-A individuals appears to be a desperate attempt to eliminate life's fundamental unpredictability. The hypercritical blaming and need to dominate others that corrode Type-A individuals' relationships seem likewise to be destructive reactions to accepting personal responsibility and being in relationship (Bracke, 1992). Table 2.1 presents these characteristic Type-A reactions to life's basic conditions.

Thus, Type-A behavior may be viewed as an existential addiction employed to eliminate the distress of anxiety and emptiness by overfilling one's life with activities such as work and/or home projects. The inevitable futility of this addiction may result in pervasive disappointment and chronic hostility. Individuals who employ the Type-A lifestyle as an existential addiction — a destructive means of avoiding life and its basic anxiety-provoking issues — suffer severely.

Table 2.1. Type-A Reactions to Conditions of Being.

Conditions of Being	Embodied	Finite	Action-able	Choiceful	Separate but Related
Confrontation	Change	Contingency	Responsibility	Relinquishment	A-partness
Existential anxiety	Pain and destruction	Fate and death	Guilt and condemnation	Emptiness and meaninglessness	Loneliness and isolation or absorption
Existential need	Spiritedness	Identity	Potency	Meaningfulness	Relatedness
Authentic response	Wholeness	Faith	Commitment	Creativity	Love
Type-A reactions	Compulsiveness Obsessiveness	Hypercontrol Ultraindividuation "Specialness" Hyperactivism Materialism	Blame others Suspiciousness (hostility) Conformity	Cynicism Alienation from self Hypercriticism	Dominance Alienation

The pervasiveness of existential addiction is the result of many powerful social, political, and economic trends. Preeminent among them is the emergence in our culture of a pervasive sense of personal emptiness. Many authors have described how economic, political, and social forces have assailed the needed experience of being oneself and having an internal locus of control (Cushman, 1990; Gendlin, 1987; Lasch, 1978). Concurrently, individuals have been increasingly expected to be self-sufficient and self-satisfied. Conventional wisdom recognized no limits to achievement and fulfillment for middle-class Caucasians born in the baby boom era. Such inevitably frustrated expectations in combination with the overvaluing of individualism only deepened the emerging sense of alienation and intensified the widespread sense of emptiness (Bugental and Bracke, 1992). Such a confusing, empty, and hostile social context dramatically amplifies existential anxiety, making existential addiction irresistible for many.

The corporation has emerged as the major "supplier" for those individuals who develop existential addictions. Wittingly or not, many corporations capitalize on alienation and emptiness and promote addiction to work as the answer to dealing with life's difficult issues and seem to promise a path to fulfillment and meaning. In short, the individual unable to confront existential anxiety becomes "hooked" to avoid life's issues and consequently is highly vulnerable to the seductive pseudosatisfactions offered by the corporate life.

We speak of this vocational lifestyle as an addiction to highlight certain critically important features: the compulsive nature, the absence of a sense of personal choice, the trend toward repetitive and mechanical quality of action, the lack of any lasting satisfaction from the activity itself, and in severe instances, the tendency for there to be a decline in quality and/or quantity of work accomplished.

Defining existential addiction in this way sets it in contrast to the healthy commitment and dedication of an individual whose work is a continually growing source of satisfaction, continually presents new and evocative challenges, and subtly or manifestly engenders a broadening of the person's horizons.

This last characteristic may take a variety of forms: more meaningful relations, the opening of new vistas in the chosen field,
the incorporation of fresh elements (often in a way that others
less devoted have not previously recognized).

For the addiction-free individual, work is only one dimension of a more balanced life. For the individual trapped in existential addiction, work *is* life. Many individuals work long
hours and are occasionally overscheduled, but they do not suffer
anxiety, guilt, and depression when a task is completed. Genuine
dedication leads instead to a sense of satisfaction and an appropriate weariness. Unlike the Type-A professional or workaholic, the addiction-free professional is able to reject or postpone the continual demands of work.

The nature and pervasiveness of existential addiction
strongly suggest that no profession is exempt. The most common instances include people in business who devote huge
amounts of time and energy to their work without concern for
the larger meaning of what they do or produce or for the costs
to themselves and other people in their lives. Individuals with
the freedom to determine their own work hours, projects, and
standards may be at increased risk. Any work is potentially an
opportunity for mind-numbing obsessive immersion. The destructive effects of existential addiction include the following:

Increased risk for stress-related disease (for example, coronary heart disease)
Loss of self-awareness or a centered awareness of being
Failure to attend to health and other maintenance needs
of self and others
Loss of meaning in personal relations; other people have
value only as they serve the addiction
Lack of satisfaction in what is already attained; continual
pressing to achieve more
In advanced cases, gradual decline in quality of work and
in relationships
In some instances, existential addiction expressed through
multiple addictions (for example, overeating, alcoholism)

In summary, existential addiction is not to be confused with genuine dedication to work or any other activity. An existential addiction exists when certain specific conditions are present. The individual's obsessive involvement in work or continual "doing" is motivated by an intense need to avoid existential anxiety. In the attempt to meet this need, self-awareness is severely reduced or eliminated. The psychological center of experiencing is displaced from within the individual's own subjectivity and resides almost totally in the work. The sense of meaningfulness in the individual's life comes almost entirely from work and "doing" and thus is so circumscribed that all other aspects of life are evaluated only as they contribute to those endeavors. Moreover, in some advanced cases, the quality of the work products (whatever they may be) decline rather than increase, as such "dedication" would lead one to expect. Here are some other common symptoms of existential addiction:

Chronically overscheduled with work demands as well as other activities

Excessive impatience with people, time, and events

Irritability, tension, anger, suspiciousness

Long working hours, even on weekends, often with relatively modest production

Various tasks and projects often completed simultaneously, that is, polyphasing or multitasking

Overly objective outlook; avoidance of subjective involvement

Little or no sense of humor

Abstracted manner, difficulty in maintaining attention on topics not explicitly related to the addiction

Work routinized and mechanical, and experimentation and innovation resisted

Case Examples of Existential Addiction

The constricting and destructive nature of existential addiction can best be illustrated by case examples and case-specific discussion.

Case 1. Charles

At forty-five years of age, Charles is a highly successful chief executive of a moderate-sized but growing retail tool company. His boyish handsomeness is striking. As he tells his story, it is clear that his rise in the corporate world has not been an untroubled one. After what he describes as an idyllic college experience that included being president of his class and an array of romantic interludes, he had "hit the real world and crashed." The demands of his first two positions had apparently exceeded his abilities. These disappointments had been traumatic to both him and his family's expectations for him. These professional setbacks seemed to have precipitated a greater determination to succeed and a perplexing chronic depression.

Charles married a college sweetheart who had been "the only girl who hadn't been easily charmed by" him. The new responsibility of marriage combined with his reaction to the previous professional failures engendered a more aggressive and dedicated stance when he made his next career move. With borrowed funds, he took over a small and rather mediocre company and proceeded in just seven years to amaze the corporate community by rebuilding it into an industry leader—a position in which it has remained for some years. However, competition in the field is challenging this preeminence more each year.

During the years after he first took the firm over, Charles "lived and breathed [his] company as [he] dragged it to the top." He formed a pattern of consistently working twelve-hour days, including most weekends. This schedule, he proudly contends, is the sacrifice that one has to pay for major corporate success. Charles is certain that the two major factors in his success are his ability to "assess what [his] board of directors wants and to deliver it" and his "commitment to work at a project until it is perfect—no matter how long that takes."

Such an intense focus on work has prevented him from spending much time with his family. Charles's wife has reacted to his consuming passion for his work by withdrawing resentfully and refusing his romantic advances. His college-age son has progressed from tolerating his father's absence from his life to currently refusing Charles's attempts at contact and generally treating him with disdain. Charles's relationship with his teenage daughter is only marginally better, and their time together usually consists of a few hours "stolen" from weekends filled with work. Though not estranged from his daughter, Charles recognizes that he really shares little with her.

When confronted with this sad state of his family, he takes refuge from his guilt by insisting that he has given them nearly all the material advantages available. Nevertheless, there is a hollowness to this defense, which he himself seems to recognize, at least partially.

Charles speaks of his relationships with his wife and children as "not as intimate" as he would like but insists that such family problems are to be expected when one "takes on the challenge of big-league corporate success." Thus, while he is bothered by his wife's lack of sexual desire and the cold responses of his children, he is at a loss as to how to resolve these "typical family problems"—while still maintaining his work pattern, of course. The notion of reducing his immersion in work does not even occur to Charles as a possibility. Bewildered, he concludes: "How can I change my life without upsetting all the people who depend on me?"

While detailing his success as an executive, Charles also confesses bewilderment at several troubling symptoms. The first is that for years he has suffered from an intermittent depression for which he is taking a currently popular antidepressant medication. He is dissatisfied with this means of holding in check what he feels is a sign of personal weakness, but he is certain that he has no choice but to continue the medication. His account strongly suggests that, at this time at least, his distress is rather directly exacerbated by the criticism he is starting to receive from his board of directors. He is aware of how vulnerable he is to any apparent faultfinding, and that irritates him because he believes he has high self-esteem and thus feels that he should not react in this way.

Charles is even more concerned about a second problem, his chronic late-night compulsion after completing work to eat large quantities of junk food. However, this pattern of overeating concerns him primarily because he thinks that his overweight appearance will be viewed by other executives as an indication that he is "not in control" of himself. In contrast, he seems surprisingly unconcerned about his elevated blood pressure and high cholesterol count.

Almost as an afterthought, Charles adds that after such a continual and intense focus on "carrying [his] company to the top," he is aware of how he nearly always experiences a nagging anxiety that he has more to do than he has time for. On the heels of this reluctant recognition comes another admission, even more hesitantly volunteered. Recently, he has begun to notice that projects that he had previously been able to complete on time and in superb fashion are now often delayed and even then suffer from what he is forced to recognize as diminished creativity and precision.

When talking about these concerns, Charles is casual, dismissing them as exceptional instances "bound to happen to anyone" and not worthy of special attention. However, his efforts to downplay them are forced and not very convincing. The decline in the quality of his work is, in fact, beginning to evoke genuine panic in him and may well be the real, although underlying, reason why he has come to psychotherapy.

Charles presents a reasonably typical Type-A pattern, but a crucial additional element, noted in the preceding paragraph, distinguishes his condition as an advanced existential addiction. Some people who show Type-A overcommitment and a heedless expenditure of their energies seem to be able to operate at this level indefinitely. Indeed, some may be said to thrive on it, if a very constricted view of life's potential is employed. However, existential addicts such as Charles are not such people.

More importantly, Charles's style of working and his relationships with family, friends, and corporate peers reveal the central existential issues that his Type-A behavior obscures and allows him temporarily to avoid. Three existential challenges seem particularly difficult for Charles to confront: responsibility, relinquishment, and relationship (that is, a-partness). In avoiding the burden of accepting responsibility for the choices he makes, Charles has adopted a broad conformity that dismisses his innate needs and stifles his true vitality to pursue a life that he would find genuinely satisfying. Sadly, such conformity is pervasive. Charles, like many other Type-A workaholic individuals, has subscribed to a deadening contemporary philosophy: "It is better to look good than to feel good" (Bugental and Bracke, 1992). Appearance and the approval of others have directed Charles's life to the nearly complete exclusion of his unrecognized needs. The essence of the existential addiction is strikingly clear: Charles has severely limited his self-awareness and choices in order to attain a pseudocomfort. Such harsh dismissal of himself may well be the source of his depression. Deeply inauthentic responses to life appropriately engender despair.

Caught in a life directly primarily by social convention and the expectations of others, Charles experiences a lack of meaning and an ambivalence in his relationships. As a means of relaxing, and attempting to assuage feelings of emptiness, Charles guiltily turns to food binging, which is immediately satisfying. While this practice creates health problems, it may also be a hopeful sign of rebellion after years of stifling conformity.

In the context of a lifestyle that he has worked so hard to build, it is understandably frightening for Charles to consider that the path to a more satisfying life will require relinquishment. As he comes to realize how much of his life has been erected to gain the approval of others, he will understand his bewildering dissatisfaction. A life built upon chronic conformity and loss of self-direction may require extensive renovation if Charles is truly to move toward satisfaction and meaning. Such re-decision will confront Charles with the necessity of relinquishing some of his personal and professional choices.

Charles's conformity also creates formidable obstacles to satisfying relationships. Perhaps in reaction to an unconscious awareness of how chronically he loses himself to the expectation of others, he has become distant and alienated from many of the people with whom he might be intimate. Until he comes to understand and respect his own needs, he will experience great difficulty in being separate from and yet genuinely related to others.

Psychotherapeutic examination of his problems is difficult. His treatment is often interrupted by the demands of his work, which are usually given precedence over therapy sessions. Gradually, however, therapy makes some progress. Charles is able to become more aware of how much others have influenced and continue to influence his choices and life. He recalls a powerful memory of his mother proclaiming enthusiastically that he, Charles, could be successful at anything he wanted to do. What gives this memory particular power in his emotions is the recognition that he had come to associate it with another early childhood yearning — to be able to fly. This was an ambition he had carried to the point of convincing himself that he could actually leave the ground by flapping a set of cardboard wings that he had eagerly fashioned. His imagination portrayed how he would impress his family and friends and how very happy with himself he would then be. Now he is flying, as a business executive, and yet he is naggingly unsatisfied still. Surrendering his ability to choose has led him to a glittering emptiness.

A parallel line of exploration in therapy brings Charles to the realization that his binge eating is very likely his only means of relaxing, of satisfying himself and at the same time rebelling against his "always having to do the right thing." Abruptly, he realizes how seldom he actually finds his work or his family truly satisfying. Reluctantly, he recognizes that by so persistently acceding to the rules of corporate culture he has lost touch with what he actually needs.

These recognitions open out into the realization that in the course of ascending the corporate hierarchy he has not developed any close friendships. Now he becomes vaguely aware of longing for companionship. Sadly, he begins to see how distant he has become from a wife who no longer understands or seems to care and from children who are ready to begin independent lives of their own. Charles finds little comfort in the observation that "no one else in my business has relationships that are much better."

Case 2. Susan

At forty, Susan is about to be promoted to vice president of a growing and successful medical supply firm. Although she has worked tirelessly in the company's behalf for the past ten years and feels flattered and deserving of her impending promotion, recent personal events have dampened her excitement. While she is keenly aware of the high pressure and stress of her work and knows that she has been "moving at the speed of a low-flying plane" for many years, she is shocked when she first experiences chest pains. The fact that a cardiological examination does not indicate an imminent heart attack does surprisingly little to assuage her fears.

Susan also realizes that, while she has recently been working at a less frenetic pace, her energy is lower and her creative vigor has decreased precipitously. In short, she has suddenly lost much of the satisfaction that she had previously derived from her work. Her initial response has been to work harder in an attempt to "jump-start her creative juices." This has only increased her general sense of burnout. The loss of energy and interest is particularly troubling to her and to her company because she has always been able to give "200 percent effort" to her work.

During her ten years with the company, Susan rose rapidly to the position of top salesperson, largely through "working as long as necessary to ensure that a project was completed on time in order to keep all customers satisfied." She realized early on that this would require her to work many fourteen- to sixteen-hour days, especially on key projects. She had eagerly committed to meet this professional demand. It seems, however, that she ends up working most evenings and weekends — even when the actual demands of work do not require it.

Because of her tendency to take on an increasing amount of responsibility for completing projects, her co-workers have come to view her with a mixture of respect, envy, and resentment. Susan's response is to reiterate that to succeed "you must always look eager, poised, and relaxed regardless of how you actually feel." Thus she has successfully created the image of a tireless, competent, hyperresponsible superstar who will never let customer or company down.

Not surprisingly, most of her personal relationships are business related. This seems highly satisfactory to Susan because such friendships have been greatly advantageous to her profes-

sional success and "people in business understand and appreciate [her] drive and ambition." Although she felt that she did
not have enough time for a traditional romantic relationship,
she met and married a man with a similarly demanding profession as a stockbroker. Their married life consists primarily of
shared commutes to work, small portions of evenings and weekends when they can put aside work, and occasional vacations
to popular ski and beach resorts, usually as part of a group of
business friends.

Susan enters psychotherapy with the goals of managing
her stress more effectively and deciding how to deal with her
impending promotion. Early therapy sessions are disrupted by
urgent calls from customers that she receives on her car phone
or via the nearly constant buzzing of the pager in her purse.
Although she learns and applies the most effective stress management techniques, she becomes increasingly distressed that
the quality of her life does not appreciably improve. Even the
most competent time and stress management strategies do not
reduce the "stress" that chronically distresses her. She gradually realizes that even when she copes exceptionally well with
the demands of her work, she is somehow deeply dissatisfied.

The basis of her dissatisfaction is first revealed in two
powerful dreams. Ironically, when Susan's burnout requires her
to rest more, she begins to have and recall dreams for the first
time in many years. In her first provocative dream, she finds
herself in a familiar childhood park, looking down a deep well
that had, in fact, existed on her grandfather's farm, a place of
childhood joy, solitude, and reflection. She recalls "asking the
well for an answer to [her] problems." The well's provocative
answer is to demand that she "leave the well alone" and "not
to come down into the well to look for answers." Rather than
being discouraged, she concludes that she needs to know herself better in order to resolve her problems.

A more provocative dream soon follows. In this dream,
Susan finds herself in a hospital, being prepared for "some operation that will help [her]." Her relief at the prospect of being
helped turns to terror when she realizes that "they want to replace
my heart with an indestructible high-tech heart so that I can

continue to work as hard as ever." In her dream, she argues against the procedure and then flees.

Together, these dreams evoke a strong commitment in Susan to examine more carefully the value and personal cost of her professional obsession. She wonders whether becoming a vice president will be worth further endangering her health. She is able to postpone her decision on the promotion. Gradually, she is also able to limit her working hours and efforts and to create small but precious hours of solitude in which to encourage the self-nurturing and reflection that she increasingly realizes she needs.

Another powerful recognition is that although she had nearly dismissed the idea of having children, her desire to become a mother is stronger than she had realized. "How," Susan laments, "can I possibly fit a child into my schedule?" As she examines her life more deeply, she is confronted with a critical but more troubling awareness: "So many people want a piece of me that soon there will be nothing left! How can I hope to take care of a child if I haven't learned who I am and how to care for myself?"

In living her life as a "low-flying plane," Susan has developed the pervasive self-ignorance that characterizes individuals with some form of existential addiction. The compulsive frenzy and excessive accommodation to the demands of others have thoroughly numbed her to her own needs and sense of identity. Her advanced existential addiction has enabled her to temporarily avoid the anxieties of responsibility, relinquishment, and mortality. Like Charles, she has temporarily avoided the responsibility of personal choice; her professional role and company excessively determine who she is and what she does. Although such conformity allows her to avoid the difficult task of becoming self-aware and the burden of making self-based choices, it has inevitably created a bewildering emptiness, superficial relationships, and chronic, gnawing depression.

Like many individuals engaged in avoiding existential anxieties through a workaholic or Type-A lifestyle, Susan enters psychotherapy with the illusion that her "stress" can be effectively "managed" without her making any significant changes in her life. Not surprisingly, her initial commitment to therapy is commensurate with the superficiality of her goals. She allows and invites her work to intrude and interrupt her therapy through phone and pager.

Susan's continuous connection to her company reveals another aspect of her existential addiction. Repeatedly demonstrating her crucial importance to the company may be her way of establishing her "specialness." A belief in personal specialness can serve to insulate an individual from many powerful existential anxieties that inevitably lurk beyond the edge of consciousness. For Susan, the talisman of specialness may help her believe that she is exempt from aging and death — an issue reflected both in her concerns about her health and in her emerging ambivalence about having children.

During therapy, Susan begins to realize the futility of stress management. For her, as for most individuals whose existential addictions are manifested as Type-A behavior or work addiction, even the most effective strategies for managing time and stress are usually impotent. As long as Susan's approach to coping with work demands does not consider her unique needs and values, she will continue to experience chronic stress and dissatisfaction. *What must emerge in her therapy is the awareness that living a superficial and inauthentic life is inevitably "stressful" — regardless of one's coping repertoire.* The apparent avoidance of conflict that seems to come from allowing herself to be directed by others and her company will continue to undermine her sense of identity and potency. Such a painful but unconscious loss of identity can only be experienced as deeply stressful.

As she begins to value her sense of self, Susan's subjectivity is powerfully expressed through her dreams. Beyond the dramatic content of her dreams, Susan's responses of wanting to know her self better and not wanting a "high-tech heart" suggest a growing desire to confront the existential dilemmas that she has desperately sought to avoid. Her stark and frightening awareness of her pervasive self-ignorance and how she is being consumed by others and her work evokes a powerful motivation to rebuild her life in a healthier way. Anything short of such an intense personal confrontation might well be inadequate to dislodge her existential addiction.

Case 3. Michael

At his first counseling session, Michael proudly brags about the excesses of his Type-A lifestyle. He boasts of his capacity to complete two or more tasks simultaneously in order to save time. While completing household tasks, he often wears a telephone headset to "stay on-line" with ongoing business deals. He is not only immersed in the intense process of starting a computer software company but is simultaneously consulting with other companies in his capacity as a marketing consultant. In many instances, he works the entire day on his start-up venture and then continues working into the early morning hours preparing and faxing reports to his consulting clients. He states that he has always worked in this manner. Although he often comes to counseling sessions without a briefcase, he always carries his cellular phone in case he "needs to call someone while walking from parking lot to office." He has created a formidable high-tech umbilical cord that ties him to his work.

Although he expresses little genuine concern about his Type-A approach to working or his chronically elevated blood pressure, he is very distressed about his inability to maintain his marriage of fifteen years. He has been divorced twice and his third marriage is in jeopardy because of his nearly total immersion in work and the stress and irritability that he brings home. Three years earlier, in the process of trying to develop another business, he had worked so much that he barely saw or spoke to his wife for weeks at a time. She had grown increasingly resentful and began to confront him about his commitment to her and their marriage. What little time they had for intimate contact became filled with attacks and counterattacks, usually ending with his asserting his dominance through intimidation or with his withdrawal to the more satisfying computer screen or fax machine. After one particularly abusive argument, she had left, demanding that he seek professional help before she would return.

During this period of marital alienation, Michael had begun an affair with a co-worker who "understood the demands of building a company and worked as intensely" as he did. Their relationship usually consisted of working long hours followed by intense lovemaking and a return to work. Although this was satisfying to Michael, he seemed regretful that he had begun the affair and expressed a genuine affection for his estranged wife. He wanted to save his marriage but felt unable to relinquish the satisfaction and intensity of his work.

Examining these issues is difficult for Michael, who is completely uninterested in understanding how his needs and reactions might play a role in his relational distress. He is, however, able to realize that he clearly finds more satisfaction and excitement in his long and intense working than in a relationship with any person. Developing his company is the equivalent of "growing a child," he says, one in whom his identity and self-esteem are thoroughly invested. Unlike the situation with his spouse, he can easily use the power of his position to impose his will on employees who disagree with him. Gradually, he also becomes aware of a decline in physical prowess at age fifty-five and expresses on several occasions the idea that when he "is gone," he will rest more comfortably knowing that his company will live on.

As therapy progresses, Michael realizes that his personal friendships are exclusively with business colleagues. These relationships are typified by business lunches during which he exchanges war stories about business or "gets information" he needs. Even more often, however, he maintains these relationships via the computer. Michael is often more comfortable with the latter than with personal contact. In the course of his self-exploration, he begins to wonder whether this might be due to his experience of growing up in a dysfunctional, alcoholic family.

While Michael understands how his total immersion in work and the resulting stress are eroding his marriage, he is unable to forego the "adrenaline high" of work in order to rebuild his marriage. This is the case even after his affair ends because of his lover's dissatisfaction with his emotional and physical unavailability. Consequently, his attempts to reduce his Type-A behavior and to develop a better marital relationship are only minimally effective until a chance event confronts him with the severity of his situation.

After several months of therapy, Michael is beginning to develop his ability to be aware of his own internal reactions to people and events. After returning from a business trip in the early morning hours, at a nearly deserted airport gate, he is powerfully moved when he witnesses the welcome-home scene of two spouses being reunited. In fact, he is moved to tears by the exquisite tenderness and joy that he sees in the embracing couple. More powerful, however, is his stark terror at somehow realizing for the first time that being married to his work has made him unable to feel any love and tenderness toward another person. He is empty and alone and unless his life changes drastically, he will die this way.

Michael's extreme Type-A behavior and work addiction are means of obscuring the anxieties of mortality and relatedness. The meaning and central importance of "growing his company" as a way of coping with concerns about mortality and contingency are apparently close to Michael's awareness. But while he rather casually reflects on the comfort he feels in knowing that his company will "live on" after his death, he uses such intellectualizations to avoid and deny his subtle, but nagging anxiety.

Further, Michael's nearly constant working appears to help him cope with the feelings of powerlessness that accompany contingency and mortality. Michael has created a lifestyle in which the intense volume of his activities prevents him from hearing and confronting these basic issues in a healthier and more effective manner. Ironically, he is risking his life in the service of avoiding anxiety related to aging and death. A predominant goal in Michael's psychotherapy will be to help him begin to experience his driven workaholism as a death-denying feat. Moreover, he, as other existential addicts, can eventually come to perceive his mortality in a life-enhancing manner. Although death destroys life, an awareness of death can be a powerful motivational force in deciding what is truly important in life and committing to the pursuit of one's authentic values.

Like Charles, Michael also appears to be employing an overinvolvement with work as a means of avoiding the difficulties of intimate relationships. His most satisfying relationships are totally embedded in his professional striving. His awareness that he finds more satisfaction and excitement in his intense involvement with his fledgling company would be useful in his psychotherapy were it not for the fact that he is apparently completely at ease with such alienation.

Existentially, Michael is experiencing the anxiety inherent in the condition of being both separate from and related to others. Subjectively, this experience of a-partness confronts one with the existential anxiety of isolation and loneliness or, conversely, of engulfment. Unable to confront and integrate his fundamental a-partness, Michael has actively created a deep interpersonal estrangement, primarily through using the demands and goals of business to distance and insulate himself from others. While he has temporarily succeeded in managing his anxiety, the cost is a nearly complete alienation from human intimacy.

Although Michael's psychotherapy has undoubtedly been difficult for both him and his therapist, it has apparently progressed enough to awaken some of Michael's subjective sense. His powerful reaction to a couple's affectionate reunion has propelled him into an agonizing confrontation with his own loneliness. More useful as an incentive to deepen his commitment to change significantly his Type-A lifestyle is his potentially transforming awareness that he will very likely die in isolation. Michael's experience may impress upon him that he cannot risk postponing the development of meaningful relationships until after his work is completed. Together, these stark confrontations with reality, made at a deeper level than that of his apparent ease with such alienation, may stimulate the concern and commitment needed to successfully change his empty Type-A life.

Case 4. Madeline

By the time Madeline was forty, she had achieved what most people can only dream of — she had founded and developed a highly successful, nationally known mail-order company. After two years as president, however, she found herself suffering from the stress of "staying at the top" and proceeded to sell her company at an impressive profit. For the first time in many years, she arranged her life in a more relaxed manner. Having decided not to have children, her return to "civilian life" was unencumbered by the demands of parenting. She allowed her husband, a prosperous doctor, to support their lifestyle and spent her time trying to cultivate neglected friendships and vacationing.

As time passed, however, she became increasingly restless, irritable, and oddly depressed. Thus, after a six-month respite, she decided that she "needed a challenge" and embarked on the development of a new company, this time in an entirely different field. Using her expertise, experience, and business relationships, she began building a business-consulting firm specializing in helping businesses develop strategic planning.

Although entering a different business field required additional training, grueling hours, and frequent nationwide travel, Madeline initially seemed satisfied by the excruciating demands and intensity of her chosen task. She felt a vague and perplexing need to prove herself regardless of her previous achievements. Her new venture required that she be away from her husband and friends for many days each month. When she was at home, she was in constant demand by clients and employees alike. She even used her commuting time to listen to professional tapes. Her entire life was essentially devoted to nurturing her fledgling company.

Although her new company clearly began to prosper, Madeline experienced the same overwhelming stress that she had encountered previously. She continued to meet the formidable demands of her position as president until she found herself becoming extremely irritable with her husband, unable to sleep, and unable to recall the names of several familiar employees. These symptoms were dramatic enough to prompt her to seek help, although the loss of her lifelong interest in art and music did not concern her.

Initially, her attempts to understand and reduce her stress and Type-A behavior are thwarted by her continual need to travel on business. When she does attend group counseling sessions, she exhibits her hypercompetitive and impatient Type-A style by talking rapidly, interrupting others to make her point, and disagreeing with the opinions of other group members, especially women. In discussing her obvious overinvolvement in her work, she defensively but proudly proclaims that her intense pace and constant struggle to achieve success are worth it because "it's my company and I make the final decision on all important matters." When group members propose that her desire to exert such control might be a means of bolstering precarious self-esteem, she cheerfully dismisses the idea as ridiculous. It is simply her role to be in charge.

As Madeline begins consciously to reduce her Type-A behavior, her perception of her "stress" begins to change. At those times when she slows her frenetic pace and reduces her work demands through prioritizing and delegating, she experiences a sharp sense of discomfort. In describing this to her group, with whom she is becoming more comfortable, she eventually identifies her discomfort as a feeling of "not being worthy or attractive." This awareness leads her to recognize a chronic sense of not feeling very special or attractive, a feeling that began during adolescence, when she was teased about her social awkwardness, homely appearance, and relative slowness in physical development. Although she is now an attractive woman, she wonders whether "those old feelings" have anything to do with her competitive drive to succeed.

After six months in the Type-A modification program, she decides to leave the group in order to meet the increased demands of her growing company and to get time for herself. She promises to return when her "schedule permits."

The progression of Madeline's existential addiction unfortunately typifies that of many individuals who manifest Type-A behavior and work addiction. Although she has achieved stellar professional success, she is apparently still unsatisfied and struggles to achieve more. Further, the paradoxical distress that she experiences whenever she attempts to relax strongly suggests that even temporarily suspending her immersion in work allows troubling anxieties to emerge. Madeline's decision to struggle with the formidable demands of developing an entirely new company further intensifies her existential addiction in an attempt to avoid the anxiety associated with relatedness, contingency, and death.

The apparent decline in the quality of Madeline's work as well as in her professional relationships indicates that her existential addiction is at a critical stage. Even as her new venture begins to prosper, she experiences increasing distress and irritability from which she can find no escape. Madeline's physical health and psychological stability are clearly being threatened.

The specific nature of Madeline's relationship to working and her relationship to others suggests that her addiction is a means of coping with anxiety about death and isolation. Like Michael, Susan, and Charles, her importance to her company is undeniable and repeatedly demonstrated. In the professional arena, her specialness is unmistakable. While her competitive drive to become prominent is undoubtedly related in part to painful feelings of unattractiveness during adolescence, her specialness serves a more fundamental purpose.

When clearly established to the self and to the world, specialness promotes a belief in personal inviolability. Specialness and inviolability create the comforting illusion that one is exempt from fate and death. Further, like most individuals caught in existential addictions, Madeline's pervasive and excessive need for control belies a powerful anxiety about the fundamental uncertainty of life. Feeling powerless in the face of contingency, the existential addict may attempt to assuage this anxiety by struggling to control people, events, and even time itself—often through intimidation, rigid scheduling, and constant activity.

Madeline's difficulties in participating in group counseling further illustrate the nature and destructive power of her addiction. While she is concerned about her symptoms of burnout, she is unable to make a strong commitment to attend group sessions. This is most likely due to the severity of her existential addiction and to the difficulties she experiences in relating to others. The classic hypercompetitive, critical, and impatient Type-A style that she exhibits is a means of establishing power, control, and specialness in her group.

In addition, the dominating style Madeline presents may be an attempt to cope with anxiety about estrangement. Like Michael, Madeline appears to experience strong anxiety in relating to others. Her total immersion in work precludes intimacy. Her strong Type-A style repels others, preventing the intimacy that she apparently finds threatening. Unfortunately, the anxiety she experiences in relating, combined with the power of her existential addiction to work, will at least temporarily prevent her from extending the meager progress she has begun to make. Madeline's typical inability to commit to and engage in treatment challenges the mental health profession to develop more potent treatments for existential addiction.

Treatment of Existential Addiction

Although a comprehensive discussion of treating existential addiction is beyond the scope and focus of this chapter, we suggest that the following are essential components of an effective treatment program.

• In the process of avoiding existential anxiety, the individual becomes severely alienated from the self. Recovery can only occur if the individual attains an awareness of his or her unique subjective domain. In developing this self-awareness, it is inevitable and necessary that the existential addict confront the anxieties that have been avoided and experience the extent to which personal choice, needs, and values have been lost.

• Before existential anxiety can be confronted and integrated in a healthy manner, the compulsive behaviors must be reduced or eliminated. That is, treatment must provide a program for helping the individual change Type-A behavior or addiction to work. Essential in this aspect of treatment are (1) an understanding of how Type-A behavior or workaholism is supported by the professional environment and (2) a specific cognitive-behavioral program designed to help the individual transform his or her relationship to frenetic "doing" (that is, to Type-A behavior) or to work from compulsive behavior to choiceful experience.

• While reducing the destructive effects of a Type-A or workaholic style requires a problem-focused approach, brief cognitive-behavioral psychotherapy will be insufficient in changing existential addiction. Modifying behavioral coping patterns without addressing and resolving underlying existential conflicts may only lead to greater disillusionment, further loss of self, and the emergence of a compulsive pattern in another area of life. An existential-humanistic approach is essential for expanding the client's subjective awareness and thus fully experiencing dreaded anxieties and unique needs. Only the recovery of this lost sense of self will be sufficiently powerful to enable the individual to confront and resolve the anxiety that he or she has been so desperately avoiding.

• With these requirements in mind, we are cautiously optimistic that existing treatment programs for Type-A behavior and workaholism may be modified to include the existential-humanistic approach and intervention necessary to treat the existential addiction effectively. The necessity of helping clients explore basic existential and spiritual questions as part of effectively treating Type-A behavior has been acknowledged and described elsewhere (Thoresen and Bracke, 1993).

Unless we develop effective means of helping individuals eliminate the destructive coping patterns of existential addiction and confront the conflicts that they dread, many, as they approach midlife, are likely to experience stress cracks in their thinly insulated selves. The inevitable anxieties of mortality will precipitate greater confrontation with emptiness, a sense of purposelessness, uncertainty about personal values and identity, and depression and anger deriving from feelings of impotence and betrayal.

The cruel tragedy of existential addiction is that it prevents individuals from experiencing the potential of successfully confronting and integrating the existential anxiety inherent in the human condition and then setting out to fulfill their unique needs with increased vitality. In addition to saving lives, helping individuals recover from existential addiction and reclaim their humanity will help infuse our corporations and society with the potent creativity and commitment that we are all capable of and so desperately need.

Part Two

Resisting the Myth
of Organizational
Perfection

3

The Search for Excellence and the Denial of Death

Thierry C. Pauchant

This chapter is concerned with the existential origin and some of the consequences of what could be called the excellence trend. I propose that the current strength of this trend in organizations is perhaps the clearest sign of the importance of the existential dimension in the organizational life. The labeling of this trend has, of course, been derived from Tom Peters and Robert Waterman's 1982 best-seller, *In Search of Excellence,* and the trend has taken corporate America and organizations in other parts of the world by storm. More than seven million copies of the Peters and Waterman book have been sold, and it has been translated into fifteen languages. Tom Peters's subsequent books (Peters and Austin, 1985; Peters, 1988; Peters, 1992) also rapidly became best-sellers in the United States and abroad. Indeed, the search for excellence has become one of the most often used buzz phrases of the 1980s and 1990s, with numerous corporations, universities, governmental agencies, and other organizations stating it as their company ideal and philosophy, as their strategic means for surviving and competing successfully in what is known today as the global marketplace.

The excellence trend is as strong today as it was in 1982. For example, Byrne, in a 1992 *Business Week* article, still identifies Peters as one of the few most influential gurus in management. Not long ago, I received by mail an advertisement invitation from Career Track Seminars, based in Boulder, Colorado, to attend a one-day $99 seminar entitled "The In Search of Excellence Seminar." Finally, consider as a last example the strength and endurance of this trend in organizations today through their continuing infatuation with the search for perfection, as expressed in programs in total quality, zero default, just-in-time, constant innovation, turnaround strategies, time-based management, and re-engineering. These programs, while more applied than the search for excellence originally proposed by Peters and Waterman, have much in common with this search, striving for superiority, purity, ideal effectiveness, total control, excitement, the absolute.

Considering this larger trend, the specific analysis provided in this chapter on the book *In Search of Excellence* should thus not be seen as an analysis only of the arguments developed in that particular book but also of the philosophical bedrock of programs, such as those just cited, much used in organizations today. My intent in this analysis is to help the reader better comprehend the existential origin of these current appeals for excellence and their dangers.

A Superficial Analysis of *In Search of Excellence*

At a superficial level, it appears that Peters and Waterman have defined company excellence through the use of financial criteria, claiming that they have chosen companies "in the top half of [their] industry" for a period of twenty years on the basis of at least four of the following six criteria of "long-term superiority" (Peters and Waterman, 1982, pp. 22–23): asset growth, equity growth, ratio of market value to book value, and returns on total capital, on equity, and on sales. In addition, these authors state that they refined their analysis by measuring the degree of innovation of the chosen companies on the basis of the ratings of industry experts. After having presented these criteria of "superiority," Peters and Waterman describe the famous eight principles (among them "a bias for action," "close to the customer," and "stick to the knitting") that, they claim, all excellent companies have learned; in subsequent writing, the number of principles was reduced to four (see, for example, Peters and Austin, 1985).

Those who have criticized *In Search of Excellence* have often missed its existential dimension, focusing instead on the financial criteria, the principles, the research methodology, or the choice of the firms included in the model. For instance, Carroll (1983) criticized Peters and Waterman's research design, lack of information about their analysis, their definition of an "excellent" firm, and the fact that they left out nonmanagement variables. The following year, a cover story in *Business Week*, "Who's Excellent Now?" (1984) mentioned that several firms included in the sample were having serious difficulties in several areas. In another article, Johnson, Natarajan, and Rappaport (1985) argued that the only "true" criterion of superior performance is the creation of shareholder wealth. Hoffman (1986), while supportive of the book, deplored the fact that the authors did not include ethical values and morality in their discussion of corporate culture. Then Hitt and Ireland (1987), in a review of the foregoing critics and based on an empirical study that they themselves conducted, proposed that Peters and Waterman had failed to integrate a number of concepts found in traditional organization theory and had used too narrow a definition of excellence, leaving out the perspectives of many other stakeholders. Based on the results of their study, Hitt and Ireland (1987, p. 91) concluded: "Peters and Waterman's work may be one of advocacy rather than science."

It is interesting to note that although these criticisms, while valid, did not address the existential foundation of *In Search of Excellence,* neither was this foundation mentioned in the reasons invoked for explaining the success of the book. Carroll applauded the book's informal style and practical tone, and Peter Drucker (cited in Hitt and Ireland, 1987, p. 91) suggested that the book offered a simple way to address complex problems. I argue that a critique of Peters and Waterman's work should go well beyond issues of research design or prescriptions taken at face value and, at a higher level, interpret Peters and Waterman's prescriptions as an expression of a deeper reality, acknowledging these authors' grounding in the existential tradition and, paradoxically, their fundamental misunderstanding of the full consequences of their prescriptions. Further, I argue that a deeper understanding of the success of the excellence trend should go as well beyond questions of style and tone and that this trend is not only directed toward the achievement of greater productivity, competitiveness, and economic success; the trend as well as the book can also be understood, or "experienced," as a tentative resolution of much deeper issues, including the existential experience of boredom, anxiety, fear, lack of meaning, and despair, and as an attempt to offer a potential resolution of death itself.

The Existential Basis of the Excellence Trend

A careful reading of Peters and Waterman's book shows very explicitly that they have attempted to answer the issues addressed by existentialists. These authors have derived their theoretical grounding from the work of existentialist-anthropologist Ernest Becker. Becker (1924–1974), a distinguished social scientist, university professor, and author, is one of the key authors, including William Barrett (1958) and Rollo May (1960), to introduce the existentialist tradition to the general public in North America. Becker was the author of several influential books, including *The Birth and Death of Meaning* (1962), *The Denial of Death* (1973) — for which he was posthumously awarded a Pulitzer Prize — and *Escape from Evil* (1975).

Becker was particularly interested in studying the diverse strategies individuals use to derive an experience of meaning, as well as the consequences of those strategies. In *The Denial of Death* and *Escape from Evil,* which form the theoretical framework for *In Search of Excellence,* Becker argues that the fundamental problem confronting individuals is the realization of their inescapable biological death. Positing that many individuals are unable to confront this inevitability, Becker argues that most humans have found refuge in a symbolic world by creating an "alter-organism" (1975, p. 3) and thereby developing a cleavage between the biological/material world and the subjective/cultural one. As he states in *Escape from Evil* (p. 63):

[M]an wants what all organisms want: continuing experience, self-perpetuation as a living being.

But . . . man [has] a consciousness that his life came
to an end here on earth; and so he [has] to devise
another way to continue his self-perpetuation, a way
of transcending the world of flesh and blood. . . .
This he did by fixing on a world which was not
perishable, by devising an "invisible-project" that
would assure his immortality in a spiritual rather
than physical way. This way of looking at the doings of men gives a direct key to the unlocking of
history. We can see that what people want in any
epoch is a way of transcending their physical fate,
they want to guarantee some kind of infinite duration, and culture provides them with the necessary
immortality symbols or ideologies; societies can be
seen as structures of immortality power.

Becker developed his argument by drawing from authors
in many different fields, including Mircea Eliade, A. M. Hocart,
and Marcel Mauss in anthropology; Sigmund Freud, Erich
Fromm, Carl Jung, Erich Neumann, and more centrally, Otto
Rank in psychoanalysis; and Søren Kierkegaard, José Ortega
y Gasset, William James, Friedrich Nietzsche, Jean-Jacques
Rousseau, and Paul Tillich in philosophy and existentialism.
He also placed great importance on the works of Erwin Goffman
and, even more fundamentally, of Norman O. Brown. However, despite these diverse influences and references, Becker
declared that his overall ambition was to apply the work of Otto
Rank to a general theory of society. As Becker states in the
preface of *Escape from Evil* (p. xvii): "In *The Denial of Death* I argued that man's innate and all-encompassing fear of death drives
him to attempt to transcend death through culturally standardized hero systems and symbols. In this book [*Escape from Evil*]
I attempt to show that man's natural and inevitable urge to deny
mortality and achieve a heroic self-image are the root causes
of human evil. This book also completes my confrontation of
the work of Otto Rank and my attempt to transcribe its relevance
for a general science of man. Ideally . . . the two books should
be read side by side."

It is interesting to note that all the critics mentioned in the preceding section have failed to acknowledge Peters and Waterman's debt to Becker's work. In fact, while these two authors have often been accused of trivializing complex problems, it could be argued in their defense that in *In Search of Excellence* they have attempted to introduce into management a theory that goes much beyond traditional organizational behavior concepts. As they state in their introduction to that book (1982, pp. xxii-xxiii; emphasis added):

> Discussions of management psychology have long focused on theory X or theory Y, the value of job enrichment, and, now, quality circles. They don't go far toward explaining the magic of the turned-on work force in Japan or in the American excellent company, but useful theory does exist. The psychologist *Ernest Becker,* for example, *has staked out a major supporting theoretical position, albeit one ignored by most management analysts.* . . . About the winning team, Becker notes: "Society . . . is a vehicle for earthly heroism. . . . Man transcends death by finding meaning for his life. . . . It is the burning desire for the creature to count."

Indeed, this statement indicates one of the inherent ambivalences in Peters and Waterman's book. On the one hand, they claim to have identified excellent companies through the use of "objective" financial criteria as specified by classical finance theory; and on the other hand, they posit that these are the companies that have given to their employees a sense of their transcendence of death, a theme emphasized by existentialists. It is clear that Peters and Waterman consider this existential perspective to be the sociopsychological bedrock of corporate excellence. Again, as they state toward the end of *In Search of Excellence* (p. 323): "The skill with which the excellent companies develop their people recalls that grim conflict . . . : our basic need for security versus the need to stick out, the 'essential tension' that the psychoanalyst Ernest Becker described. Once again the paradox, as it is dealt with in the excellent companies, holds. By offering meaning as well as money, they give their employees a mission as well as a sense of feeling great. Every man becomes a pioneer, an experimenter, a leader . . . [and] at the same time he is part of something great: Caterpillar, IBM, 3M, Disney Productions."

However, while Peters and Waterman state that they have used Ernest Becker's work as their theoretical framework, they have shied away from Becker's in-depth analysis of the illusive escape of death as well as his warning that an extreme denial can lead to evil actions.

Comparing Peters and Waterman's Argument with Becker's Argument

To compare Peters and Waterman's argument with Becker's argument as precisely as possible, I have used part of the method advocated by Toulmin (1958) for analyzing complex arguments, thus going into much more detail than I did in an earlier analysis (Pauchant, 1993). Toulmin's method has already been used successfully in the context of business policy and the identification of strategic assumptions (Mitroff, 1983; Mitroff, Mason, and Barabba, 1983). As part of his method, Toulmin distinguishes between the claims, evidences, and warrants that constitute an argument. *Claims* are the argument's outcomes, *evidences* are statements made about the nature of the world, and *warrants* are the links that allow one to move from an evidence to a claim. Using this analytic framework, I propose that the existential argument developed in *In Search of Excellence* consists of two claims, two evidences, and four warrants, each of which is discussed below and summarized in Figure 3.1.

Claim 1

The first general claim made by Peters and Waterman is that the individual can transcend death, that he or she can resolve once and for all the issues related to existential meaning. This claim is particularly evident in Peters and Waterman's citation

Figure 3.1. Comparison of Peters and Waterman's
Argument with Becker's Argument.

	Peters and Waterman	Becker	
C1	Individuals can transcend death through work in organizations.	Individuals cannot transcend death, and denial of death leads to denial of life.	**Claims**
C2	Transcendence of death is associated with economic prosperity.	Denial of death can lead to evil actions.	
W1	Excellence[a] is assured through heroism.	Although illusory, heroism is necessary but can lead to lack of authenticity and evil actions.	**Warrants**
W2	Excellence[a] is assured through meaning produced by organizations.	Meaning is personal, leading to authenticity.	
W3	Excellence[a] is assured through rituals.	Life enhancement through rituals is temporary and needs to be connected to the cosmos.	
W4	Excellence[a] is assured through visions established by top management.	Although illusory, visions are necessary and need to be grounded in ecological reality.	
E1	The nature of the world is social and consists primarily of organizations.	The nature of the world is ecological: humans create a subjective and social reality.	**Evidences**
E2	The forces governing the world are those of competition among organizations.	The forces governing the world are cosmological.	

[a]A sense of immortality and the achievement of economic prosperity.

of Becker's statement that "man transcends death by finding meaning for his life."

Becker's view is much different, however. He (1973) argues first that individuals cannot triumph over death and second that the *fear of death* is *also a fear of life*. While it is true that Becker states that individuals have attempted with all their strength to transcend the experience of death through symbolism, he also acknowledges that all attempts have failed and that "the terror of death still rumbles underneath the cultural repression" (p. 5). It is important to note that, despite this final impossibility, Becker never minimizes the importance and the necessity for individuals to develop a symbolic reality. However, and thus relativizing the claim made by Peters and Waterman, he is also very aware of the inherent impossibility of winning over death: "Each society is a hero system which promises victory over evil and death. But no mortal, nor even a group of as many as 700 million clean revolutionary mortals, can keep such a promise: no matter how loudly or how artfully he protests or they protest, it is not within man's means to triumph over evil and death" (1975, p. 124).

Further, while Peters and Waterman (1982, p. 323) propose that the individual who creates a symbolic reality produces "more life" through meaning, becoming "a pioneer, an experimenter, a leader," Becker argues that the denial of death leads to a denial of life itself, to mediocrity. Drawing from the concept of the Jonah syndrome introduced by Abraham Maslow (1971), Becker (1973, p. 49) stresses that many individuals have a "lack of strength to bear the superlative, to open oneself to the totality of experience." Following existentialists such as Kierkegaard and Tillich, he emphasizes the necessity but the rarity of the "courage to be" (Tillich, 1952) or, as Rollo May (1975) puts it, the "courage to create." According to Becker (1973, p. 56–57):

> We flirt with our growth, but also dishonestly. This explains much of the friction in our lives. We enter symbiotic relationships in order to get the security we need, in order to get relief from our anxieties,

our aloneness and helplessness; but these relationships also blind us, they enslave us even further because they support the lie we have fashioned. . . .
We seek stress, we push our own limits, but we do
it with a screen against despair itself. We do it with
the stock market, with sport cars, with atomic mis-
siles, with the success ladder in the corporation or
the competition in the university. . . . It was not
until the working out of modern psychoanalysis that
we could understand something the poets and religious geniuses have long known: that the armor of
character was so vital to us that to shed it meant
to risk death and madness.

In another context, Zaleznik (1989, p. 15) has similarly
argued that current business education encourages the wish for
mediocrity, or a life lacking in the "courage to be," because that
education emphasizes narrow self-interest as opposed to mutual
obligation, commitment, responsibility, and a view that places
business and work in the larger context of life. Echoing Becker,
Zaleznik also proposes that mediocrity is very popular as it is
much easier to achieve than is the courage to be.

Claim 2

The second general claim Peters and Waterman make is that
the organization that allows its employees a sense of the transcendence of death will be more profitable and a leader in the
global marketplace. This second claim springs from the ambiguity the authors introduce about the dual nature of excellence, that is, as generating both superior financial results and
the (illusive) capacity for the transcendence of death. While we
cannot be sure which comes first in their model, it is clear that
these two notions are meant to be closely related and that the
sense in the transcendence of death is seen as the explanation
for the "magic of the turned-on work force" (1982, p. xxii).

While it is true that Becker emphasizes that to embrace
the symbolic reality proposed by the utilitarian culture of a so-

ciety or an organization can lead individuals to perform "more," he also emphasizes that an enduring or extreme denial of death (and life) can bring several negative results and evil consequences ("more" in this sense lead to "less"). We will examine several of these negative consequences as presented by Becker for society and for the individual shortly. For now, it will suffice to stress that for Becker the search for the transcendence of death and economic prosperity is not without drawbacks because it can lead to very destructive actions. As he argues (1973, p. 85; emphasis added): "Modern man's defiance of accidents, evil and death takes the form of skyrocketing production of consumer and military goods. Carried to its demonic extreme this defiance gave us Hitler and Vietnam: a rage against our impotence, a defiance of our animal condition, our pathetic creature limitations. *If we don't have the omnipotence of gods, we at least can destroy like gods.*"

Finally, it is important to emphasize that the claims made by Peters and Waterman that organizations can provide *immortality* and *prosperity* are, according to Becker, the two classic promises made by religious and revolutionary groups, building on people's psychological hunger for reassurance about death and their need for life aggrandizement. Indeed, Peters (1992) continues to emphasize this revolutionary aspect, claiming today to lead a "management revolution."

However, Becker (1975, p. 132) points out the dangers of such heroic ambitions as attempting to provide immortality and prosperity, or as commonly expressed, "eternal progress," "always more," or (even more in fashion) "sustainable development":

> Each society elevates and rewards leaders who are talented at giving the masses heroic victory, expiation for guilt, relief of personal conflicts. It doesn't matter how these are achieved: magical religious ritual, magical booming stock markets, magical heroic fulfillment of five-year plans, or mana-charged military megamachines — or all together. What counts is to give the people the self-expansion in righteousness that they need. The men who have

power can exercise it through many different kinds
of social and economic structures, but a universal
psychological hunger underpins them all; it is this
that locks people and power figures together in a
life-and-death contract.

We now turn to another part of Peters and Waterman's
argument, their basic assumptions about the nature of the world.

Evidence 1

The first evidence that Peters and Waterman propose is that
the world, viewed from a business perspective, can be reduced
to a world that consists primarily of organizations. Although
this specific conception of the world may seem trivial at first,
it carries with it a host of consequences. For example, the idea
of an organizational world gives supremacy to the concepts of
corporate culture and corporate top management's power and
vision. Further, this particular view of the world can lead individuals to reify the concept of organization, considering an organization to be a living entity and referring to it by a specific
name, such as IBM, rather than considering the individuals
managing it or working in it. In this view, individuals become
mere "objects" of a larger and impersonal system, denying the
existential reality of the subject.

This organizational perspective of the world also sets the
organization as the final guarantor of individuals' values, needs,
and happiness. For example, if we define the world as mostly
organizational, the wish of individuals to feel part of something
great or something larger than themselves must be fulfilled by
their association with a corporation such as IBM, as proposed
in *In Search of Excellence,* and as opposed, for example, to their
association with other institutions, organizations, communities,
formal and informal groups, or causes. As we have seen, Peters
and Waterman have been criticized for not integrating into their
definition of excellence the views of such stakeholders as governments, other groups or institutions, communities, or the public at large.

Becker adds another constituent to this list of stakeholders: nature itself. Conscious of the necessity for human beings to invent and share a symbolic reality, he agrees that the illusion of culture is beneficial; but he also warns that this illusion can become fatal if it leads to the denial of the biological nature of human beings and the denial of the biological nature of the planet. It is rather evident that a view of the world as an organization is quite different from a biological view of the world as a planet or human beings. The former leads individuals to view the world from a restricted social science perspective, evaluating reality by means of concepts drawn primarily from economics, political science, corporate strategy, finance. It seems that today we are dearly paying the price for this supremacy of the sociocultural perspective over the biological-natural one, considering the extent of current problems such as stress and burnout at the human level (see, for example, Aubert and Pagès, 1989; Bracke and Bugental in this book) and the current ecological crisis at the ecosystem level (Hawken, 1993; Smith, 1993; Shrivastava, 1994).

Although it might seem somewhat surprising to link existentialism and ecologism, this linkage is central in the work of many existentialists, such as, for example, Heidegger (Zimmerman, 1983). To put the matter another way, Becker's argument about the denial of death, that is, the denial of the biological nature of the human body, is also a powerful argument for explaining the denial of the biological and ecological nature of the planet; to realize the reality of the first often leads to the realization of the other because both address the biological reality (Bohm and Edwards, 1991). Because Becker does not present a specific section on this topic but rather provides several remarks in different parts of his work, I present a composite of his comments in *Escape from Evil* (1975):

All truths are part-truths as far as creatures are concerned, and so there is nothing wrong with an illusion that is creative. Up to a point, of course: the point at which the illusion lies about something very important, such as human nature [p. 147]. Man

is first and foremost an animal moving about on
a planet shining in the sun. Whatever else he is,
is built on this [p. 1]. Today we are living the
grotesque spectacle of the poisoning of the earth by
the nineteenth-century hero system of unrestrained
material production. This is perhaps the greatest
and most pervasive of all evil to have emerged in
all history, and it may even eventually defeat all
of mankind [p. 156].

Elsewhere I have discussed the degree and some of the
effects of this *anthropocentric view* denounced by Becker, that is,
of the exclusive perception of nature through the perspective
of human utilitarianism grounded in the social domain (Pauchant
and Fortier, 1990).

Evidence 2

The second evidence that Peters and Waterman posit is that,
since the world is supposed to consist mostly of organizations,
the forces governing the world are competitive forces among
organizations. Such a conception of the world legitimizes in turn
the necessity for constant research and development, innovation, competition, higher performance, perfection. In this conception, where the globe becomes a global marketplace, where
the environment is only a social-political-industrial environment,
where human beings are viewed as human resources for the survival of organizations, and where ecosystemic forces are replaced
by competitive ones, the social reality of organizations gains still
more power, leading to a single strategy: more of the same.
Thus, if an organization's market is large, it needs to become
larger; if an organization has the capacity to move quickly, it
should move more quickly; quality should be replaced by total
quality; regional competition needs to become global; social and
moral values need to be replaced by fast opportunism and quick
turnarounds; good management principles need to replaced by
time-based management and nanosecond decision making.
    It is interesting — and frightening — to note that in this con-

ception of the world, the denial of the death of the individual is perfectly achieved, at least temporarily, having been replaced by the collective defense of the survival of the organization. In that sense, as suggested by Sievers (1986a; in this book), for example, the organization becomes a powerful symbol of immortality: if the individual cannot survive, the organization will. Moreover, in this conception, the force to be combated is no longer the biological clock that governs the body because everybody senses that in the final analysis the result of this combat is doomed. Rather, the new force to be combated is the competitor, the external force that can jeopardize the survival of the organization; and if competitors are not always perceived as bluntly evil (after all, competitive forces can sometimes rightly stimulate), they are nonetheless often greatly feared, and this leads to a host of different corporate strategies, from combat to alliances.

Becker's conception of the world is obviously different. As already noted, his conception includes the biological reality, and the overall force governing the world is the cosmic dance of life and death. Further, for him, the fundamental problem concerning human beings does not emerge from an outside force, such as a competitor, but the inner tendency to deny one's own mortality. This commonly observed shift from an inner issue to an outer one led Becker to propose that the denial of death induces human beings to use the mechanism of *projection*. Arguing that many individuals are unable to confront their mortality, Becker suggests that individuals project onto others what they cannot stand in themselves, that is, what they perceive as evil. Or they may even wish to kill the other in an attempt to save their own life. Echoing Sartre's motto that "hell is other people," Becker (1975, p. 111) writes that "man is bloodthirsty to ward off the flow of his own blood." He sees in the mechanism of projection the origin of ethnocentrism, scapegoating, racism, genocide, and war and thus emphasizes again that the denial of death can lead to evil actions: "If there is one thing that the tragic wars of our time have taught us, it is that the enemy has a ritual role to play, by means of which evil is redeemed. All wars are conducted as 'holy' wars in a double sense then — as a revelation of fate, a testing of divine favor, and as a means of purging evil from the world at the same time" (1975, p. 115).

Although business competition need not lead to a bloodbath, I invite the reader to read Robert B. Reich's 1992 review of several books that fiercely assert that Japan has become "a new evil empire" directed against the United States and threatening its economic security.

Proposing the evidences that (1) the world primarily consists of organizations and (2) the forces that govern the world are competitive ones, and making the claims that (1) excellent organizations are the ones that provide a sense of transcendence of death and (2) are also the ones that strive economically, Peters and Waterman suggest a number of warrants or means for moving from their evidences to their claims; that is, they prescribe different mechanisms for the concrete realization of excellence. I will discuss in particular four warrants that are central in *In Search of Excellence*: the search for heroship, the creation of meaning, the use of rituals, and top management's formation of vision.

Warrant 1. The Search for Heroship

Peters and Waterman propose that the search for heroship transcends existential issues. They argue that individuals will be willing to commit, or surrender, themselves to the purpose of an organization if this organizational purpose provides them with a sense of greater meaning and that at the same time individuals will wish to stand out in the organization and strive to satisfy their own ambition. As the authors state (1982, p. xxiii): "Men willingly shackle themselves to nine-to-five if only the cause is perceived to be in some sense great. The company can actually provide the same resonance as does the exclusive club or honorary society. At the same time, however, each of us needs to stick out — even, or maybe particularly, in the winning institutions. So we observed, time and again, extraordinary energy exerted above and beyond the call of duty when the worker . . . is given even a modicum of apparent control over his or her own destiny."

   Although Becker speaks of the quasi-necessity for human beings to engage in "earthly heroism" (that is, heroism springing from the culture in which individuals are immersed) and "personal heroism" (that is, a creative act separated out of the common pool of shared meanings), he also speaks, as we have seen, of these heroisms as a denial of death and as an escape from human authenticity. Further, he stresses that the task of authentic individuals is to challenge the sources and the validity of these heroisms and to realize their dangerous illusions, to understand the final perils of mediocrity or heroics, as well as the necessity for the courage to be. In Becker's words (1973, p. 6): "[H]uman heroics is a blind drivenness that burns people up: in passionate people, a screaming for glory as uncritical and reflexive as the howling of a dog. In the more passive masses of mediocre men it is disguised as they humbly and complainingly follow out the roles that society provides for their heroics and try to earn their promotions within the system, wearing the standard uniforms . . . allowing themselves to stick out, but ever so little and so safely, with a little ribbon or a red boutonniere . . . not with head and shoulders."

   Echoing Becker, Aubert and de Gaulejac (1991), as well as Aktouf, Aubert, and Morin (in this book), have similarly proposed that this search for heroship can increase human despair because it obliges individuals to become (pseudo) constant warriors and constant winners. Becker also warns that each victory in heroism, because it is based on a denial of mortality, takes its toll, potentially widening the gap established between the biological and social realities: "Every heroic victory is two-sided: it aims toward merger with an absolute 'beyond' in a burst of life affirmation, but it carries within it the rotten core of death denial in a physical body here on earth. If culture is a lie about the possibility of victory over death, then a lie must somehow take its toll on life, no matter how colorful and expansive the celebration of joyful victory may seem" (1975, p. 121).

   Finally, Becker warns of the potential negative consequences of striving for heroics. Again, he emphasizes the potential for evil results. In particular, he comments on the size and danger inherent in the technologies now used in modern societies, such as atomic power, chemicals, and biogenetics. He argues that the heroism of primitive man was much less problematic than it is today because it was "small scale and more easily controlled" (1975, p. 96). Along the same lines, in a study I conducted with Ian Mitroff, we found that managers in large, powerful companies that define themselves as excellent companies have a tendency to deny the need for preventive and systemic crisis management programs and to deny even the possibility of their own company's involvement in a major industrial accident (Pauchant and Mitroff, 1992).

Warrant 2. The Creation of Meaning

One of the other methods that Peters and Waterman propose for propelling the workforce toward greater competitive capabilities is the creation of meaning, allowing people to become "heroes." According to these authors (1982, p. 239), excellent companies turn "the average Joe and the average Jane into winners." Contrary to this view and fully embracing the existentialist tradition, Becker argues that the search for meaning is a *personal* experience; individuals must come to feel and believe, from their own life experiences, that what they are doing is truly meaningful, even though, paradoxically, this feeling can emerge from a genuine encounter with others. He describes (1973, p. 73) unauthentic individuals as those who "do not belong to themselves, are not 'their own persons,' do not act from their own center, do not see reality on its terms." Emphasizing the negative consequences for individuals of attempts at the "engineering of meaning," he presents (1973, pp. 77-79) a continuum of "unauthenticity"; at one end are "depressive psychoses," that is, individuals who are afraid of being themselves and fearful of exerting their individuality, and at the other end are "schizophrenic psychoses," that is, individuals who experience a sense of inflation of inner fantasy and symbolic possibility. Thus, far from advocating that the sense of the transcendence of death is for an individual to be "made heroic" by society or an organization, Becker stresses that healthy, true, real individuals are the ones who have actualized themselves by realizing the truth of their situation, by dispelling the lies of their character and of their cultural heritage, by realizing their own mortality (1973, p. 86). In this sense, the transcendence of death is no longer a denial but a genuine realization of both the necessity of death and the requirement for a human being to assume his or her life, as is argued by Morin, Bracke, and Bugental in the first two chapters of this book.

Echoing Becker's views on the negative consequences of the denial of death, a number of diverse authors who have conducted studies in "excellent" companies in both Europe and the United States have concluded that these organizations have a tendency to become "religious systems" (Pagès, Bonetti, de Gaulejac, and Descendre, 1979) and have a dangerously increasing tendency toward totalitarianism (Schwartz, 1987b).

Warrant 3. The Use of Rituals

It seems that Peters and Waterman have also too quickly operationalized their version of Becker's work in emphasizing the importance of ceremonies and rituals for developing a sense of heroship and meaning: "Ritual is the technique for giving life. [Man's] sense of self-worth is constituted symbolically; his cherished narcissism feeds on symbols, on an abstract idea of his own worth. Man's natural yearning can be fed limitlessly in the domain of symbols" (1982, p. xxiii). As an example of this symbolic management, so much in vogue in organizations today, Peters and Waterman describe a team of IBM salesmen applauded by executives, colleagues, family members, and friends as they emerge from the players' tunnel of a stadium.

Contrary to this view, Becker warns of the dangers of a "compulsive character" building extra-thick defenses against existential despair and anxiety. Quoting Kierkegaard and echoing Sartre's concept of bad faith, he stresses that "for a partisan of this most rigid orthodoxy, truth is an ensemble of ceremonies" (1973, p. 71). Moreover, in the entire first chapter of *Escape from Evil* (1975, pp. 6–25), he describes the process and functions of rituals as practiced in primitive societies. He emphasizes, as Peters and Waterman do, that the technique of rituals is a life-enhancing mechanism and argues that "rituals generate and redistribute life powers" (p. 14), although in a temporal fashion. However, Becker also stresses that originally rituals were not directed toward the accomplishment of specific individuals, as proposed by Peters and Waterman. According to Becker, if individuals can draw a temporary sense of life enhancement from rituals, it is because these rituals are directed toward a person's and a community's participation in nature, as well as their (perceived) control of the total cosmos, the perspective emphasized by the pre-Socratics and Heraclitus of Ephesus (as discussed in the introduction). As Becker writes (1975, p. 16; emphasis added):

> It is only in modern society that the mutual imparting of self-importance has trickled down to the single maneuvering of face-work; there is hardly any way to get a sense of value except from the boss, the company dinner, or the random social encounters in the elevator or on the way to the executive toilet. Primitive society was a formal organization for the apotheosis of man. Our own everyday rituals seem shallow precisely because they lack the cosmic connection. Instead of only using one's fellow man as a mirror to make one's face shine, the primitive used the whole cosmos . . . *it related the person to the mysterious forces of the cosmos, gave him an intimate share in them.*

Warrant 4. Top Management's Formation of Vision

While Peters and Waterman advocate both a "tight" and "loose" corporate culture, that is, a strong inculturation of employees and also a degree of relative freedom for each (1982, p. 106), they also attribute the responsibility for this inculturation to top management. In particular, they insist that top managers and leaders are responsible for defining an organization's core values through the development of a "vision," a theme very much in fashion in current management's practice: "In the excellent companies . . . values are clear; they are acted out minute by minute and decade by decade by the top brass; and they are well understood deep in the companies' ranks" (1982, pp. 97–98).

Again, Becker's views differ considerably. As we have seen, he emphasizes as an existentialist that meaning should be discovered by oneself and also stresses that leaders often convince or charm their audience through an additional escape into the social reality, promising both immortality and prosperity. According to Becker (1975, pp. 166–167):

> The problem has always been that the leader is the one who usually is the grandest patriot, which means the one who embraces the ongoing system of death denial with the heartiest hug, the hottest tears, and the least critical distance. . . . [T]he leader lives with his head full into the clouds of the cultural symbols; he lives in an abstract world, a world detached from concrete realities of hunger, suffering, death; his feet are off the ground, he carries out his duties much like funeral directors and men who perform autopsies or executions — in a kind of emotional and psychological divorce from the realities of what he is doing.

Becker's judgment may seem overly harsh. Many executives do have a sense of the concrete and can judge the results of their actions on the day-to-day living conditions of employees and community members and on the environment. However, it also seems true that other managers are often not aware or at all concerned with the daily reality of the living conditions of others and blindly apply the corporate rationality or strictly protect the interests of the very few. Johns Manville's managers during the asbestos drama, ITT's managers during the scandal in South America, and Ford's managers during the Pinto crisis are cases in point (Hills, 1987; Pauchant and Mitroff, 1992). Enriquez (1989), in a study of other "excellent" companies, similarly concludes that employees in these organizations were forced to deny their own bodies, thinking, and psyches, often becoming the "cool killers" of their competitors or the public at large.

In any case, it seems that leaders' tendencies to focus primarily on the positive, on the great deeds, or on winning carry their own shadow by further widening the gap between the social reality and the biological one, which seems to be, at bottom, Becker's argument. In Chapter Eight of this book, Schwartz emphasizes the need for acknowledging this shadow.

Addressing the Search for Existence

Despite the foregoing shortcomings, Peters and Waterman have contributed to a better understanding of the cardinal importance of cultural issues in organizations and have at least introduced some existential notions in management theory and practice. However, — in their two evidences, four warrants, and two claims — they have also greatly denatured the theoretical foundation upon which they originally grounded their argument.

To be fair to these authors, I should note that they do very briefly mention some of the negative sides of the search for excellence about which Becker warned. For example, they state that managers can be tempted to do almost anything in the search for excellence and that this quest can lead to abuse (1982, pp. 59, 78) or, as Peters (1986) suggests, to a "search for arrogance." Nevertheless, as suggested in this and other chapters of this book, the strength of the excellence trend and its emphasis on more of the same have entrapped many workers and managers alike in destructive vicious circles that become stronger and faster with each turn. Because these vicious circles need to be addressed and modified, I will discuss briefly in this last section of the chapter a number of potential avenues toward change as well as the present conditions that hinder their possibility.

There seem to be at least three general barriers to change. The first one is obviously economic. Because many organizations around the world use techniques derived from the excellence trend to accelerate the overall competitive movement, addressing the vicious circles would require strong political courage and a more global view of the purpose of work and production. The second barrier is existential. As argued in this chapter, the strength of the excellence trend is partly derived from a denial of death, which is at the very basis of societal and organizational cultures and the individual character. Further, as we know from psychology and psychoanalysis, to confront defense mechanisms is difficult and potentially dangerous. On this subject, Becker (1973, p. 23) warns that "people have psychotic breaks when repression no longer works, when the forward momentum of activity is no longer possible." The third barrier to change is scientific. Simply stated, we do not presently have — and perhaps will never have — an overall understanding of the interdependent forces that animate the cosmos, societies, communities, organizations, and individuals. The risk of worsening the situation through misguided interventions is therefore important. However, despite these formidable barriers, there seems to be several avenues that would at least lead in the right direction.

The first avenue toward change is the conscious realization of the existential origin of the excellence trend in organizations in particular and society in general. This objective is one of the goals of this book and the function of education. However, its full accomplishment through education seems doubtful because the denial of death goes much beyond the conscious level, springing from the subjective/existential realm. Perhaps therapy could help in this direction, but it is problematic — to say the least — to treat literally millions of people. It seems that a review of the function of education, in organizations, universities, and other schools, as proposed for example by Carl Rogers (1983), could be very useful in that direction. That is, the function of education could become less oriented toward scientific knowledge and more oriented toward the full development of one's personality or what others have called "personal mastery" (Senge, 1990).

The second avenue toward change is a better realization of the subjective functions of cultures, at the societal and organizational levels (Bohm and Edwards, 1991). While this necessity has been emphasized by many existentialists, expecting one to realize one's culture is akin to expecting a fish to jump out of water and survive. The best chance of achieving this realization is for those in organizations and universities alike to take

seriously the contentions made by such authors as March and
Olsen (1976) that decisions in organizations are "random interpretations" and Weick's (1979) "enactment theory."

A third avenue toward change involves changing the
criteria of leadership. Following the lead of Chester I. Barnard
(1968), several authors have already called for a different kind
of leader. For example, Warren Bennis (1989) and Abraham
Zaleznik (1989) have emphasized that a leader should have the
capacity to face the human condition bravely, including the fear
of death and life; to have the existential and political courage
to address issues such as concreteness, morality, responsibility,
and commitment; and to become a role model for others. However, the problems involved in finding such leaders and in their
ability to effect change are substantial.

Fourth, an effort should be directed toward reintroduc-
ing the biological and cosmological dimensions in business. Because the possibility of canceling out the social reality is doubtful for many individuals — since it is at the basis of culture, and
most people need to feel that they at least partially "manage the
dream" (Bennis, 1989) — a complementary myth needs to be
rediscovered. It seems that the current emergence of ecological
concerns in and out of organizations could be powerfully used
toward that purpose. That is, more ecological concerns in organizations would not only potentially benefit the ecology of the
planet and stimulate innovation in new markets, services, and
products but could also benefit and broaden the sense of existential meaning by finding another, more basic connection with
nature — with the danger, of course, of wishing to "manage the
planet" (Fox, 1990; Morin and Kern, 1993; Serres, 1990).

Fifth, and addressing the same general issue, an effort
should be made to reintroduce in business the importance of
future generations. Already, concerns about children have been
raised in organizations on issues as diverse as the effect of workaholism on employees' children, pension plan payments by future generations, the poor state of children's education, and the
present and long-term threats of ecological problems. While these
concerns may seem very diverse, they all reconnect humans with
elements of their biological reality that reflect a longer time span.

Sixth, attempts could be made to rejuvenate the importance and nobility of working in more direct contact with matter. Mechanical advances and other factors have allowed a dramatic increase in what are called information workers, those specifically involved in the subjective domain, or what Peters (1992) calls "brain-work." Authors as diverse as Fritz Schumacher (1979), Alfred North Whitehead ([1933] 1961), and Simone Weil (1949) have viewed a more direct contact with matter and its relationship to the spirit as one of the fundamental functions of work.

Seventh, the current dangerous idealization of technology needs to be lessened somewhat. In particular, technology should be placed in its proper context, and individuals should better comprehend the cultural and subjective underpinnings of technology, as well as its potential dangers (Barrett, 1986; Bohm and Peat, 1990; Heidegger, 1972).

Eighth, and related to the previously suggested avenues toward change, a new generation of crisis management approaches needs to be developed in enterprise. Although crisis management has certainly gained recognition in the last few years in organizations (Pauchant and Mitroff, 1992; Shrivastava, 1993), the purpose of new approaches should be to anticipate the potential disastrous effects of goods, services, and more generally, the "wish for heroship" in multiple domains, including the existential and ecological ones, that affect many diverse stakeholders. Globally, these approaches should attempt to operationalize in organizations Becker's call for better understanding the origin of evil (1975, p. 126); they should address *both the productive and counterproductive sides of organizations* and thus inform strategic decisions in a more concrete and global manner (Dupuy, 1982; Pauchant and Morin, 1994; Pauchant and Cotard, in press).

Ninth, it seems, paradoxically, that one of the most significant approaches for addressing the search for existence in organizations would be to allow employees and managers alike to gain more distance from these organizations, thus going in a direction opposite to that advocated by Peters and Waterman (1982). By doing this, individuals could also embrace other causes represented by such diverse groups or institutions as consumer groups, communities, ecological groups, families, political parties, religious groups, and so on. As a result, individuals would be better prepared to relativize the cultural dimensions of their organizations in particular and business in general by placing them in a larger context. On this point, it also seems that the increasingly multicultural and multiethnic composition of today's organizations could help individuals realize their own cultural heritage through a process of genuine dialogue (Bohm and Edwards, 1991; Cayer, 1993; Isaacs, 1993; Senge, 1990).

Finally, perhaps one of the strongest incentives for change will be a repeated experiencing of crises, be they existential, industrial, economic, social, or ecological. While this last avenue does not belong to the panoply of traditional strategies for "planned change" and carries with it the possibility of great destruction, it seems the most likely to trigger change by at least challenging traditional defense mechanisms and fostering a consensus for change, as some studies conducted after the experience of an industrial crisis have shown (Pauchant and Mitroff, 1992).

As is evident, the means for change that I have proposed, which are drawn from the existential tradition in general and Becker's work in particular, are different from the classical techniques currently advocated and derived from the excellence trend. However, it is not necessary to agree with the totality of Becker's work in order to relativize these more traditional practices; nor is it necessary to posit, as Becker did, that the denial of death is *the* key concept for fully understanding the entire process of human history and the working of evil.

Nevertheless, it seems rather evident that the "fear of death" is a major factor in our society, when defining this fear more globally than Becker did. While Becker emphasized the fear of biological death, other authors have defined this fear in different ways. For example, James Bugental (1976) stresses the experience of the unrealization of one's potential, Albert Camus (1947) the lack of responsibility, Heinz Kohut (1985) the fear of change in the subjective experience of self, Rollo May (1975) the experience of nonbeing, Max Pagès (1984) the fear of loneliness, Erich Fromm (1973) the experience of impotence in actions, and Simone Weil (1949) the lack of spirituality. In the fields of organization theory and organization behavior, what managers are often said to fear the most are experiences of uncertainty (Galbraith, 1977) or ambiguity (Weick, 1979).

The point I have tried to make in this chapter is not that Becker's arguments are superior to those of others. Rather, I have used Becker to show that the excellence trend in general and Peters and Waterman's (1982) attempt to address deepseated existential issues in organizations are currently backfiring; they are prompting even more suffering in and out of organizations. I have tried to sensitize the reader to the view that the issues involved in managing organizations and those that derive from the search for excellence include but go well beyond the issues of productivity, competitiveness, and shareholder wealth. They also get at a more fundamental, and often hidden, level. It seems that a reworking of management principles in the future will not be possible without that insight.

4

The Management of Excellence: Deified Executives and Depersonalized Employees

Omar Aktouf

My attention was first drawn to the links between the power position of managers, their self-deification, their fantasies of omnipotence, and their illusions of immortality by the very strong language used by numerous employees of the organizations in which I carried out my research during the 1980s (Aktouf, 1983, 1986, 1989). In reference to their bosses, they used such derisive terms as *pharoah* and *god on earth* and spoke of them as people who "think they are descended from extraterrestrials." Several years later, the works of authors such as Becker (1973), Berle (1957), Sievers (1986a), Kets de Vries and Miller (1985), and Enriquez (1983, 1989, 1990) led me to a more systematic theoretical investigation of this phenomenon.

Over and above my numerous references to Greek mythology, to philosophy, metaphysics, and particularly psychoanalysis and existentialism, which are inevitably derived from these studies, I would like to explore a particular form of so-called archetypical power: that of being king (Berle, 1957). From the absolute power of the tyrant to constitutional monarchy to the republican form of government, the status of king has been the epitome of human greatness and misery throughout history. In addition, this archetypical power has had a marked influence on another form of power that is currently on the way to becoming archetypical: that of the manager, of the corporate leader in a world increasingly dominated by organizations (Perrow, 1979). Perhaps unconsciously, our business leaders at times tend to behave as organizational monarchs. All forms of power lead to the temptation of absolute power, as is abundantly clear in the organizational world. Howard Hughes, Harold Geneen, Alfred Krupp, and Henry Ford all illustrate this monstrous and compulsive quest for omnipotence in which the organization is primarily used to support fantasies rather than as a production tool (Kets de Vries and Miller, 1985; Enriquez, 1983; Pagès, Bonetti, de Gaulejac, and Descendre, 1979; Miller, 1992). Moreover, the management literature is replete with examples of the total and rapid bankruptcy of small organizations that were not able to survive their owners' obsessive need for power and control beyond the famous three- to five-year horizon (although these bankruptcies could obviously be attributed to a large number of other factors in addition to the behavior of their managers).

How can power lead to such suicidal acts? This type of behavior, best exemplified by Louis XVI of France, can be found in all the dynasties of human history. Could it be akin to the blindness of so many managers of gigantic Western organizations that are facing the threat posed by Asian competitors (Morgan, 1986)? On a more modest scale, could this type of behavior also be akin to the apparently irresistible drive toward "organizational republicanism," in which the corporation tries to bridge the gap between the "king" and his "subjects" through participatory management, semiautonomous work groups, and total quality and in which the human capital willingly contributes its intelligence to increase productivity? Why, then, are there so many failures, so much ill will, and so much resistance to change? Why are there so many delays and so many problems in the attempt to make the manager and the employee act as partners in what is increasingly called a common endeavor?

In this chapter, I explore the paradoxes, perils, and dilemmas of the archetypical absolute power of king in order to provide a better understanding of the underlying reasons for the

prevailing situation in the vast majority of modern Western organizations. I draw upon the works of one of the keenest observers
of the human condition, William Shakespeare, to reveal the hidden aspects of modern organizational power through his meticulous dissection of royal power. In the first section, I analyze the
bases and dilemmas of the archetypical existential condition of
royal power in reference to some of Shakespeare's most famous
plays. In the second section, I attempt to highlight the hazards
and major issues associated with all power positions (particularly that of the corporate manager) in which absolutism is a
risk, as well as deification, omnipotence, or illusions of immortality. Finally, in the third section, I suggest possible solutions
to the apparent impasse of the current management of excellence (Pagès, Bonetti, de Gaulejac, and Descendre, 1979; Aubert
and de Gaulejac, 1991), based on an examination of a number
of different systems of actual "republican management" that draw
on "human capital" through effective partnerships that go beyond
the jargon of excellence.

Royal Divinity and the Corporate Manager

Throughout the last decade, the management of "excellence" has,
perhaps unintentionally, led to a new form of deification and
"heroization" of the manager and a commensurate depersonalization of the employee (Aubert and de Gaulejac, 1991; Linhart,
1991). This in turn raises the basic question of the relation of
the "being" of man to this deification phenomenon and its concomitant alienation of the employee (Pagès, Bonetti, de Gaulejac,
and Descendre, 1979). I will make a few brief abstract and
speculative references to existential questions in order to better
define the existential paradox of man before discussing one of
its historically favored means of escape: power.

This paradox is rooted in the fact that human beings are
condemned to live with the permanent and inescapable knowledge of their own mortality. According to Becker (1973), "Man
is a God with an anus"; according to Sartre (1945), "The future
is the makeup of life as the vacuum is the makeup of matter";
and according to Hegel (1966), "Man doesn't have an essence;

his essence is his action." Ancient philosophers, not to mention theologians and philosopher-theologians, have repeatedly insisted that human beings are nothing but fallen God, banned in time to underscore their expulsion from eternity, or from deity and immortality. This summarizes the whole question of "contingency" and of the nonnecessity of the being of humans in front of the absolute being, which humans cannot really apprehend — or of the notion that, by accepting their own negation as beings, the nonbeing of humans would support the idea of an absolute being that transcends time and individuals, if only by contrast or by reference.

One of Hegel's (1966) major concerns was that of alienation, which he calls "the loss of man in the world of objects." This reification is obviously the ultimate downfall since the last attribute of the last trace of transcendence in man is his free will as a subject, which is then destroyed in a process of self-estrangement. Man's own degradation then relegates him to the status of a quasi-object, or an object bound by external determinism and subject to the laws of objects. In the famous parable of the master and the slave, alienation and "the loss of man" will set in unless the slave achieves the "negation of the negation" of his generic being (this negation is temporarily imposed by the necessity of submitting to the order of objects) through the self-creative act of work, which allows him to contemplate the reflection of his own rationality in the work he has created. In an obviously simplified sense, this Hegelian philosophy is the very heart of existential anxiety, which man has always tried to alleviate in a manner appropriate to his nature as a thinking being: magical, mythical, metaphysical, or phantasmal.

Until the triumph of the scientific rationalism and positivistic materialism of the nineteenth century, the preferred manner of dealing with this anxiety was essentially religious in nature, at least in the Western world. Man set out to accomplish rites and rituals (concrete acts) in appropriate places and at appropriate (and equally concrete) times that allowed him to participate in the life of the founding myth (in reference to the absolute being); this granted him access to part of his own "sacredness" and, thus, on a symbolic level, to his own timeless and transcendent dimension. This was the price to be paid for the illusion of participating in eternity: man devoted a great deal of his life to learning to die. In the case of kings, however, the claim to the throne can rightfully only be based on the claim of being above the common human condition, which makes it difficult to reconcile the king's humanness with the necessary transcendence of the common condition. This suprahumanity is difficult to live with as a human being. The perenniality of the royal person, and hence of its participation in the absolute being, can only be justified by the timeless permanence of the royal institution regardless of the individuals involved. The Chinese dynasties claimed to have a mandate from heaven; the Egyptian pharoahs were human gods; the kings of France ruled by divine right. However, the gold medal of this legalometaphysical game probably goes to the legal scholars of the British monarchy under the Tudors, who from the fifteenth century onward developed what came to be known as "the fiction of the two bodies of the king" (Kantorowicz, 1989).

This example is unique in the history of Western monarchies; this fiction conferred upon the British monarchy the exceptional quality of having the body of the royal political monarchy, which transcended the physical person of the king, and the body of the "natural" individual, who lived and died as a man although he had been king. The "celestial-immortal" body had the property of being transmittable to another physical individual (the successor) when the king's human earthly incarnation died. In fact, scholars talked of dismissal rather than death: the fallible body (which was subject to the flaws, suffering, and death of mere mortals) was dismissed from the king's infallible, eternal royal and divine body. As long as the king lived, these two bodies were united in his person. Depending upon the circumstances, his behavior would alternatively emanate from his earthly body or from his political-celestial one. Thus, the monarchy accomplished and legitimized the superhumanity of the royal institution through its political-celestial body, whose members were subjects of the realm. As king, the individual thus acquired royal immortality.

The main interest of these notions is, of course, the narrow and inescapable link that they created with power, its nature, legitimacy, practice, and consequences. In this respect, Shakespeare's meticulous autopsy of a number of royal tragedies offers particularly rich and accurate insights into the rending, intolerable existential ubiquity of kings who are forever torn between their human ego and their divine ego. The pathetic destiny of King Lear or Richard II offers a wrenching testimony of the unavoidable and painful interdependence between power and fantasies of omnipotent deification on the one hand and mortality and earthly relations with oneself and one's fellow men on the other. King Richard II, who suffered defeat at the hands of the nephew whom he had unjustly despoiled and banished, had to his own despair realized the extreme vanity of the "royal name and body" as he had to personally shed the "trappings" (the crown, the scepter, and so on) of his apparent immortal royal condition. As he remembered the tragic fate of his ancestors, King Henry V lamented the fact that the king was deprived of the makings of the simple and happy life of his humblest subject: the clear and peaceful knowledge of being only a natural body, sheltered from the illusions of remoteness of a divine body, which is in fact vulnerable to the "breath of every fool." For his part, King Lear naively believed that he would be able to live the life of a "simple" father under the benevolent hospitality of all of his children after he had given them the wealth and material means of the royal condition. However, Lear also intended to retain the signs and the trappings of his royal body. He believed he would still be treated as a king with his court and courtiers. After he had been rejected and abandoned to the fury of a devastating storm, he realized that his royal-celestial body would have been much better treated if he had retained the material instruments and the power that would have allowed him to redress the wrongs that his ungrateful daughters had inflicted upon him; this would have allowed him to render "justice" and to deserve the love and the respect he would have "earned" through the accomplishment of his royal *duties*.

Berle (1957) proposes an interesting parallel between the absolute power of the Norman and British kings and that of the leaders of modern corporations (owners and managers alike),

who as sovereign lords and masters are free to make whatever
decision it pleases them to make (particularly in the current context of neoliberalism and government noninterference). This new
absolute power linked to the right of ownership is used in ways
that are very close to its archetypical model; it is then subject
to conditions, uncertainties, and risks that are very similar if
not identical to that of the original model. Briefly, Berle's hypothesis, which I support, is that *all forms of absolute power,* be
they royal or corporate, *are threatened with self-destruction* if they
are not protected by a system of checks and balances to coun-
teract their absolutism, impose a degree of moderation, and
make them more humane. Absolute power must therefore be
tempered by *a system of accountability,* such as the obligation to
deliver justice or to account for one's stewardship, that forces
the individual to behave according to *a certain notion of common
good* and to redress injuries (caused by the king or some other
powerful person). Justice, then, goes hand in hand with power.
Otherwise, totalitarianism sets in and paves the way for conspiracy, rebellions, riots, and ultimately chaos. In fact, this had
already been noted by the great and largely unknown fourteenth-
century North African historian and sociologist Ibn Khaldoun
(1978), who noted a three-generation cycle that inevitably led
to the downfall of the Arabo-Bedouin dynasty. After the first
generation had conquered and consolidated its power, the second and the third generations set out to live in the lap of luxury, thus squandering the wealth of the realm before robbing
their own subjects. This initiated a process of rebellion and destruction that in turn led to the arrival of a new dynasty.

The way to salvation, according to Ibn Khaldoun, is strikingly close to what emerges from Shakespearean plays and from
Berle's analysis: the king must take care of using power along
with the material means at his disposal to provide for a mini-
mum of justice and equity, for the redistribution of wealth, and
for the security of his subjects. This implies a modicum of ethical behavior and concern on the part of the king, who must look
after the welfare of his weakest and humblest subjects. Long
before Jean Rostand, Ibn Khaldoun understood and advocated
the claim that the degree of advancement and stability of a civili-

zation is a function of the way in which it treats its weakest elements. For the sovereign (or the holder of power) to truly accomplish his duties in the area of justice and equity, he must make himself available and implement a system that will enable him to hear the unbiased requests, criticisms, and complaints of his humblest "subjects." In this respect, Chinese emperors were watched over by a group of censors who were responsible for the just interpretation and implementation of their heavenly mandate. In terms of Western medieval history, Berle (1957) demonstrates how the Norman and English kings provided a form of direct justice in which every subject could petition the king through the expression *"Haro!"* (which is derived from "Ah! Rollo!" in reference to the name of the Norman duke and then king Rollo, the predecessor of William the Conqueror). Berle traces the origin of English common law to this custom, which he also believes to be the origin of the *Curia Regis* (king's court). The possibility of petitioning the king is probably one of the indirect explanations for the famous fiction of the two bodies. At the beginning of the thirteenth century, it became necessary to establish a specific location in which the subjects could appeal to the king's conscience; until then, it followed the Curia Regis as it traveled along with the king. The first English courts were established at Westminster to provide the material means of appealing to the king's conscience. Through their continued presence at Westminster, the Curia Regis and the lord chancellor (who was the bearer and the repository of the king's conscience) are probably at the heart of the permanence and transcendence of the institution of royal justice, which could function without the physical presence of the king because it represented what was to become its political and celestial body.

The tragedy of Shakespearean kings, however, illustrates the painful renunciation that goes along with the possession of the celestial body: kings are banned from the simplicity of the human condition expressed in reciprocal relationships with one's fellow men; they therefore lose the essential "mirrors" of their human condition. This is what troubled Henry V (*King Henry V,* act IV, scene 1 [Wells and Taylor, (1600) 1989]) as he cried:

O hard condition, Twin-born with greatness:
subject to the breath of every fool,
. . . .
What infinite heartsease Must kings neglect
That private men enjoy?
. . . .
What kind of god art thou, that suffer'st more
Of mortal griefs than do thy worshippers?

This, according to Kantorowicz (1989, p. 35), "constitutes the human tragedy of the twin condition of the monarchy which Shakespeare highlighted," in the sorrow of Henry V as he brooded over the destiny of Richard II or in Richard's despair in confronting his own treacherousness as a natural body toward the political body of the king (*The Life and Death of King Richard II,* act IV, scene 1 [Wells and Taylor, (1597) 1987]):

Mine eyes are full of tears; I cannot see.
. . . .
But they can see a sort of traitors here.
. . . .
I find myself a traitor with the rest,
For I have given here my soul's consent
T'undeck the pompous body of a king

In an earlier passage (act III, scene 2) Richard evokes the long tragedy of kings, who are tormented by their own destiny:

For God's sake, let us sit upon the ground,
And tell sad stories of the death of kings —
. . . for within the hollow crown
That rounds the mortal temples of a King
Keeps Death his court . . .
. . . .
Infusing him with self and vain conceit, —
As if this flesh which walls about our life,
Were brass impregnable. . . .

As Kantorowicz (pp. 39–40) explains, this passage clearly illustrates the fact that Richard II has come to a painful realization: "It is not only that the king's human nature triumphs over the divine nature of his crown and that mortality succeeds over immortality, but even worse . . . the king suffers an even more cruel death than do other mortals."

This brings us back to the anxiety of being versus nonbeing, which is part of our existence as humans. However, it also highlights the tragedy of the dual condition of kings. The blatant illusion of their immortal, sacred body and the immense downfall that accompanies the realization of this illusion cause kings to suffer a "more cruel death than do other mortals." This is all the more tragic for King Lear, who deliberately unleashed the forces later harnessed against him. The power instruments of his political body had been entrusted into hands that eventually used them to kill this same political body. In addition, Lear had the illusion of retaining the symbols, trappings, and privileges of this political body in a sense *in abstracto*.

In his detailed analysis of *Hamlet* and *King Lear,* Bonnefoy (1978) rightly draws our attention to two words that Shakespeare uses in the most intense moment of each play: *readiness* and *ripeness.* For instance, as Hamlet is preparing to fight Laertes, he declares: "readiness is all"; Edgar, the son of the duke of Gloucester, declares toward the end of *King Lear:* "ripeness is all." Bonnefoy argues (p. 20) that *readiness* and *ripeness* are unequivocal references to the idea of preparing or *ripening for the acceptance of death.* This is the fate of mankind, which man in his wisdom must accept. However, the process of gradually achieving readiness and ripeness is inordinately wrenching and painful for the king as an archetype of the human god. Moreover, there are also other conditions that man must accept in order to achieve this lucidity and wisdom. Basically, these conditions could be described as the need to accept a modicum of obligation toward one's fellow men, who then become the preferred method of confirming one's existence and identity. For kings as well as for those who hold absolute or near absolute power, these conditions are expressed as the obligation of using power for noble purposes and of being accountable for their power by providing for justice and fairness. Omnipotence and absolute power are only viable when they are applied for humanistic purposes or when those who hold such power are closely attuned to the voice of their *conscience,* that is, when they are aware of the concerns of their lowly fellow men and are devoted to making life under their stewardship fair and equitable. We shall return to these notions, but the point to be made here is that these checks and balances — or this counterpower, this constant questioning of established authority — are the first condition of their capacity to endure as well as the best guarantee of the humanness, wisdom, and disalienation of their holders. As we shall see later on, they are also the basis of the recovered productivity of contemporary organizations. Indeed, the relationship between the dual condition of kings and their two bodies and the current situation of corporate leaders and managers is far from evident. Nevertheless, as Berle (1957, p. 60) rightly submits: "From the Norman dukes and kings to the managers of modern corporations [there is] a form of power [that] is a permanent phenomenon [and that], in spite of its limitations, is essentially absolute." This proposal is hard to dispute in the face of the boundless power of the leaders of some of our large corporations and institutions, not to mention the "owner-manager" who enjoys the "inalienable right" to manage "his property" as he sees fit, regardless of its size. Indeed, the Geneens, Fords, Morgans, and Krupps are not the only examples of boundless power, of the illusion of immortal omnipotence, and of the archetypical dilemma of kings (Kets de Vries and Miller, 1985; Morgan, 1986; Miller, 1992). This is precisely what I intend to cover in the second part of this chapter: how CEOs and managers in general live with the explosive mix of the existential anxiety common to all men and their absolute or near absolute power and what the consequences of this process are.

Structural Obstacles to the Personification of the Employee and to the Establishment of Partnerships

I use the word *structural,* in its economic sense, in reference to the concepts discussed in this section because I believe that these phenomena are inherent in the diachrony and fundamental relationships between the actors involved in intraorganizational as well as interorganizational relations. In addition, the choice of this word deliberately refers to the notion that these phenomena are deeply rooted in the organization's mentalities and "structures" (physical premises, social systems, and interpersonal relations within the organization). Because these phenomena are also durable, they cannot be adequately understood or even discussed within a framework limited to the apparent modus operandi or the existing situation at any point in time. I am discussing basic principles and fundamental concepts. I will try to illustrate how (on a phantasmal rather than a political and legal level) corporate managers are trapped in the same deeply rooted illusion of omnipotence, immortality, and corporal duality as the English kings of old. We must first consider the historical and diachronic reasons whose consequences are still felt in the sociocultural foundations of our management systems. Bear in mind that the largely dominant (not to say monopolistic) "Anglo-Saxon" management model applied during the first seven decades of the twentieth century was materially born in Great Britain and that it prospered theoretically and doctrinally in the United States. Its founding principles are central to our discussion: the modern manager and current theories of management are heir to the principles that drove and justified the Anglo-American industrial barons of the eighteen and nineteenth centuries. In a nutshell, it is a very smart and very appropriate mix of various elements of Calvinist puritanism, Adam Smith's "invisible hand," Darwinism, and Spencerism. The adoption of *The Book of Common Prayer,* the dogmatic foundation of the Anglican Church, became the Calvinistic Foundation of the future Protestant ethic, which Weber (1964) later described. It represents a very convenient amalgamation of the concepts of calling, predestination, and individual achievement in which the individual receives concrete signs of his predestination and election through the success of his "earthly vocation" (Braudel, 1980, 1985; Weber, 1964). This effectively legitimized individualism as a value, whereas it had previously been regarded as a sin. (It is still seen as a sin, or a near sin, in Confucianism and, less clearly, in Lutheranism and Catholicism.) From then on, nascent individualism was no longer regarded as a flaw or sin but was about to be justified, reinforced, and even glorified through the successive ideological sedimentation that derived from specific elements of the works of Calvin, Smith, Darwin, and Spencer. Calvin advanced the notion that material success and wealth are signs of divine election; Adam Smith, through his concept of the invisible hand provided the near divine absolution for all injustices, inequities, inequalities, and human miseries; Darwin's works were used to advance the very appealing notion that natural selection would complement divine election; finally, Spencer postulated that personal election-cum-selection contributes to the advancement of the most evolved societies.

This, in itself, would be quite sufficient to kindle the megalomaniac inflation of many egos and to generate countless hagiographic and glorifying theories of leadership and entrepreneurship. A substantial part of the traditional managerial literature is nothing but the cult of the exceptional individual, of the hero (etymologically, the demigod), the creator, and the builder of organizations of all ilks (who have now become media stars after being business school stars). This literature also offers abundant examples of the deeply rooted notion that humankind is blessed with a few exceptional individuals who are (virtually innately) the incarnation of the "entrepreneurial" phenomenon. They are presented as privileged beings who embody the entire organization, along with its attributes and modes of operation. These attributes are then actualized and materialized through the creation and then launching and the management of organizations. This is the "fundamental managerial myth" (Sievers, 1994) that presents the manager as a kind of godlike creator-organizer, who alone knows how to manage. This hero worship of the manager is far from a mere matter of style and even less an exaggeration. One only needs to look at the term *self-made man,* which is so dear to the entrepreneurial mind. What could be more deifying than this self-creation followed by the creation of an organization, of jobs and wealth? What follows is almost too good to be true. I refer the reader to an article published in the *Wall Street Journal* on March 22,

1993 (cited in "Classics in American Business Schools," 1993) in which the following comparisons were made: Henry V would come back as Lee Iacocca at the head of Chrysler Corporation; Agamemnon as James Duth at Beatrice Foods; Karl Von Clause-witz as Michael Quinian at the head of McDonald's; Cordelia, the heroic daughter of King Lear, as Christie Hefner at the head of Playboy Enterprises; and Ulysses as Kenneth Olsen at the head of Digital Equipment Corporation. These somewhat incongruous but highly revealing parallels were developed at Hartwick College. They were then presented as case studies (complete with guest speakers and professional moderators) in universities and businesses throughout the United States. The article also indicates that institutions such as the Harvard and Stanford business schools are considering "the introduction of classics in management courses." (Although I would enthusiastically support the teaching of "classics" in business schools, I sincerely hope that it will not be done according to the Hartwick model.) Nevertheless, the reader will agree, this provides an extremely eloquent illustration of my main argument: the deep and durable hero worship of managers, particularly in the place where modern management was born and bred, the United States. As we have seen, the primeval stew is made up of the amalgamation of Calvin, Spencer, Smith, and Darwin. This deification also rests on other foundations, which I will list very succinctly here, albeit at the risk of theoretical simplification or an unwarranted epistemological leap.

First of all, I submit that there is indeed a parallel to be drawn between the immortal political body of the English king and the identification-incarnation of the manager (particularly of the owner) within "his" organization, which becomes immortally immanent by transcending its members. (In fact, all management textbooks draw profusely on Fayol's famous analogy, in which the manager is the "brain" of the "social body" of the organization, while employees are its "limbs" and "organs.") Thus, according to Sievers (1986a) managers endow themselves with this transcendence and immortality through their identification with the organization and, particularly, with the actors who have the power and the knowledge to manage it because the "organization" and its "omnipotent management actors" both transcend the humble condition of the mortal human being who "is managed." This phantasmal construction of omnipotence and immortality is to be found in the immortal and demiurgic character of the inseparable duo of "organization-management." As we all know, however, there is no identification without projection; the leader can therefore only be the organization and the hands-on manager if there are others who from the start cannot be the organization and cannot manage themselves. This, of course, refers to subordinates, particularly the employees, who are there to be organized and managed as passive, obedient, and interchangeable objects. Ultimately, they come to be seen as mobile cultural vacuums, devoid of (the correct) values and beliefs because the management of excellence repeats ad nauseam that, over and above managing and organizing, one of the main tasks of the manager-leader is to build, change, remodel, and transmit the symbols, beliefs, values, and culture of the organization (Deal and Kennedy, 1982; Peters and Waterman, 1982; Schein, 1985).

It seems as though the omnipotence-immortality of the leader (and his phantasmal participation in the absolute being) must be matched by the necessary reification, by the existential vacuum and the "nonbeing-nonperson" of the employee. Employees surrender their time and their own control over time (thus, all of their significant "capacity of being" in reference to the organization) to the leader, who will organize and manage them. In so doing, the leader gives up his freedom, his free will as a subject, and by extension, his own faith in the generic mode of being of humankind: work as the ultimate creative and self-creative act that shapes both the environment and the self. In addition, the manager's self-deifying demiurgic fantasy of omnipotence will be magnified because he has now been invested (through Calvin's, Smith's, and Darwin's heritage) by the management of excellence with an even more grandiose role, that of the creator of all that is "sacred" in the organization: myths, symbols, beliefs, values, and so on.

In delving more deeply into this process, one must come to the conclusion that for the manager, the identification with the organization will necessarily take place in a mode in which the "object" of the organization will be fantasized as a "good object," or as much as possible, as a systematically gratifying object (I would add, without any mandatory reference to any particular school or particular psychoanalytic dispute); otherwise, what good is it to be the leader? Self-gratification through the organization generates and maintains a whole array of concrete facts, gestures, and signs that allow for the reification and the actualization of the fantasy of omnipotence and immortality, all of which concretely cast the leader as the one who plans, organizes, decides, and controls. From the leader's point of view, the organization (even if it is only a subdivision of the whole organization, such as a subsidiary, department, or unit) cannot be seen as a frustrating or disappointing object. The dangers and dysfunctions of this type of process are obvious: collusion, cleavage, reactionary formation, transformation of reality, censorship and self-censorship, the systematic search for scapegoats, and so on. The boss will be less and less tolerant as his fantasies take root and "his" organization fails to behave according to his visions and desires; he will then seek to eliminate all that he sees as opposition to or disappointment with his leadership and even everything that does not glorify his leadership. The process is well known: the megalomania of the leader is reinforced until it degenerates into collective delirium, madness, and meticulous self-destruction. There is no shortage of examples, from Napoleon and Hitler to Hoover, Geneen, Henry Ford, and Howard Hughes (Kets de Vries and Miller, 1985; Miller, 1992; Mitroff and Pauchant, 1990). Along the same lines, Morgan (1986) proposes that the deep-rooted reason for the long-standing blindness of American automakers vis-à-vis the Japanese threat was that their "organizations" could not stop being gratifying by providing them with concrete evidence that the cars they produced were increasingly outdated and shunned by consumers.

If we add to the picture the unquestionable "anality" of organizational life and of most of its leaders, we encounter another worrisome (and hidden) aspect of the work of most managers-organizers: they tend to actualize in their daily lives a form of relationship to others based almost exclusively on the notion of give-and-take, accounting, controlling, classifying, supervising, ordering, dominating, standardizing, filing, and keeping. (Looking at the symptoms of the anal-obsessive characteristics described by Abraham [1970], one cannot fail to be impressed by the similarity of these symptoms to what many management textbooks describe as the ideal personality traits of a leader.) This list is virtually complete, including self-sufficiency; obsession with time and order, numbers, control, written communications; and predictability, dominance, authoritarianism, and compulsive possessiveness. This is hardly surprising in view of the fact that one of the founding fathers of modern management, Frederick W. Taylor, exhibited a particularly striking case of obsessive anal neurosis (Kakar, 1970). This would ultimately be amusing if it were not for the considerable pain and damage that these mechanisms inflict in the workplace. In fact, they often result in the destruction of entire organizations or even of whole industrial sectors, geographical areas, local economies, and communities (Pauchant and Mitroff, 1992).

In the course of my field research, I had the opportunity to meet and observe the manager of a group of factories who was deeply convinced and claimed — erroneously, as it turned out — that he spent a couple of hours every morning in "his" shops — to "get a feel for the morale of my troops" and to "look into everyone's problems." Nobody among his immediate colleagues, his secretary, or the shop managers had ever dared to make him realize that, as a rule, he hardly ever met anyone and that he never listened. As several of his colleagues told me, "You just don't contradict him." But the fact remains that the boss, probably in all good faith, believed that he knew his employees, shops, and machines very well. The negative consequences of this type of belief are not difficult to imagine when the time comes to make decisions, manage, and decide on trade-offs, in sum, to direct what's happening on the production floor.

From this perspective, the situation is in fact rather gloomy: demiurgic fantasies, omnipotence and immortality, focus of the leader's status on the pleasure principle and of the organization as a gratifying object, anal obsessiveness, collusion, transformed reality, and collective and mutually reinforced rationalizations (the famous groupthink that Janis [1972] has emphasized). As Berle, Sievers, Kets de Vries, Miller, and Morgan, among others, have indicated, this is unfortunately the price to be paid for the continued growth of the organizational universe of Western industrialized societies. Modern Western organizations have become hotbeds of absolute power and have given birth to a race of demigods and a system that contributes to their ever-growing glorification and deification (perhaps with the exception of Scandinavian and German organizations). Ultimately, the situation becomes a mirror image of the pleasant harmony portrayed and frenetically called for by the bards of corporate excellence. Now more than ever, our organizations are cleft and polarized universes in which employees are simultaneously mellowed with flowery discourse (the "priceless human capital that will provide total quality") while being treated as objects of management to be adjusted according to anticipated short-term profit or deficit levels.

In other words, the "employee-ambassadors" that Peters and Waterman (1982) so ardently called for more than ten years ago are still far from being treated as ministers with full powers but are more than ever regarded as profit fodder. In most "advanced" countries, GDP per capita productivity and production are on the rise (because of new technologies) while middle managers and other employees are forever more vulnerable to unemployment and poverty. The employee as a variable cost (as a factor to be adjusted according to the needs of production and financial requirements) is still the necessary condition to the continued position of the leader as a "fixed cost" (not even considered in production costs, as in the case of so-called direct labor costs). This results in the protection of the leader's position and privileges regardless of the situation and also affords the manager a truly royal form of treatment. In the United States, executive "salaries" have gone as high as $80 million dollars, even though some timid attempts have been made to reduce the level of executive compensation ("Executive Pay . . . ," 1992).

The increasing deification of the manager is matched by the growing relegation of the employee to an "input," a production factor; workers, in other words, are regarded as totally expendable. During a prolonged recession, for instance, a CEO may be paid an exorbitant salary while swelling the ever-growing ranks of the unemployed through his rationalizations and compressions. This represents a glaring contradiction that the management of excellence has vainly tried to solve over the past twelve or so years through its pseudo-humanist gymnastics (Aktouf, 1992). The worker is depicted as the (necessary) object to be valorized by the leader-hero–living legend and simultaneously as the dedicated and enthusiastic partner of the excellent corporation in which he will constantly demonstrate his correct acculturation to the values of the leader, who is only a "fixed cost" (immortal), because the worker is a "variable cost" (mortal). This "human resource" can never really be admitted in the sanctum sanctorum of the immortals precisely because his status as an expendable, interchangeable variable cost is the very foundation of the attributes and existence of the members of this sanctum sanctorum. The worker is then not merely a mortal, virtually subhuman because he lacks vision, reflection, ideas, knowledge, and the correct values, credos, and so on; from a managerial point of view, he is also a nonperson and a nonentity because he is only a cost/resource, which necessarily makes him a passive, heteronomous object to be managed. In hard economic times, this worker even becomes the most "strategic" of all management objects, and the manager will be all the more heroic because he will have to rationalize, cut expenses, cut the fat, make hard decisions, and produce more with fewer resources. In the management of excellence, however, this same worker is also invited to participate, to contribute to innovation and total quality, and to be mobilized within the framework of objectives, strategies, vision-mission, culture, and values, all of which are defined elsewhere by omnipotent and omniscient leaders. From an existential point of view, this situation is even more intolerable than that of the silent employee who only had to contribute his energy and his obedience. Today's employee is asked to participate, to echo and parrot what the boss wants to hear while being fully aware that despite whatever he does or says the decisions will still be made at the top (Linhart, 1991; Aktouf, 1990b and 1992).

If we agree that the human being's status as a subject and as a person is articulated through the "I" who is allowed to define himself or herself and speak as an "I," it is easy to realize the glaring depersonalization that employees suffer in the workplace. Historically, assembly line employees have been asked only to be quiet and obey. (According to Morgan [1986], 87 percent of American service and industrial workers have to deal with more complexity in getting to work than in the work itself.) Moreover, a number of authors, including Ronald Laing (1970), have clearly illustrated the psychic damage caused by "collusion" and "double constraint" situations in which workers are requested to act as if they are not even aware that they are playing a role. This is the silly game called for by the management of excellence. To survive, the omnipotent hero-manager needs to maintain armies of impotent nonsubjects in a childlike dependence condition; because of their impotence, these people will then refer all the difficult issues and decisions to the "top." This is the only way for the hero-manager to use the organization as a base for permanent status as an overworked, harried hero, that is, to live in a state of nonlucidity. (See, for example, Mintzberg's [1984] description of such managers, who are constantly on the move dealing with different problems, roles, decisions, and tasks, to understand that they are in a constant condition of myopic nonlucidity with respect to the situation at hand. See also Mitroff and Pauchant [1990], who refer to this situation as "busyness" instead of "business.") I intentionally use the word *nonlucidity* because, as the English word *workaholism* clearly indicates, the process is akin to the artificially induced escape mechanism common to all forms of drug abuse. In addition, the mountainous piles of papers, bulging attaché cases, and countless meetings and telephone calls are particularly useful in the sublimation of existential anxiety.

And the vicious circle goes on: the manager of excellence can only be a superperson if the rank-and-file members of the organization become nonpersons, and just as the victim needs a torturer, the subhuman creates the superperson. Of course, the discourse of excellence claims to make a superperson out of everyone. I have personally seen disciples of Peters and Waterman who attempted to apply these "principles" by trying to convince a receptionist that she was the most important member of the entire organization because she was the first point of contact with the customer. Apparently, those who use this type of discourse are not even embarrassed by the daily contradictions of its soothing rhetoric. The most pernicious aspect of this vicious circle on rank-and-file employees (who must face their own existential anxiety and who are also confronted with the profound absurdities of human destiny) is that they have no choice but to contribute to their own reification by behaving and by asking to be treated as objects; this is the only escape from their own anxiety because the other possibility, admittance to the sanctum sanctorum of thinking subjects, is "structurally" closed. Linhart (1991, p. 174) relates the reaction of some team members in a context of so-called team management: "We're here to work, not to manage. *They manage.*"

The concept of participation and mobilization also meets with the same unambiguous answers: "Let those who get paid for that manage the problems of the organization"; "just leave me alone with my job, and at five o'clock, I'm out of here"; "it's all been planned and decided ahead of time" (Aktouf, 1986 and 1990a). From Simone Weil (1964) to Robert Linhart (1972) to Beynon (1973) and Terkel (1976), the literature of industrial field studies is replete with such examples. All seem to refer to the same basic suffering: *in a large majority of cases, there is no room at the bottom of the organizational pyramid for people to be treated and to act as people.* To add insult to injury, this situation is then used to support the idea that part of humankind (rank-and-file employees) "is not prepared to face any challenges . . . or doesn't like to participate" (Laurin, 1973). There is also the argument (still in vogue in certain quarters — for instance, see Simon, 1973a, 1973b) that the self-fulfillment of the worker must take place outside the firm, because what the firm needs is his "productive capacity." The individual of the nondemiurgic and nonheroic variety is increasingly attempting to escape from the organization and its concomitant in order to come to terms with himself, as best he can, "elsewhere," a process that Mintzberg (1989) describes with surprising candor.

Where, then, will the management of excellence lead us? Its depredations and human costs are already formidable (Aubert and de Gaulejac, 1991), and its attempts to create a working partnership between managers and employees, between capital and labor has met with dismal failure. So why is this policy still the order of the day in management circles? Is there a way out of this dilemma? These are the issues I discuss in the concluding section of this chapter, where I also present a number of hypotheses and possibilities, along with a few concrete examples, of "renewed management."

Negotiated Finalities,
Empowering Actions, and Shared Benefits

It is highly significant that whenever the idea of bringing radical change to Western organizations is raised, it is immediately met with scepticism and accusations of utopianism and of cultural genocide treacherously fomented by the invasion of the "Japanese model." In fact, now more than ever, the proponents of the management of excellence are calling for a revolution without revolutionary change. How else could we explain the incredible flight into rituals and symbolism that is constantly advocated by the ideology of excellence; this is an outright refusal to see the productivity problem (in the United States in particular) for what it really is: a gigantic and growing material gap between managers and employees.

The situation is even worse if we consider that rival models (particularly in Germany and Japan) provide constant training in the workplace, for an annual average of 240 hours per employee (versus two hours in the United States), or when we consider that one German CEO out of four began his career as a rank-and-file worker, or when we consider that nepotism is not a factor in the Japanese promotion system or that a forty-five-year-old Japanese worker and father of three can be paid three times as much as a young single manager (even one who graduated at the top of his class from one of the major universities). When these factors are taken into consideration, the true nature and importance of the gap between the American manage-

ment model and its German and Japanese counterparts become
readily apparent. Why, then, do organizations devote so much
attention to the symbolic and cultural? Why do they try to foster
the pipe dream of attachment to the organization through the
fanciful and disembodied quest for the fusion of the self into
the organizational ideal (Pagès, Bonetti, de Gaulejac, and Descendre, 1979)? To be clear on this point, the issue at stake is
nothing less than the preservation of the status quo at all cost.
  The employee is still treated as an input and a production cost, the only difference being that, with the ideology of
excellence, he will "whip himself" as a production tool and strive
for his own compression as a financial cost. When it comes to
employees, the management of excellence obdurately refuses to
see them as an investment rather than a cost or to train and
valorize them instead of cutting and rationalizing them, which
would have an adverse effect on the pursuit of maximum profits
in the short run.
  The result is an increasingly anxious, frustrated, suffering, and undertrained workforce, one that is on the receiving
end of an ever-growing form of doublespeak. Such employees
will never become enthusiastic partners who are ready to be
mobilized in the cause of greater productivity. Moreover, they
are fully aware that the new technologies allow the organization to produce on a greater and greater scale with fewer and
fewer employees (see "Le travail partagé" [work sharing] in the
March 1993 edition of Le Monde Diplomatique). The problem,
however, is that this workforce is the only source of constant
innovation and improvement (the famous Kaizen system), which
is at the root of improved productivity and quality and is ultimately essential to the prosperity and survival of modern organizations. It is therefore just as essential to allow individual
workers to become enthusiastic and committed partners with
a personal interest in the success of the organization. This transformation, however, must be accompanied by conditions that
managers refuse to recognize because they are threatening the
status quo: corporate leaders, regardless of their "high" position, must henceforth accept their status as mere mortals among
mortals. The absolute power whose attributes and trappings they

would like to keep puts them in the same dilemma as Richard II and King Lear: if they want to secure the commitment of their employees and the survival of their organizations, they must accept transparency, personal examples, profit sharing, accountability, fairness, ethics, a commitment to the common good, and the possibility of permanently appealing to their conscience. This obviously represents a radical change; the battle will involve the transformation of statuses and identities, which implies that from now on the worker must be treated as a person instead of an object.

There are several ways of achieving this objective. First, managers must agree to step down, symbolically and materially, from their pedestals as superpeople who "manage" others. Second, they must try to embody the actual attributes of the hero according to Greek mythology: that is, transgressing for one's fellow humans and forgoing, at the peril of one's life, the taboos that mere mortals cannot transgress; accepting in full lucidity the idea of one's death and demonstrating one's status by performing truly heroic acts; and finally, as Jupiter in the guise of Amphytrion, realizing that to deserve the love and devotion of human beings they must also accept their mortal condition. This form of leadership and heroism, however, is very different from that advocated by the management of excellence and the cult of individualism. Now more than ever, *the organization must become a collective adventure whose leaders have as many duties as rights.* In particular, they must be seen as providers of justice, fairness, and security in a framework within which the individual's place is secured in collaboration with his colleagues rather than against them. *The respect and the satisfaction of the employee and of the customer must come before the payment of dividends to select shareholders.* This approach calls for a total change in the organizational perspective and logic. Satisfied, respected, and confident clients and employees are the best guarantee of longevity for the organization and satisfaction for the shareholders.

The management of excellence must stop portraying its leaders as stars and heroes and start fostering the collective appropriation of the organization and a new form of sharing in which all members of the organization enjoy the attributes and the status of the acting subject: thinking, expressing oneself, reflecting, deciding, managing, exercising one's free will, and so on. Putting an end to the deification of the manager and repersonalizing the employee within the framework of negotiated, understood, and accepted finalities and strategies supported on a daily basis by empowered, decentralized, and autonomous actions are the order of the day. Implementing the fair, open, and apparent sharing of all management acts and of the results of common efforts is the nonnegotiable condition.

The famous ownership-obligation and joint-management aspects of the German model, as well as the *Wâ, ringi* and *Ie-amae* of the Japanese model, are essentially nothing but effective manners of curbing the temptation of demiurgic and omnipotent behavior and of fostering within the workplace the emergence of solidarity, a shared human condition, and freely consented, accepted, and benevolent authority whose main role is that of providing for material as well as existential fairness. I believe that these methods are largely responsible for the success and originality of new forms of management, notably in Quebec, where numerous organizations are successfully implementing a more humane and "attractive" form of management marked by transparency and sharing in all aspects of organizational life. (Among these are large corporations, such as Cascades, which now employs eighty thousand people in sixty-five subsidiaries on three continents, and smaller firms, such as the dynamic small- and medium-sized businesses of the Beauce and Eastern Township regions.) In a sense, we are now witnessing a certain resurgence of Aristotelian and Thomistic values that tends to downplay the individualism and mythical omnipotence of the entrepreneur and to foster the common and shared appropriation of the workplace in which all members enjoy the freedom of speech and are *all* regarded as mere fallible mortals who are aware of their condition (Aktouf, 1991b; Aktouf, Bédard, and Chanlat, 1992).

All this being said, however, we must realize that such an evolution cannot be imposed from above. Corporate leaders will not willingly forsake their fantasies of immortality for the wise acceptance of their own mortality or modify their behavior accordingly no matter how intensely we may desire such changes.

I would submit that there are two preferred places in which to remind business leaders of their mortal condition so as to free them from their fantasies: the organization itself and the business schools that train future leaders. In the organization, bosses must realize that they cannot achieve anything without the cooperation and willing participation of all those involved. This realization leads to more humble behavior and to a more respectful attitude toward others in order to secure their cooperation. This humility and respect are expressed in every aspect of daily life. For instance, leaders such as Lemaire at Cascades and Stayer at the Johnsonville Sausage Company will readily admit that they do not know everything and that the lowliest employee can also express his or her opinion on the management of the organization (Aktouf, 1992).

Renouncing fantasies of omnipotence and immortality cannot be achieved through a logical and rational process. Rather, it entails a painful relinquishing process, a reexamination of the self in which privileges and other trappings of the "divine body" are given up. For business leaders, the road back to mortality first involves a series of concrete and material renunciations: their exclusive information, secrecy, exclusive privileges, unwarranted luxury, astronomic salaries and bonuses, countless benefits, and monopoly on decision making. This is how Richard II, King Lear, and Henry V learned to live with the intolerable dilemma of their twin bodies: the painful "undecking" (in Shakespearean terms) of the external trappings of the "royal body." This, in effect, entails the obligation of providing for common good and justice, or assuming an apparent and temporary form of transcendence toward mere mortals in order to better serve them.

Moreover, in business schools, it is high time to put an end to the implausible cult and glorification of the manager, the entrepreneur, or the leader as an exceptional individual far above the hoi polloi. The example of Hartwick is a case in point, but the same phenomenon is present at several other schools, even the most prestigious ones. This overdose of the case method causes students and future business leaders to act on a daily basis as if they were Agamemnon, Cordelia, Ulysses, Wellington,

Napoleon, or Rockefeller. In the MBA programs, this goes on for two full years. In addition, while these case studies devote a great deal of attention to the attributes, qualities, talents, and rites of managers, their flaws, eccentricities, and most of all their *duties* receive far too little attention.

Our organizations must follow the same paths as the states that evolved from monarchies to republics. Just as the city-state of old, the organization must become a "public thing" for its members. This, in fact, is the main characteristic of today's efficient models, in which a certain type of *republicanism* prevails in the form of joint decision processes, across-the-board consultation. The survival of our organizations, our economies, and ultimately our societies is contingent upon this evolution.

5

Organizations as Existential Creations: Restoring Personal Meaning While Staying Competitive

Nicole Aubert

Before discussing the potential contribution of existentialism to an improved understanding of organizational phenomena, I would like to explain my understanding of its major axioms. For me, the underlying element that unites the numerous authors within the area of existentialism is the tendency to emphasize *existence* over *essence,* or to quote Sartre's famous formula, to accept the notion that "existence precedes essence." In this respect, existentialist philosophies are fundamentally opposed to the essentialist philosophies that were prevalent until the nineteenth century.

Conversely, for me, existentialism is not interested in essences, potentialities, and abstract notions. It is interested in what exists and conceives of existence as an act, not a condition. As its etymology indicates, *to exist* implies leaving what is (*ex*) to establish (*sistere*) something that has previously been only a possibility. To the atheistic branch of existentialism, the primacy of existence implies that humans exist first—that is, become aware of themselves, emerge in the world—and only after this define themselves. According to Sartre (1970, p. 22):

Note: Unless otherwise indicated, the translations in this chapter are the author's.

From an existentialist point of view, if Man cannot be defined, it is because he is nothing at first.
He will only be afterwards, and he will be what he
has made himself to be. Hence, there is no such
a thing as human nature, because there is no God
to define it. Man is . . . not only what he conceives
himself to be, but what he wants to be. . . . Man
is nothing but what he makes of himself. . . . Man
exists first, which means that Man is first and foremost what plunges into the future, and what is conscious of projecting himself into the future. Man
is first a project which is lived subjectively . . . there
is nothing before this project; nothing that makes
sense in heaven, and Man will first be what he will
have projected to be.

From this perspective, the destiny of human beings lies
within themselves, and there is no reality outside action. They
exist only insofar as they accomplish themselves and are nothing but the sum of their acts. This concept of existence as a permanent project does not imply that the choice of what humans
decide to be can be made once and for all; to exist, they must
constantly choose the being that they wish to become. They cannot establish themselves in a permanent position in existence.
Existence implies a form of transcendence, of improving upon
one's personal best. Individually, human beings can only exist
through the free accomplishment of this *surpassing of themselves.*
    The Sartrian concept of transcendence is defined as a con-
stituent element of the individual, no longer as an external element. The constant surpassing of the self results from the individual's existential quest. According to Sartre (1970, pp. 92–93,
emphasis added): "Man is constantly beyond himself; it is only
by projecting and losing himself beyond himself that Man can
exist, and, moreover, it is through the pursuit of transcendent
objectives that he may exist. . . . This definition of transcendence, as a constituent element of Man — not in the sense in
which God is transcendent, but in *the subjective sense* of surpassing oneself, in the sense that Man is not enclosed within himself — *is what we call existentialist humanism.*"

The popularity of Sartrian existentialism in France and abroad fits within the general framework of the development of individualism that has marked our society since the beginning of the century. By rejecting the concept of suprahuman transcendence and by defining transcendence as the surpassing of the self within the limits of human finitude, the existentialist current has contributed to a definition of the individual as a subject who is his own referent. For each individual, this raises in extremely acute terms the question of the meaning of his existential commitment and establishes the necessity of pursuing his own self-accomplishment and constructing his transcendence in his daily life and on an earthly scale.

The general weakening of the values and finalities that more or less governed social existence until the end of the Second World War, as well as the collapse and gradual bankruptcies of the major political and religious systems, resulted in a type of *vacuity* in the possible avenues of existentialist construction of the self. The way was then paved for the emergence of new actors who blithely tried to "harness" for their own benefit this enormous unused energy potential by providing meaning for the inner demand for existential commitment and self-transcendence. I would submit that the organization is one of these new actors of existential construction. It has been all the more successful in this new mission in that it has appropriated for its own use the previously dominant solutions regarding work and professional success as means of existential success.

The Organization as a New Actor
of Existential Construction

In his analysis of the influence of the Protestant ethic on the origin and development of capitalism, Max Weber demonstrated how incessant work and material success were regarded as both means and evidence of personal salvation "in the next world." Very early on, the companies that have been strongly marked by the Protestant ethic (particularly multinationals, such as IBM, Procter & Gamble, American Express, and Digital Equipment) adhered to the ethic of excellence that flows directly from this philosophical current. At the corporate level, the search for excellence is the moral foundation of a kind of system designed to encompass the whole individual by establishing unbreakable bonds between professional and personal requirements and molding personal values to corporate values. Such a system constitutes a particularly powerful form of domination because its logic of professional success is rooted in the inner core of the individual. It postulates indissoluble bonds between the ethical and the economic dimensions, which makes it all the more powerful because professional success then becomes a moral as well as an economic necessity.

The concept and the value of excellence have become so important in the organizational world during the last decade that the corporate system on which they are based deserves close scrutiny. In fact, because of the ever-growing intensification of competitive pressures, an increasing number of organizations are affected by the issue of excellence, although the degree of its implementation varies substantially from one firm to the next. Moreover, although this tendency does not affect all organizations, it has gradually become an inescapable reference model in the organizational world. As a result, its importance goes well beyond the number of firms that are directly affected by it. In particular, I will attempt to demonstrate how the positioning of the organization as an actor of existential construction is now a deliberate and organized activity.

The Obligation of Excellence: The Ideological Functions and the Evolution of the Concept of Excellence

The search for personal excellence advocated in the organization is simultaneously a vector of existential construction and one of the safest ways for the organization to achieve its objectives. This is probably the main reason why the concept of excellence has gradually appropriated the values of aggressiveness and competitiveness implied by the logic of economic survival. Indeed, as we look for the profound significance of this search, we soon note that it rests on a deeply rooted existential requirement unrelated to its economic aspect. Contrary to the traditional Protestant ethic described above, the excellence ethic is no longer interested in what might be called salvation in the next world or in suprahuman transcendence but rather in material success as the sole guarantor of meaning and self-accomplishment in a world in which spiritual references have evaporated and in which existence, along with its concomitant finitude, has become the only certainty. "You are nothing but your life!" cries Inès, one of Sartre's characters in *No Exit*, to express a concept of life narrowly linked to the limited temporality of human existence. Similarly, the modern organization has advanced its own existential proposal: *You are nothing but your professional life!* One's career has become the central organizing element and the source of meaning in one's life.

The economic necessity of excellence therefore goes hand in hand with the need to define the meaning of one's life in the temporal horizon of existence so as to confer upon excellence the status of ultimate finality in the organizational philosophy. Excellence becomes comparable to Christianity's kingdom of God or communist ideology's classless society (Landier, 1988). It appears as both the instrument of economic survival and the source of existential meaning. For the organization, excellence becomes a way to tap individual energies, to project them into an indefinite quest, and to channel them into its own projects. Among the reasons that explain the general and rapid acceptance of this concept of the organization is the fact that it is also an individual and collective "life project." It makes up for the current lack of meaning by providing individuals with a framework and an instrument to define the meaning of their life and to pursue their existential quest. The Procter & Gamble employee manual is a case in point; it defines the corporation's major principles through the title "What We Want to Be: Excellence Through Total Commitment and Innovation."

All the other concepts that underlie the implementation of a renewed form of management through excellence, such as motivation, mobilization, participatory management, and so on, have finally been combined with the notions of quality, excellence, and more recently, vision. They are now part of the required reading of official management regardless of their context. They figure prominently among official management buzzwords in the discourse of most top managers and senior consultants (Landier, 1988).

However, the concept of excellence itself has undergone a major evolution during this process. As one looks at the changes in the meaning of the word *excellence* over the years, one realizes that the "excellence" of old was a concept related to *duration* and *being*. It has now become an essentially ephemeral notion related to *doing*. Excellence was formerly defined as the capacity to endure over the years, or "what emerges from the flow of time" (Van Der Meersch, 1987). It is now defined by a radically different logic, one marked with the seal of modern technology, mass production, and rapid communication. In its original meaning, the notion of excellence implied the consecration of time, which made it a value so close to perfection that it represented the intrinsic quality of what is so good and perfect in itself that it can resist the passage of time. In its second meaning, excellence still implies the capacity to stand out, but it has lost its temporal connotation. It has become a mere scale, dedicated to the glorification of its upper levels. As such, it is an essentially ephemeral concept in that excellence is always open to the challenge of a better, more spectacular performance. It implies the notion of always doing more, faster, and better. Excellence is now a *process* rather than a *condition*.

Being excellent is now defined as having the capacity to triumph over others as well as over oneself, with all the precariousness involved in such a concept. According to Perrenoud (1987, p. 67), "Pursuing excellence implies the will to surpass oneself, to approach perfection, to improve upon one's personal best, as the mountain climber who is always reaching for higher summits, the athlete who is always trying to break his own record, and the researcher or the artist who is always trying to get closer to what he believes to be truth or beauty." This type of excellence, articulated around the concept of personal triumph, is an accurate reflection of our society and its prevailing individualism. It expresses the "ultimate stage of individualism" (Roman, 1987, p. 69), which we have now reached.

Being the best has become "the absolute necessity of our times, without, however, any particular prescribed field of excellence. . . . '[E]xcellence' has become another word for self-accomplishment, which is the only remaining finality" (Roman,

1987, p. 69). This new meaning of the word carries no transcendent finality: the life of the individual has become an end in itself. The individual is thus "the entrepreneur of his own life" (Ehrenberg, 1987) and is responsible for the sound investment of his own capital. The quest for this ultimate form of success and accomplishment justifies whatever efforts are needed and gives a meaning to existence.

The present concept of excellence also retains traces of the various nuances the notion has acquired over the years. It does not only refer to what's going on at the top. Regardless of the field in which it is used, it is not only a direct expression of the underlying values of competitiveness and global competition in social relationships. At a deeper level, it also retains the meaning "a need to symbolize a certain type of transcendence through exception" (Guillaume, 1987, p. 86). The current success of the concept of excellence as well as its wholesale adoption may therefore be attributed to the fact that it makes up for something, such as the need for an absolute, the absence of God, the lack of an ultimate reference, and so on. Through its advocacy of a permanent quest to surpass oneself and others, excellence then becomes a form of an absolute. This phenomenon is at the heart of the existential question described earlier because the absolute that is so pursued is in fact an absolute of the self, a quest for self-accomplishment carried to its outer limit.

Psychic Consolidation:
Harnessing Desires and Channeling Passions

As the organization makes extensive use of the value of excellence to meld its own objectives with those of its employees, it consolidates its new role as an actor of existential creation by appealing to individuals at the level of their deepest desires. To do this, the organization developed a type of management whose sphere of influence gradually increased over the years. Whereas Taylorism represented the triumph of the management of *bodies,* with its accompanying repression — which Foucault (1976) calls a disciplinary system — it was succeeded by Elton Mayo's school of human relations, which attempted to manage *hearts*. The current model of management is primarily concerned with the psychic dimension of individuals and is attempting to manage their *fantasies*.

The term *fantasy* refers to the products and processes of the imagination, be it in its cognitive dimension (ideas, thoughts, concepts, and creativity) or in its affective dimension (defense mechanisms, sublimation, desires, ambitions, and beliefs); the two dimensions are inextricably intertwined. I use the term *managing fantasies* to highlight the sometimes irresistible temptation to harness and domesticate fantasies for the purposes of the organization. I submit that all of the individual's cognitive and affective elements (ideas, fantasies, desires, ambitions, sublimations, defense mechanisms, and so on) may be used and abused by the organization to orient behaviors and influence personalities with the ultimate objective of maximizing efficiency and productivity. Vincent de Gaulejac and I (Aubert and de Gaulejac, 1991) have suggested this concept of fantasy management in reference to the attempt *to manage fantasies and to manage through fantasies*. Fantasies have now become an object to be managed toward greater efficiency and productivity, as was previously the case for the individual's physical energy and, more recently, for the individual's affective dimension.

The appearance of this new management system signals specific consequences for the new relationships between the individual and the organization. Earlier, in the conventional corporation, nothing more was expected of the individual than the proper accomplishment of his assigned duties. There was no attempt to take over the employee's inner world. Employees were free to think whatever they wished of their employer, and the organization made no existential promises whatsoever. Conversely, in the fantasy organization, the individual and the organization are no longer distinct entities. Individual commitment must be secured through the internalization of the company's values, objectives, and logic. Messine (1987, p. 93) summarizes this new concept in an eloquent manner: "The distance between the worker and the organization, which had been unduly widened by scientific management, must first be abolished. . . .

This represents a minor Copernican revolution: if the worker is not to be against the organization, he must stop being in front of it; it's not enough for him to be with the organization, he must be part of it; he must become the organization, and he must feel that he is part of its substance, that he is subjectively involved, as a part of the whole, as an atom in matter." For this to occur, the organization must be seen as the arbiter of personal destiny, as the craftsperson of individual development, as an object of love, and *also* as the only source of self-accomplishment and as being able to provide for the individual's need for immortality by addressing his anxieties. The organization accomplishes this by capturing desires and by addressing the individual's "passional" potential.

A quick glance at the careers section of any major newspaper reveals some of the ways in which the organization appeals to the individual's desires. "What if commerce meant love!" reads the job advertisement of a large French corporation. The ad portrays a little Cupid, with bow at the ready; the caption features the name of the corporation and the line "For those who want to succeed." It doesn't take a great deal of imagination to interpret the ad's meaning as, Choose company X to be loved . . . and successful.

Apparently, a growing number of organizations are attempting to portray themselves as being able to provide for the individual's need to be loved, desire for self-accomplishment, and need for immortality. Some companies conduct this process in a perfectly conscious and controlled manner. IBM, for instance, came to the conclusion that it had at best a mixed image among young college graduates. On the one hand, it was seen as a powerful and prestigious company that could offer job security, but on the other hand, it was viewed as a cold, standardized, and ultimately inhuman organization. In the early 1990s, IBM initiated a corporate recruitment campaign aimed at attracting young graduates and at facilitating their identification with the company. It published an ad portraying a smiling graduate with the caption "IBM, the shortest way between me and what I want to become." Here, the organization is attempting to take over the individual's quest for self-definition.

The Nietzschean prescription "become what thou art," which calls upon the individual to assume his own future, has now been co-opted by the organization, which offers an effective way of doing it: the individual can (and must) become himself with the help of the organization and through the organization. Other ads by other companies refer to the organization's alleged role as an agent of immortality through the legacy it allows the individual to leave behind. Working for company X is the first step toward an immortality of sorts. "You will be gone in the year 2000," reads another job advertisement, "but your actions will remain."

The organization does not only attempt to capture the individual's desires, however. It also portrays itself as an object of passion and demands a personal investment on the part of its members. Employees are now virtually compelled to channel their passions into the service of the organization. The organization wants driven people who will be totally committed to corporate objectives. This dimension was particularly striking in our study on the cost of excellence (Aubert and de Gaulejac, 1991). Some people talked of their "troubled love affair" when describing their career problems; others talked of their "passionate" relationship with their company.

In some companies, this requirement goes hand in hand with an attempt to manage passions. Not only do these companies demand an impassioned commitment from their employees, but they also expect to control it. "Control is everywhere," says one manager; "are you a little committed, a lot, passionately?" She adds, "It's in everybody's interest to be passionately committed." At the same time, on the individual level, people must not be seen as trying too hard to possess the object of their passion because passion must be kept under control. "The cornerstone of the system," explains another manager, "is the ability to play with your passion but also to leave it aside as soon as it becomes too intense, although it hurts to walk away, as in a love affair." An older manager adds: "Those who identified with the organization, who lost themselves in it, were then left aside because they were no longer interesting. They had become empty shells, mouthpieces of the organization; they were no longer able to contribute any living flesh. The organization therefore thrives on your rebellion."

These examples illustrate that the dialectic opposition between commitment and frustration, fascination and rebellion is what generates the psychic energy to drive the system. Why, one may ask, does the company maintain such meticulous accounts of its employees' ever-growing personal investment if not to increase and improve production? In fact, this amounts to *the virtual enslavement of the being in the service of production.*

Managerial Man: An Anxious "Hero"

We have seen in the analysis of the concept and value of excellence that the organizational and the individual processes involved are in fact highly congruent. We have also seen that the search for excellence and the pursuit of total quality, which have become necessary as a result of the dramatic intensification of global competitive pressures, also address the individual's narcissistic needs for self-accomplishment and for overall performance and that these two forces strengthen each other.

As a result of the social evolution that followed the collapse of the major traditional systems of meaning and the economic evolution that followed the growth of increasingly devastating competitive practices, the organization is no longer limited to its traditional role of accumulating capital; it is also at the core of a new way of being within society. It spreads its own values and develops a cultural behavior model and a style of living and acting that are centered around such values as action, triumph, performance, and excellence. Consequently, people now manage their private and individual lives as entrepreneurs who marshal their resources and their limited time to achieve their objectives efficiently. The organization then becomes the forum in which this pursuit of self-accomplishment and this quest for a "self-referred absolute" can take place.

This being said, however, we must also consider that this movement is a two-way street. We will now examine the ways in which individuals "invest" in the organization and expect it to provide answers for their existential anxiety. I will also attempt to sketch a brief picture of managerial man as a product and an actor of the "existential" organization just described (Aubert and de Gaulejac, 1991).

Homo Psychologicus

It would be impossible to draw a picture of managerial men
and women without first describing the general rise of narcissism, which has been extensively analyzed by sociologists and
philosophers, such as Lasch (1978), Sennett (1979), and Lipovetzski (1983); and by psychoanalysts, such as Anzieu (1985),
Bergeret (1974), Grunberger (1975), Kernberg (1970), and
Green (1985). While the rise of narcissism in contemporary societies must be linked with the collapse of the major systems
of meaning described above, it is also the consequence of the
personalization process that promoted and embodied the basic
value of self-accomplishment, in which "the systematic elimi-
nation of all transcendent positions generated a purely present
and subjective form of existence, devoid of meaning or of objectives, and abandoned to the giddiness of its own self-seduction"
(Lipovetzski, 1983, p. 69).

The personality that emerges from this process, which
Lipovetzski calls *Homo psychologicus,* is that of an individual
forever interested in his own being and welfare, wrapped up
in himself in a perpetual quest for his own accomplishment, and
increasingly indifferent to others; of a person with whom it is
impossible to establish a relationship. To paraphrase Sennett
(1979), one could say that *Homo psychologicus* has developed a
vision of reality in which the other is nothing but a mirror of
the self.

However, this description does not consider the emergence
of new providers of meaning that allow the individual to project
his existential quest. Lipovetzski's description of modern man
"lost in a vacuum," in a desperate narcissistic pursuit of himself, is far from being applicable to all human beings. As we
have seen in this chapter, the organization reacted to this existential quest by becoming a transcendent entity, a provider
of values, culture, morality, and goals and by offering a way
into the future. The organization has evolved from its traditional role as an agent of production and a place to work to become the focus of fantasy investments, the pursuit of pleasure,
and the fight against anxiety.

When *Homo psychologicus* invests himself in the existential firm, he encounters an organization that is apparently able to allay his fears and to provide for his desires. He then becomes what I have called *managerial man* (Aubert and de Gaulejac, 1991), whose fantasies are regarded as an object of management by the firm. Managerial men and women place their hopes and expectations in the organization; this becomes the place where they look for values and self-accomplishment, for meaning and significance.

The organization becomes an actor of existential creation as a result of two parallel and complementary dynamics. First, in his search for meaning and self-accomplishment, the individual invests himself totally in the organization, which he perceives as the only agent that can provide him with meaningful signs, landmarks, beliefs, and so on. Second, the organization develops a very seductive discourse to attract the individual who can be so mobilized and to marshal his energies in the service of its own objectives. Managerial man is the result of these dynamics. He is the producer of the first dynamic, which drives him to the organization in the hope of finding an answer to his existential anxiety, to project and pursue his need for meaning, and to satisfy his need for self-accomplishment. He is, however, the product of the second dynamic, in which the organization "works" and "acts" on him, shaping his values, beliefs, ideas, inner images, and so on, in sum, his fantasies.

In the first sense, managerial man is one version of the narcissistic personality. He is the actualization of this personality when, instead of operating in a vacuum, he chooses the organization as the focus of his projections and the object of emotional investment. In the second sense, managerial man is the product of the organization, the result of the mobilization of fantasies.

The Characteristics of Managerial Man

I will now attempt to describe the characteristics of managerial man. The first, as briefly noted above, is his narcissistic quest for the absolute. Managerial man adheres to the organization, in which he sees a way of satisfying an inner requirement beyond him. One manager describes the process that made him join his current company as follows: "In a sense, I needed to become a fanatic by making a personal commitment to something which went beyond me. I liked that requirement, that attitude, the fact that people were saying, 'Listen we're trying to do better and we're trying to do very well; now it's up to you to define what very well means.' That was very neat, very motivating. I was like a mussel in search of its rock, and my rock was the fact that I had a requirement which went beyond me. It was the possibility of living what I really am in my flesh and bones, of sublimating the whole lot and of presenting it to this God, this instant God, this God within me, who was not something cold, remote, and inaccessible; it was a very concrete vision which mobilized the whole lot and made it meaningful. It was a form of alienation, but a pleasant one, because you drown in a kind of objective inner principle, which in a certain sense, addresses existential anxiety."

This message underscores the important notion of *fanaticism*. Managerial man has an inclination toward fanaticism or will develop one. Indeed, if the individual is not sufficiently imbued with the desire to be fanaticized by a personal commitment that goes beyond him, the corporation will take care to nurture his desire. Survival and combat management training, in which candidates are expected to walk on red-hot coals and to jump from an airplane, are good examples of what Edgar Morin (1990) has called "corporate fanaticism."

The second important element is the narcissistic quest for self-accomplishment. The requirement involved in the manager's foregoing description of the process that led him to join a certain company is not a transcendent requirement but an inner God. Here the absolute is no longer a transcendent, external force to which the individual would submit; it is an inner demand for total self-accomplishment, for the accomplishment of the inner absolute in which the individual will drown in pleasure, just as Narcissus drowned in his own image. The organization becomes the instrument of self-absorption, which Sennett (1979) describes as the mainstay and the danger of narcissism. According to Sennett, the meaning of the myth of Narcissus is not to denounce the perils of self-love but rather those of self-projection, of apprehending the external world as if its reality could be captured through the images of the ego.

The third important characteristic is a narcissistic ethic. In such a circumstance, contrary to Lipovetzski's (1983) schemes, narcissism does not operate in a vacuum. It becomes an *ethical* form of narcissism. In this sense, we can extrapolate on Sennett's formula and suggest that the narcissism that underlies the "morality" of excellence is the Protestant ethic of our day. Here, narcissism and the Protestant ethic obey the same logic. The Protestant entrepreneur invested in his work to escape God's silence and to see in his success the signs of his election and salvation. His counterpart, the managerial man, invests in his organization to escape the social vacuum, the absence of a referent, the absence of meaning and to find in his work and career the signs of his personal self-accomplishment. Self-accomplishment at work is now, as in early capitalism, the only way to the conquest of an absolute and to a form of personal salvation that is no longer related to an external transcendent God but to the instant internal God of the self, the "narcissized" God described above. The ultimate referent is no longer in the next world but is now an earthly referent because self-accomplishment has become the sole justification of existence. The Protestant work ethic and the narcissistic quest for self-accomplishment are driven by the same engine: existential anxiety and the silence of God.

The final characteristic of managerial man is the peculiar nature of his relationship with his own anxiety, which far from being paralyzing is rather a very motivating force. Managerial man must live like a "winner" to feel sure of his own existence. He looks for challenges and thrives on adversity because the satisfaction of overcoming obstacles is his source of pleasure in existence. As one manager explains: "You must find ways of improving upon your personal best, you must find the growth you need, you must find the right challenge. I personally don't like it when the goal is too easy. I have no tolerance for what I call the equality of mediocrity. I don't like mediocrity. I like it when the bar is a little higher. In negotiations, I always tend to ask for a little more."

However, the level of anxiety in existential organizations can be far more radical. It derives from the obligation to be strong; from the impossibility of losing or even of giving the appearance of weakness; from the absolute necessity of reaching objectives at all cost, which is even more compelling because these objectives are self-imposed; and ultimately from the impossibility of existing beyond the boundaries of the organization without being banished to the vacuity of one's own existence. Just as the hero of Sartrian drama is "condemned to be free," managerial man is condemned to success. From an individual or an organizational point of view, success is the only acceptable form of existential accomplishment, the only solution to existential anxiety, and the only justification for the considerable efforts that are demanded within the organization.

Existential Perversity

The condemnation to success, in which managerial man is a willing participant, is at the very heart of what might be called a process of existential perversity. Instead of leading to an authentic form of self-accomplishment and transcendence in a meaningful existential projection, this process actually leads the individual to a certain form of self-destruction and existential "non-sense." When this occurs, the source of life becomes the source of death, regardless of the symbolic or real nature of this death.

On a strictly economic level, the demand for excellence and total quality has become an absolute requirement of survival. The logic of "economic world war" (Esambert, 1991) involves a need for permanent progress that confines the individual to an inescapable process of acceleration, the intensity of which may vary from one sector to the next but that is generally impossible to stop. The paradox facing managers is vividly expressed in the words of an executive who is speculating on the consequences of this mode of operation: "One of our problems is getting people to understand that from the moment you stop moving up, you start moving down. All of our current actions are geared to the continuation of this permanent progress.

But as we try to achieve this permanent progress we are literally cut in two. Permanent progress means going faster and faster, until you crash. We are absolutely convinced that the end of progress means death, but the pace is constantly accelerating."

Let's briefly look at the following elements of this speculation:

If we stop moving up, we start moving down.
We must therefore act continuously to achieve permanent progress.
But this action cuts us in two.
Permanent progress implies the necessity of going faster and faster.
The risk of crashing then becomes more important (it would then be advisable to stop).
But stopping leads to death.
Yet as the pace accelerates, the risk of crashing does also.

This passage offers an eloquent illustration of the "death anxiety" that is so common to a large number of organizations and that affects virtually all of their members. Indeed, the manager's deeply-rooted belief that permanent movement, constant action, and intentional creative disorder are the only means of not being overtaken by competitors, and thus of avoiding economic death, apparently drives the *vicious circle of permanent progress* that paradoxically leads to another form of anxiety: "the risk of crashing" and "being cut in two."

The lifestyle induced by "permanent action" is in a sense comparable to the action of drugs because it generates a form of deplorable but also highly addictive dependency. People have become used to this kind of acceleration and hectic activity; they complain about it, but whenever it stops, they wonder what's going on. In fact, it seems as though one part of an executive may be totally committed, both rationally and emotionally, to the necessity of permanent action and progress (the source of life, pleasure, and progress), while the other part has the feeling of no longer being in control of the constant acceleration and is afraid of succumbing to its deadly momentum.

On a more personal level, the search for excellence as the pursuit of a self-referred absolute is obviously frightening, dangerous, and in certain cases deadly. It becomes frightening as soon as it is seen as a didactic and prescriptive standard. It is dangerous because it is related to what Aragon (1944) calls the "taste of Absolute" and describes as a horrible disease, a devouring passion that eats its "beholder" and takes "those it has trapped." Finally, it is also deadly because the cult of the self (the heroization of the self) that it involves condemns the individual to a narcissistic love for his own image. In Rosset's words (1976, pp. 113–114), "The deadly mistake of the narcissistic individual is the fact that he prefers his own image to himself when comes the time to choose. The narcissistic individual suffers from a lack of self-love: he doesn't love himself, only his image."

This is probably what Georges Dumezil (1987, p. 21) had in mind when he declared in an interview a few months before his death: "The ideal man is quite the contrary of the excellent man; [he is] the man who is aware of his ephemeral nature and of his limitations, who knows that he is not excellent." However, this balanced ideal is far from the ideal of managerial man. In fact, the extreme demands that the ideal of the self makes upon managerial man lead him to believe that he should pursue his own personal accomplishment through a wholesale commitment to the organization's ideals. This leads to a form of existential patchwork that takes its toll on him.

While the efficiency of the system with respect to short- and medium-term productivity has long been demonstrated, it is nevertheless important to look at what might be called its mendacious aspects. The system is incredibly efficient as long as the individual and the organization operate in tandem, but it becomes problematic when for one reason or another (lowered performance, personal problems, and so on) the individual is no longer really adequate for the organization either because he cannot maintain the pace, deliver the required performance, or keep up with the (very high) required level of "passional" investment. In such a circumstance, the person who used to be totally committed to the organization and operated at a very intense level no longer receives the gratification and the rewards

that he had come to expect. This loss, even if it is only symbolic, is particularly difficult to accept when the bonds between
the individual and the organization had become too strong, when
the symbiosis had become too intense, or when the individual's
self had finally merged with the organizational ideal. These circumstances lead to episodes of brutal depression in which the
person "cracks up," either suddenly or gradually. The phenomenon is particularly intense in those individuals who had a very
high self-ideal and who had invested in a cause, a career or an
organization in which they believed and which "let them down"
when they could no longer deliver what was expected of them.
These individuals then feel empty, consumed by this immense
self-commitment whose futility and vanity they now realize. This
is a classic example of the phenomenon known as burnout,
which leaves the individual devastated from within, as in the
case of a fire (Freudenberger, 1985).

I have seen numerous cases of this devastation. For instance, Naomi, who had happily "worked herself to death" for
nine years, was gradually pushed aside and slightly less rewarded.
She describes the collapse that preceded her depression this way:
"It was worse than if somebody had died in front of me . . .
somebody who had been very dear to me. My whole self-esteem
then went down the drain. It was as if I had taken somebody
and then broken him." These comments clearly illustrate the
inner cleavage that occurred in this woman's mind. One part
of Naomi's self, her ideal self, which she had identified with the
organization, just collapsed, while the other part of her self contemplated the disaster. Although the process is not always as
devastating and profound as this, the inner splitting is indicative of the subtle discomfort that goes on within the individual
and is expressed in such declarations as, "I feel simultaneously
good and bad about myself."

What is the attitude of the organization when it becomes
aware of this essential perversity? The issue is complex because
this process is precisely the one that drives the operation of the
organization (stress as the "fuel" of performance, idealization
as the mainstay of emotional investment, and so forth). This
is probably why organizations are reluctant to discuss the matter.

This is also probably the reason why some organizations take care of the individual "until the very end." Some of them even take care of selecting the clinic in which the affected individual will be treated for his depression.

It is legitimate to ask how far we can go in this logic of frantic competition that demands greater and greater exertion on the part of the countries and organizations involved. Be it a case of physical exhaustion, as in the case of the Japanese *karoshi* phenomenon of sudden death due to excessive work, or psychic exhaustion, as in the case of burnout, the symptoms are in fact indicative of a breakdown that becomes the only way of escaping the vicious circle in a constantly accelerating society bent on a frenetic and neurotic quest for economic success and narcissistic self-accomplishment.

How, then, can the individual manage the personal commitment that the organization demands? The individual must learn to keep his distance, to avoid "losing himself" totally in the organization, to strike a balance between what I would call the hard and soft dialectic. The soft part is the enticing aspect of the organization, the ways in which it stimulates and addresses the individual's desires for communication, profit, togetherness, and so on. "I can actually touch the chairman of the board," exclaimed a star-struck manager at Hewlett-Packard." Conversely, the hard part is the the obligation to be strong, the impossibility of losing, which is dictated by the tyranny of win/win logic. To avoid transforming his necessary self-commitment into enslavement of his being in the service of "production," the individual must apparently learn to preserve his inner world, his reference to himself; he must strike a balance between *being* and *doing,* and he must learn to resist the siren song of symbiosis.

What are the individual or collective implications of the foregoing observations? The Sartrian perspective helps explain the new mentality of modern man, that of an individual who no longer defines his existence (life) project or measures the meaning of his life in reference to a mythical "other world" but rather chooses to do so with respect to an effective realization of his project or purpose. This perspective, however, offers no insight into the way of fighting the existential perversion just described, which effectively leads to the alienation of the individual rather than to the accomplishment of a meaningful professional project.

I will formulate my concluding remarks in the general framework of the question of individual and collective meaning. If the meaning of life currently advocated by modern management theories consists of "identifying with the combative and efficient, not to say omnipotent, nature of organizations" (Palmade, 1988, p. 118), it can then be asked what meaning we are talking about. Is it a meaning that advocates an emotional investment in the idea of progress, defined as economic and technical development? Is it a meaning that advocates an overinvestment in new technologies (aimed at controlling time, space, and people), along with the accompanying notion of omnipotence? Is it a meaning that is exclusively derived from the joy of power that follows victorious battles? Then the question that must be asked is whether the "fantasy" system described in this chapter does not actually rest on an appeal to what Enriquez (1990) calls the "enticing fantasy." According to him, organizations now have a choice between two forms of fantasies in their attempts to shape the thoughts of the individual, penetrate his inner psychic world, and generate the forms of behavior that are essential to their dynamic: they can resort to motor fantasies or to luring fantasies. Motor fantasies are those through which the organization allows the individual to make full use of his creative imagination and to draw on his psychic resources to drive his own actions. Luring fantasies are those through which the organization attempts to ensnare the individual in the web of his own desires by addressing his anxieties, desires, and fantasies. Ultimately, the organization then substitutes its own fantasies for those of the individual. According to Enriquez (1990, p. 213):

> The organization thus poses as a divine, omnipotent institution, as the sole reference, as being able to deny time and death; on the one hand, it is also the overprotective and smothering mother and the benevolent and nourishing mother; on the other

hand, it is simultaneously the castrating and the
symbolic father. In this view, the organization is
forever threatened by external and internal enemies
bent on preventing it from fully accomplishing its
ascribed mission; it is rent with specific fears, fear
of chaos, fear of the unknown, fear of uncontrolla-
ble love impulses, etc. As it appears simultaneously
over-powerful and extremely fragile, the organization intends to occupy the entire psychic world of
its individual members, who are no longer able to
imagine any other form of behavior.

For the time being, however, it seems that the main problem of the organization consists in navigating as well as it can
between the two forms of fantasies, that is, capitalizing as much
as possible on motor fantasies without falling prey to enticing
fantasies. As we have seen, the limitations of this system and
the breakdowns it generates in individuals clearly indicate that
the most advanced societies in the performance race are also
the first victims of the system's intrinsic contradictions. The
"resignation neuroses" that are more and more frequent in Japan
(that for a growing number of young managers are indicative
of an infernal system they refuse to enter, a system of an existence solely devoted to the pursuit of professional and economic
performance) are the first indications of a healthy individual reaction to the excesses of a lifestyle entirely devoted to the necessi-
ties of productivity.

Refusing to accept the concept of the organization as a
new form of transcendence, identifying the pitfalls of enticing
fantasies, and becoming aware of the risks of a productivity race
partly based on the use of anxiety and stress as engines of economic performance are some of the prerequisites for the restoration of the creative powers of motor fantasies within the organization. They would allow the organization to become a true
actor of existential creation in the positive sense of the word,
that is, one that would allow for the full expression and accomplishment of the individual.

Part Three

Rediscovering
Responsibility and Courage
in Organizations

6

A Private Journey:
Uniting the Fragmentary Self
Through Contradiction

Kenwyn K. Smith

The format I have chosen for presenting my ideas in this chapter is a little unusual. The issues I wish to explore are relatively easy to relate to when presented in story form but become elusive when packaged in regular academic discourse. For this reason I am going to tell a story.

The narrator, Douglas, is an executive who lets us peek at a few entries in his personal journal from a time in his life when he is involved in inner wrestling normally kept private. The struggle is really between different parts of himself. However, Douglas comes to understand the contours of these contesting forces in the context of a relationship.

The relationship is atypical. It takes place down at the river, at a private spot where Douglas often stops for a few moments to meditate in the early morning after his five-mile run. Occasionally, a character called Gaelin visits this sanctuary at the same time. Over the years Gaelin has become Douglas's confidant.

Gaelin usually says little, but he listens in a very knowing way. Whenever Douglas is troubled, he finds solace in having this confidant. Douglas knows little about Gaelin, which is probably what makes him especially useful as a reflective device. He appears to have no agenda. Thus, as the echoes of the executive's inner struggles are returned to his own ears by Gaelin, Douglas can hear an underlying drumbeat to his experience, often discovering the music contained within the seemingly bland text of his daily life.

In Douglas's journal entries, we find numerous existential themes. Despite the fact that the journal consists of conversations that Douglas has been diligent enough to write down verbatim, a road map into the scholarly literature from whence the topics come is offered in note form at the end of the chapter. The reader is encouraged to turn to these notes only after reading the whole story. The narrator now begins the story.

Prologue

Whenever I feel lost, I stop down at the river after my early morning run and sit on the embankment. There I watch the ripples pulsate from the pebbles I toss and inspect the corrugated reflection of myself in the water. Often a path that I have never contemplated before suggests itself to me. The water always contains a message, no matter how confused I am, no matter how invested I am in solutions destined to fail.[1]

Often, while I am sitting there, an old man comes and joins me. He has been a wonderful presence in my life. I know very little about him. I suspect he is a street person. But he has a depth of insight I truly respect. He refuses to answer my questions about his life, dismissing my inquisitiveness as inappropriate. I have grown to honor his privacy and to be open to the lessons he offers me. In fact, he reminds me a lot of an imaginary friend I used to have in my childhood, an old man with a long beard whom I used to call Gaelin. I would talk to him whenever I was upset. He was my comforter. I think, in hindsight, that I have loved my times with this wise old man because they pull me into a childlike frame and open me to possibilities the adult in me normally rejects.[2] I told my riverside friend about my imaginary childhood figure. He responded, "Then I would be privileged if you would call me Gaelin."

Mostly Gaelin spends his time with me simply listening to my laments. Often he says nothing. Occasionally, he offers me a story with a relevant lesson when I need it the most. He has become such a wonderful presence in my life that I always look for him when I am at the river and feel a sense of longing when he is not there.

Three years ago I became CEO of my company. This has provided me with internal challenges that have been both torturous and exhilarating. Within months of my taking this job, the bottom fell out of the regional manufacturing base that was our bread and butter. We faced problems life had never prepared me for. We were forced to scale back 20 percent, which we did reasonably successfully. Now we have somewhat stabilized, and I believe we are a more robust and resilient company as a result of this crisis. I am optimistic enough to believe we will survive and maybe even thrive again some day.

In the midst of this crisis, Gaelin suggested that I start keeping a journal. He wisely implied that I was about to shift my way of thinking about the workplace totally and that I would appreciate the lessons ahead much more if I systematically recorded the changes I was facing. I took his advice. Now as I look back and read through my journal, I can see the central feature of the shift that occurred in me. I have moved from being an "either/or" thinker to one who sees things in "both/and" terms.[3] That has been a truly significant and liberating shift for me.

I will show you a little of what I recorded in my journal to illuminate the transition in my thinking and at the same time to pay tribute to a wise old man whose insights this forty-six-year-old now treasures deeply.

To set the scene, I should tell you that when I was younger I had the fantasy that someday I would be in *the* senior position and I would then feel independent, powerful, connected, confident, clear minded. The opposite has proved to be true. In this senior role, I constantly feel dependent, powerless, isolated, tentative, and confused. It has taken me a while to accept the latter feelings as the necessary complement of the former ones, to see that such contradictions come bound together, each defining the other.[4]

It has also been hard to appreciate that these feelings are not necessarily a good indicator of my external reality. I can feel very powerless even when I am holding enormous power in my hands. I can feel confused and shortsighted even when taking actions others experience as decisive and far reaching. I have at last learned to recognize these seemingly contradictory things for what they are and not to be thrown off by them.

Extracts from the Private Journal of a CEO

Living in the Midst of Paradox[5]

July 24, 1990

"Good, you are here today, Gaelin. I want to talk to you more about the troubling ways my organization has got itself caught in the grip of two opposing forces. On the one hand, it is consumed by an endless appetite to grow. As it expands, it devours enormous resources, often unintentionally destroying other smaller organizations in our environment. On the other hand, it seems trapped in a fear that it will be destroyed by forces it cannot control. We even fantasize that we will be gobbled up by some other giant, constantly saying, 'If *we* are not the acquirer, we'll become the acquiree.' Yet every time my organization operates on this eat-or-be-eaten maxim, it becomes less of what it strives to be. It fends off one threatening force only to make itself more vulnerable to another hidden within it."

"I have a story for you," said Gaelin. "Frederick was a man determined to defeat, once and for all, the twin burdens that plagued his existence, his all-consuming fear of death and his equally paralyzing fear of life. For years he kept himself so busy that he had no time to notice how afraid he was of dying. He became very influential and developed such immense powers that others feared him. The fear others had of his power taught him to fear it himself. So he halted his frenetic existence, thinking that if he were weaker there would be less to fear. Ultimately, he became so disengaged that he spent several years sitting around exerting minimal energy, hoping to conserve his strength so he would have a longer life. However, this gave him too much time to think about dying. Since he never did anything, he was actually getting weaker by the day. He feared he was wasting away and started to be as anxious about his existence as he was when he was powerful. He was trapped.[6]

"Frederick, seeking a way to dull the pain of his self-aware-ness, asked others for help. Everyone told him to go to the local cultural library and borrow from the shelves one of their many illusions designed for situations like his. The library had an excellent collection of illusions developed across hundreds of years to anesthetize people who felt as Frederick did. On his arrival, the librarian assured him that everyone needs such illusions because they offer us a shared way to cope with the anxieties that the reality of existence brings.

"Frederick borrowed illusion after illusion and tried each one. Initially, he faithfully believed what he took from the shelf, treating it as though it were *the* reality. But in time, each illu-sion failed him. He did body-building exercises, assuming that if he were very strong he would no longer feel weak. However, the stronger he got, the more he tried to lift, making him feel even weaker for he now understood the actual limits of his strength. He went to sensitivity school to learn how to em-pathize with others' feelings, and then he noticed how much sadness there was around him. He empathized so fully that he was always overwhelmingly sad. The list of his endeavors went on and on until, in exhaustion, he concluded that these cul-tural illusions were simply not effective for him. He still felt the immense anxiety associated with the twin burdens of the fear of death and the fear of life.

"Having learned to recognize the delusive nature of his cul-ture's illusions, Frederick resolved to live a life based only on the truth as he understood it. No longer would he accept as real what society deemed as true. Nor would he accept the illusions that the community offered him to deal with the disil-lusion he felt about society's hidden lies. He was already out of step with all the other people around him, and now there seemed to be only one option, to go it alone. However, this 'solution' created a new illusion that he never did come to recog-nize. He started to believe that human existence could be lived in isolation. Frederick did not see the illusion tucked away in this belief and therefore chose this path. The result was that henceforth he felt the daily pain not only of being unconnected to others but also of having no shared way to deal with any of the pain that his own existence invented. He ended up creating his own individual illusion that left him so totally out of align-ment with others around him that they thought he was crazy and came to call him neurotic.

"The dilemma for Frederick, the neurotic, was that his at-tempts to negate what the society was doing did not help him affirm his own life. Rather, they heightened his own negation, turning him into an even more extreme version of what he so desperately wished to avoid. Rather than merely partaking of established illusions on an occasional basis, he dedicated his life to creating new ones that occupied all his time. Feeling not free, Frederick willed himself free. However, this excessive willing actually willed his self unfree. It was like a rebellion gone wrong. What was designed to be against others got redirected against himself. He could never allow himself to see this truth, how-ever. He had to defend himself from ever recognizing it, thereby fueling further anxiety that in turn increased the demand for more illusions.

"Frederick found himself in the midst of one of humankind's most familiar and illusive paradoxes. *Overwhelmed by exces-sive awareness about both the creative possibilities of life and the seeming meaninglessness of life in the light of death, we all gain relief from cultural illusions. But the neurotic rejects these and creates his or her own illusion and becomes blind to the illusory nature of this escape from the truth about truth.*"

"Are you suggesting, Gaelin, by telling me Frederick's story, that our organization is caught in that same bind? *That every day our collective striving to preserve the organization's life merely hastens the very death we all want to avoid?*"

"Exactly," replied Gaelin. "At an organizational level, you seem to do many things to ward off the extinction you fear is inevitable and never allow yourselves to be what you are in that moment, namely, an organization consumed by the fear of extinction. You sound like you have come to believe that your own illusions are *the* truth. Have you not concluded that the bigger you are the more likely you are to survive? Now there is a myth. Even in the biological world, creatures the size of dinosaurs and elephants have no greater survival rate than that of the gnat and the cockroach. You seem determined to be something different from what you fear you might become in the future. Your organization constantly sacrifices the living available to it on each particular day so that it might be able to live more fully the next day. However, on the next day, it merely repeats the cycle. It is so focused on what it is becoming that it never allows itself to actually *be* what it is."

"If you are right, that is very disappointing to me," I told Gaelin. "I thought we were on a different path, especially after we went through all that agony adopting a developmental culture. Yet I am now beginning to see that we might have fallen into this same pattern in how we treat our senior executives."

"How is that?" asked Gaelin.

"Well, we spend enormous resources developing our people. We promote those whom we view as having potential, but as they reach the potential expected of them, they mostly get discarded. We have got so fixated on being a developmental culture that if some people are not still growing at the rate that they once did, we treat them as though they are in decline and not worthy of the same status once afforded them. A thirty-eight-year-old who might someday *become* what we want is treated as more important to us than the fifty-five-year-old who is no longer on a sharp growth curve but has already gone beyond what is ultimately projected for that younger person. We are so invested in developing the capabilities of our workforce that we underutilize the capabilities already developed."

"Yes, that is another good example of what I am talking about," said Gaelin.

"Actually, Gaelin, if I take all your comments seriously, our dilemma may be even larger than how you stated it. It is probably more accurate to say *we are so determined not to become what we fear is possible, that every day we fail to be anything of substance. And it is this failure to be anything of substance that we are so desperate to avoid. So we have already become in the present what we most fear we could become in the future. However, while we work so hard not to become that in the future, we fail to recognize we are already in that condition in the present."*

"You are right!" exclaimed Gaelin. "You are caught in the double negative helix."

"The what?"

"In algebra, when you multiply a negative by a negative, you get a positive. However, in the emotional world, when you strive to overcome a negative by trying to negate it, you create the black hole of negativism into which it is so easy to fall."[7]

"Oh, is that what we have done to ourselves? Is that what a double negative helix is?"

"I have no idea! I just made up a fancy-sounding term to get your attention. Isn't that what you corporate types do?"

Changing by Preserving the Status Quo

February 3, 1991
"For weeks, Gaelin, I have been hoping you would have something to say to me about the issue of change. My organization is in the midst of so much of it that we all feel overwhelmed. Some people are even digging in their heels and refusing to change any more."

"That's a good sign!" replied Gaelin with a mischievous smile.

"What do you mean? This resistance to change is so hard to deal with," I replied.

"That's because of the way you think about it."

"What?"

"When resistance occurs that's not the time to start feeling despair. Resistance is the beginning of the change, not the end of it. In fact, you will not have change without it."

"Oh, come on, Gaelin; you are not going to treat me to another one of your impossible riddles are you?"

"I guess you are like most people and think of change and stasis as being each other's opposite, right?"

"But, of course. Is there some other way to think of it?"

"Yes, but it is a hard lesson to learn," answered Gaelin. "You might find it useful to start by considering physical movement. Ever since Heisenberg and Einstein, we have been aware that our knowledge of movement is dependent on our relationship with what is staying still. As you sit here on this riverbank, you probably are not aware that you are traveling at a thousand miles an hour. But you are. Every day we all go one rotation of the earth. That's twenty-four thousand miles in twenty-four hours. And scientists tell us our galaxy is catapulting through space at more than one million miles an hour, being pulled by another galaxy with which we will collide in a few million years. However, since everything is moving, we have the sense that nothing is moving."

"OK," I said, "but what has that got to do with change?"

"This is hard to recognize, but change and stasis codefine each other. Each accompanies the other. Change without stasis is not change. Stasis without change is not stasis," replied Gaelin.

"So you are saying that to experience organizational change some things must remain stable?"

"Yes; *if everything is changing, then nothing is changing.* In recent years, most organizations have changed so often that nowadays *the greatest change in our organizations would occur if they were not to change.* Many have even become addicted to change. Most of us hardly even get ourselves settled from the last change before we bounce ourselves into the next."

"That's us," I said to Gaelin. "The other day I even commented to my staff that we have restructured ourselves so many times over the past decade that I think it would be very therapeutic to have a few months, even a few weeks, with no change, just the chance to enjoy a little stability."

"That reminds me of a story," said Gaelin. "PETROCom was an organization forever restructuring itself. Whenever the people there ran into a new problem, they always tried to fix it with the same old solution: restructure. The result? PETROCom was always structurally unstable. The PETROCom people had only one answer for every predicament. Thus, their repetitive attempts to create a meaningful infrastructure assured the opposite—a permanent instability that cried out for yet another new infrastructure—fueling a vicious cycle."

"Are you talking about PETROCom or us, Gaelin? That's exactly what we do."

"One thing I saw them do over and over was to tinker with their informal structures. Someone would comment that the formal communication system didn't work but that the informal system that had emerged to compensate for the inadequacies of the formal one ultimately enabled communication to occur. Whenever a structure freak heard this, the wheels would begin to grind: let's formalize the informal! In no time, they would go down that terrible path of making the informal into the formal, and it always turned into a disaster."

I looked startled, and Gaelin continued, "Very few people understand this. *The informal works precisely because it is the informal.* Were it not for the formal, the informal would not exist. The informal acts like a shadowy counterpart that compensates for the formal's inadequacies. It does not have a skeleton of its own, however. Its structure is like a scaffolding that is attached to the formal structure to give it stability. The scaffold itself is totally inadequate to hold anything like the weight the formal structures are designed to sustain. So it simply collapses the moment the burdens of the formal are placed on it. That is, the informal, when formalized, becomes as ineffective as the formal had been before it."

"Gaelin, we do that all the time."

"That is folly. If you respected the informal for what it is, you would never do that. Everything has both a formal and an informal facet. They are opposite sides of the same coin, not two different phenomena. They exist as each other's complement. Each requires the other to have a life of its own. The formal feeds off the informal and vice versa. If you formalize the informal you will always kill it off."

"Until this moment, Gaelin, I have looked at change as a linear process. Therefore, anyone who *resisted* change represented a force I had to overcome. For me, the biggest problem with change has always been *overcoming the resistance.* Those opposing the change have to be confronted with an equal or greater force."

"Yes, and I know the story as it unfolds," said Gaelin. "You then have to deal with the fact that your very fighting with the resistance warriors is what makes them strong: the more you fight them, the more formidable they become. Let me show you another way to look at this.

"When resistance emerges, the conditions within which

change can occur begin to get created.[8] Change requires the augmented presence of the unchanging for it actually to be *change*. Those who resist change efforts are making an essential contribution to the change process. Without the vigor of their resistance, without their deep dedication to preserving the status quo, our change efforts would actually come to naught. Resistance can be made the sign that the status quo forces have been mobilized and the foundation is being laid for the anticipated change to occur. Ultimately, change is an expression of the relationship between the changing and the stable. It may be experienced as change, but that is only the visible part of the process. The process is rooted in the interactions between change and stasis."

"What would you have me do then, Gaelin?"

"In a way, it's simple. Start with the question, What am I attempting to preserve by this change? Look at change as a relational phenomenon. If you begin that way, many of those who feel they are for the status quo will see that you are too, that you are invested not only in the change part of this process but also in the stasis."

Growth Requires Constant Cutting Back

December 15, 1991
I have been trying to deal with some unexpected changes that are occurring in our industry. It looks like we are facing another downsizing of 5 percent. This promises to be devastating given the massive cutbacks we have already made. I have been looking for a way out and hoping to hear Gaelin's thoughts during one of my visits to the river. He has not been saying much of late.

"I was thinking of the term *getting fired*. What a violent image, like going before an execution squad. On other occasions when we had to make cutbacks, I did what others had recommended; I hired a consultant who goes by the title "downsizing specialist" to do my dirty work. We executive leaders would huddle behind closed doors, determine the number of people who had to go, designate the individuals to be dismissed, and then get this henchman to do our execution work for us. He would make a deep and speedy surgical cut first thing Monday morning. By lunchtime it was all over. Security guards would seal the files, hand out cardboard cartons, instruct the people to pack their personal effects, and escort each one to the parking lot.

"It is cold, brutal, unfeeling. No one ever had a chance to say goodbye, let alone express shock or start the grieving process. And we would all go on about life as though nothing had happened. It has become a sign of our times; we decision makers avoid all emotional contact with those we are wounding, I suppose, to protect ourselves from the pain we inflict."

"That is all true, but you also rob yourself of the chance to recognize the constructive possibilities that accompany a person's moving on," said Gaelin, finding his voice again after many months of silence.

"Nice to hear from you, Gaelin," I said. "Why have you been so silent while I have been going through all this agony?"

"I was waiting until you were ready to listen."

"Well, I am listening now. Tell me what you think. I have been considering making the dismissals myself this time around, face-to-face. By having to look into people's eyes while inflicting this pain, I might learn how to remain a little more emotionally connected to what we are doing as an organization."

"Yes, I can see that you are again ready to listen to what I have to say," responded Gaelin. "People in positions like yours act as if cutting back is always bad. You are so busy trying not to see its destructive face that you fail to ever recognize its rejuvenating side. Losing one's job is horrible but so are many of the jobs people try so hard not to lose. Many an organization benefits greatly by its downsizing. And so do those who are downsized. If the surgical incision is clean, the wounds can heal and prompt rejuvenation will occur."

"Are you saying, Gaelin, that it is all right to cut back?"

"No, I am saying it is *essential* to cut back on a regular basis. Organizations create so many problems for themselves by refusing to prune adequately during the good times. We act as though we believe that bigger is better. We seek ever-increasing incomes and accumulate so much stuff that our lives become cluttered with possessions, making us feel excessively encumbered. We grow and grow our organizations until we wake up one day and discover that they are really fat. Getting the growth under control takes enormous effort. And it often requires truly hard times to turn things around. Then in the bad times, we do this devastating pruning and adopt slogans like getting lean and mean. We have put our organizational life very out of balance. We cut when we should be growing because we grow when we should be cutting.

"Have you not tried to grow a garden?" continued Gaelin. "You know that you must prune on a regular basis. It is a basic principle of nature. To grow, cut back! However, we rarely reduce our organizations in the good times. And we start to cut back right at the point when it makes most sense to increase."

"I hear you, but I don't think I understand you yet, Gaelin. Are you telling me I should be constantly firing people? If so, that feels particularly brutal, especially given the economy!"

"Well, I think cutting needs to occur at an earlier point in the process. I am not focused so much on cutting people, though that is clearly necessary on some occasions. I am actually talking about cutting our jobs. Let me ask you: When did you last prune your job? When did you last consciously and deliberately stop doing things that you and everyone else know are absolutely pointless? What I am talking about is cutting the processes that generate the need for an excess number of people in the first place."

Gaelin had me going now. "You mean I should stop doing a lot of what I do each day?"

"Exactly. I think it is time for us to put as much energy into pruning our jobs as we do into growing them. What I see is that you people grow and grow your jobs and clutter them with activities that are thoroughly pointless. You get yourselves totally overwhelmed by all you have to do. And then you hire someone to pick up what you can't handle, and that person repeats the pattern.

"You start coming to work earlier and staying later. You

are already at the point where none of you can do your jobs between 9:00 and 5:00 anymore. During these hours, you are doing all those pointless things. How many times do you say, 'I can only get things done between 7:00 and 9:00 in the morning or after everyone has left in the evening; it is impossible to do my job during the day—there are just too many distractions'?

"It has got to the point where no one can find you between 9:00 and 5:00, and so they now call your office at 7:30 because that's when they know they can catch you. So you now have to come in at 6:00. Next year it will be 5:00 in the morning because this pattern is spiraling out of control! When will you reach your breaking point and stop this insanity?"

Gaelin had a lot of emotion on this one. He was on a roll. "Let me tell you the story of Marcy, who worked for a company in South Carolina that was under remarkable stress. Everyone was coming in earlier and staying later but getting less and less done during the day. The CEO was furious about this. He tried to get the employees to stop this pattern, for it was out of control. Their families were paying a very high price. Every day Marcy would go home totally drained. Like her fellow workers, she counted on her family to replenish her and then she would return to the office only to have her job suck her dry again. The work stress was unbelievable, and what was worse, it was all of their own making. It was contributing nothing to productivity.

"The CEO made speech after speech about wanting to turn this around. He implored the workers to go home at a reasonable hour. He hired consultant after consultant to figure out how to break this pattern. He became a champion of the workers' family lives. All for nothing. Then one day he took a bold initiative. He put one electric light switch in his office that controlled power in all the buildings. At 5:15 every afternoon, he simply turned off all the lights. There was nothing anyone could do. The place was in darkness. None of the machines would work. So the employees all went home. The electricity was turned on again at 8:45 the next morning.

"The net result was that the workers all became civilized.

Marcy reported that they all started doing their jobs in the day-time and spent the evenings with their families. They simply had to work out ways to get their jobs done in the allocated hours. It was amazing how efficiently they began to use their time. Meetings took less than half the former time. And the employees got back hours that they had previously spent complaining about how overwhelming their jobs were.

"The next quarter this company turned in a healthy profit, and it increased consistently over the next several quarters. By doing less, the workers achieved more. So my advice to you, if you are interested in what old Gaelin thinks, is to find the courage to cut back constantly. That way you will benefit from the natural growth as opposed to cluttering up your organization and having to attack with a machete when the underbrush has grown out of hand."[9]

Becoming What I Am by Affirming What I Am Not

May 11, 1992
"So many of the things you say, Gaelin, seem so obvious when you say them, but they would never have occurred to me. I know deep down I have difficulty accepting that each creative act brings with it the destruction of something old.[10] I have wanted to be a leader who did not inflict injury. Now you are suggesting that to be creative I must be willing to accept that I am also being destructive. That runs counter to my self-image.

"However, I have just begun to see how my blindness to this reality creates some destructive forces in my senior management group. We are always searching for new ideas as a standard part of our executive group life. Yet when innovation emerges, I tend to laud the individuals who come up with the ideas, acting as though the novelty actually resides in them rather than their being the mere expressers of the group's creativity.[11] In the process, I imply that the others are not as valuable. That is wrong.

"Looking back, I can also see another destructive motif. Any innovation upsets our equilibrium as a group, and one or more of our members ultimately expresses this. I have been equally prone to locate that destructiveness in the members who give voice to it. However, they likewise can be seen to be expressing this counter perspective on behalf of the whole group. The disruptiveness they communicate is not really an attribute of them at all. What I am just learning to see is that any group's creativity automatically contains destructiveness within it. Whenever I deny this or window-dress it to make it appear as something other than what it is, somebody gets hurt. I have never seen the link between this destructiveness and my behavior before."

"It would be easy for you to blame yourself," said Gaelin, "and that would be silly. It would be more useful if you were to recognize that leadership takes courage and that this courage can only be found in the midst of one's own self-doubt. The kind of self-doubt in which you are engaging at the moment is the very stuff that gives birth to real courage."

"What on earth are you talking about, Gaelin?"

"I am sure there are times when you have been very effective as a leader and have felt the enormity of your impact. However, I am equally sure there are times when you are very influential but have no awareness of this. The latter occasions are the ones that interest me more."

"Why is that?"

"At times, you must feel totally uncertain and be filled with self-doubt, especially when the path to take is ambiguous. On these occasions, you somehow find it in you to take action that makes a difference. That requires enormous courage."

"You have completely lost me."

"Many people think courage is predicated on certainty, on a conviction that what one is doing is correct. It is the opposite. One is only really being courageous when one is floundering with all the uncertainties of not knowing what to do and yet acts anyway, believing that it may work out but that it could fail. It is a lot like faith. One cannot believe unless one has doubts. Faith is not built on certitude but on a foundation of simply not knowing.[12]

"It is often when we feel despair that courage surfaces most strongly. Many people think courage is the opposite of despair. It is not. Courage is the capacity to move ahead in spite of despair."

"It sounds like there is truth in what you say, Gaelin, but this is hard for me to grasp and difficult to apply to myself."

"I would like to tell you another story.[13] Andrew decided he wanted to be a hero. He had this desire because he knew he wasn't a hero. So Andrew thought he had better start by learning. He went looking for a school that would teach him this ancient art form. There was only one school available, and he failed its tests. He was proving himself emotionally closed to learning the school's first principle, that one cannot *plan* to be heroic. It taught that heroism is not an attribute of the self that one can actively know in advance. Rather, it is an expression of the self to which one is blind. Although Andrew failed his course, he learned enough to conclude that no such school should exist, for if the school honestly applied its lessons to itself, it would have to abolish itself. He concluded he could never be a hero.

"Andrew became consumed by the self-doubts that he had initially tried to deny by seeking to be a person without such doubts in the first place. He sought to affirm his own worth by presenting himself as someone who knew what he was about. That was false. When that failed, he resorted to thinking of himself as having no worth. That posture was equally false. In time, Andrew came to see that his striving to be heroic in the eyes of others was an attempt to overcome an unacknowledged deficiency in himself.

"Andrew wanted to become master of his fears for he was worried that ultimately his fears would master him. After striving for a long time to overcome them, he resolved to accept that these fears, irrespective of whether they were based on reality, were real enough to him. He would embrace them for what they were and not continue to strive to overcome them. He saw these fears as his negative side and came to realize that his striving to negate them was consuming him in what he called the clouds of negativism. Instead, he began to celebrate the existence of his fears, trusting that he had them for good reason and that he should embrace them, not obliterate them. That is when life began to change for Andrew. His fears never went away, but his relationship to them did. In no time, he used his self-doubt as the basis for the actions he took."

"Gaelin, why did you tell me that story? What were you driving at that has relevance to me?"

"Well, I see you constantly going toward those things that one naturally wants to avoid. You take risks that are counterintuitive. You do things that you cannot possibly know in advance are right. And even afterward, when others praise or condemn you for what you did, you stand up and take the heat for what went wrong and give credit to others for what went right. You are also willing to wait and see the longer-term implications of your decisions before claiming success or failure. And you do not try to window-dress your actions or to make them appear right if they are not. That takes courage."

"It's funny but I don't see it that way. What I see myself as trying to do is to give form to the formless[14] because so much of organizational life seems to be emptiness, a void waiting to be contoured. The problem is that I must never forget that once we have organized the emptiness the void has not been removed. We have simply packaged it in forms that make us see it as no longer empty. But emptiness it still is. Were the structures of our organization to collapse, we would just have nothingness again. When we are in the midst of our organizational activity, we can feel that we are doing something meaningful, but the meaning is very ephemeral and it can vanish like a puff, for it is predicated on nothingness. So in a strange way, the structures we produce to manage the emptiness merely keep the emptiness contained. They do not take it away. In fact, they fold the emptiness into itself, guaranteeing that each system will harbor within it the seeds of its own destruction.

"When I am struggling to give form to that which yet has no shape, I am filled with anxiety lest my molding actions create the very problems we feel compelled to avoid, problems that would not exist were it not for what I am doing. Sometimes that anxiety is almost paralyzing, but I feel I must act even in the light of it."

"And that is what takes courage," said Gaelin. "You could ignore your anxiety or displace it onto others. Or you could act with premature confidence about your decisions. Or you could let yourself do nothing in the light of your anxiety. You don't do any of those things. Instead you continue to feel the uncertainty and act in the face of it. That, by any definition, is courageous."

"But I never feel courageous," I retorted.

"And that's the base upon which such courage stands. It is your very affirmation of what you are not, in this case feeling not courageous, that actually makes you into what you are, namely, courageous."

Beyond the Binary Mind

August 3, 1992

"You know, Gaelin, I think I am now at the point of being willing to accept what you have been teaching over the last two years."

"What is that?"

"I have always been striving to be one thing *or* the other. Believing that one can be excellent or mediocre, I would strive to be the best; believing that one can be good or bad, I would strive to be noble; believing that one can be positive or negative, I would strive to be affirmative; believing that one can be full or empty, I would strive to be abundant; and so forth.

"Now I recognize that this 'either/or' world has been diminishing me as a person and all of those around me. What has changed for me is that I am seeing my experience in "both/and" terms. I am neither excellent nor mediocre; I am both excellent and mediocre. I am neither good nor bad; I am both good and bad. I am neither positive nor negative; I am both positive and negative. I am neither full nor empty; I am both full and empty. Learning to embrace these things I made into such polar opposites has brought a kind of wholeness to me that I have always craved but never thought was possible."

Gaelin nodded his assent. Then he said something that startled me, perhaps because I had simply never thought of it before. It was, after all, a very Gaelin thing to say: "You learned something for both of us. Thanks for learning this. While I know you did it for yourself, it was for all of us at the same time."

"What are you talking about, Gaelin?"

"As I see it, your knowledge and my knowledge are the same thing. What you learn I learn, and what I learn you learn. Your knowledge increases me and my knowledge increases you. How did John Donne say it? 'Any man's death diminishes me.' I would add, Every person's life augments me. As you get to be more whole so do I. Your growth was for both of us and for many others, too."

Beyond the Fragmentary Self

For a long time now, management thought has been captured by the rationalistic. Every conceivable logical solution has been applied to the complex situations that envelop us. However, we all continue to feel that something is missing. We sense that we contain within us some deeper insights that we have been unable to access. Through this story I have been pointing to the binds that get created by how we think about what perplexes us. We have become so fixated on understanding with our rational/digital brains, the world of the either/or, that we have overlooked the wisdom contained in our other, analogic brains, the world of the both/and.

How we think can fragment our experience of the world, leaving us the onerous task of having to integrate what we have artificially divided. Yet we all have in us the necessary equipment to think in more holistic ways from the outset. Here, in our right brains, the challenge is not so much integration as expanding our minds sufficiently so as to encompass patterns that stretch beyond the limits of our everyday vision.

The journey from the fragmented to the holistic may be taken in many ways, and the terrain that must be traversed can differ from one person to the next. However, one central obstacle for all who have been fully indoctrinated by the logic of rationalism is learning to see the both/and contained in every either/or. In this chapter, we have witnessed one person's voyage and some of the stumbling blocks he encountered along the way.

Notes

1. There is something very special about water. It is eternal and immediate. Even though it is essential for survival, we

take it for granted except when it is scarce. Water has often been used by existential writers as a motif for capturing truths that are both immediately relevant and transcendent. Hesse's *Siddhartha* is the most eloquent of this that I know.

2. Carl Jung, in his autobiographical book *Memories, Dreams, and Reflections* (1961, pp. 19–23), provides wonderful evidence of how many insights we glean in later life were actually known to us in childhood but not understood because we did not have the context by which to encode the character of our knowing. He makes a powerful argument that to access these insights during adult life, we need to take a childlike posture. The most profound is the truly simple.

3. This is the heart of the distinction between left- and right-brain thinking, commonly referred to as the digital versus the analogical. The digital is equipped to operate in either/or terms and is the seat of classic reasoning we know as causal. The analogical represents everything in both/and terms and undergirds the artistic and the creative. For a full description, see Wilden, 1972, pp. 155–170, and Smith, 1982, pp. 339–343.

4. Smith and Berg (1987, pp. 58–66, 78–82) elaborate on how concepts codefine each other. That which presents itself as contradictory is often the articulation of the opposite, which must be coexpressed for a sense of the whole to become clear.

5. For a formal definition of paradox, see Smith and Berg, 1987, pp. 11–18.

6. The ideas expressed in this section are based on the conception of neurosis elaborated by Rank (1945, pp. 46–59; [1941] 1958, pp. 176–189) and Becker (1973, pp. 176–189). The central argument is that we are all engaged in a struggle between our two selves, our creatureliness and our consciousness. This stirs great anxiety, which society tries to ameliorate by offering us illusions. These are temporary and fragile. Those who see through these illusions become overwhelmed by the anxiety of existence and seek their own path, crafting their own individual illusion while never recognizing that it is as problematic as the ones being spurned.

7. See Wilden, 1972, pp. 152-154, and Smith and Berg, 1987, pp. 50-54, for a discussion of negation as a psychological versus a mathematical phenomenon.

8. This is also the heart of the change process as Rank formulated it for the psychoanalytic community. See Rank, 1945, pp. 14-15, 19, and Leiberman, 1985, pp. 356-360.

9. Mitroff (1987, pp. 136-147) offers a discourse on the paradox of "more leading to less and less leading to more."

10. May (1975, pp. 61-64) points out how all creativity is predicated in part on destruction. Anything that will be new exists as a threat to that which has been. Sarason (1972, pp. 27-37) makes a similar argument: all new organizations are automatically embroiled in conflict, for their very existence highlights the inadequacies of the established order.

11. See Wells, 1980, pp. 180-185, and Smith and Berg, 1987, pp. 68-72, 145-146, for a discussion of how individuals can get filled up with attributes of the group.

12. This argument about courage is spelled out most eloquently by Tillich (1952, pp. 25-27).

13. This story is based on the existential principles espoused so powerfully by Tillich (1948, 1952, 1966) and May (1973, 1975, 1983).

14. May (1975, pp. 133-148) speaks to the importance of setting limits, of putting boundaries around the unlimited in order for both action and creativity to occur. In many ways, it is the organization of the unformed that makes both action and meaning possible. This does not take the emptiness away. It simply locates it within the structures where we live our lives. Thus all organization contains emptiness within it.

7

Carl Rogers Meets Otto Rank: The Discovery of Relationship

Robert Kramer

"All management is people management, and all leadership is people leadership. It's all people," says Peter Vaill, author of *Managing as a Performing Art* (1989, p. 126). The evidence is overwhelming that the way managers *think* about the nature of human beings affects the way they *relate* to people in organizations. Therefore, ideas about people matter for managerial practice — and great ideas matter greatly. Consider, for example, the fruitful thought of Carl Rogers, a pioneer in the applied behavioral sciences who did as much as anyone else to influence the current generation of thinking about people in organizations. Even though managers may not recognize Rogers by name, his spiritual presence hovers over the entire field of organizational behavior and development (OBD). Almost every introductory textbook in OBD heralds active listening or some variant of Rogers's nondirective, or client-centered, approach, as a prerequisite for employee empowerment, team building, or humanistic management.

According to Richard Farson, former president of the Esalen Institute (quoted in Evans, 1975, p. xl), "His [Rogers'] ideas are the main ones used to support efforts toward democratic or participative management in industry. There has probably not been a single organizational development or management training program in twenty-five years which has not built on his

theoretical foundations." Unfortunately, however, management
professors and consultants have often reduced the revolutionary thought of Rogers to simplistic slogans, trivializing it in the
process.

Contributing to the lack of understanding about Rogers
is the incredible fact that almost no one in OBD knows, or
has been curious enough to discover, *how* Carl Rogers came
to formulate his fundamental hypothesis. In what soil was the
seed planted? When did the breakthrough come? Who was his
inspiration?

This chapter tells the forgotten story of one of the semi-
nal ideas in management. It tells of a deep sharing in 1936 between a young American therapist and a famous Viennese psychologist, excommunicated a decade earlier from Freud's inner
circle for heresy. It tells of a relationship between Carl Rogers
and Otto Rank — an empathic attunement between two kindred
souls — that gave birth to a powerful idea that, if fully integrated
into a manager's way of being, would change forever how he
or she relates to people in organizations. It is an idea, at bottom, about the meaning of relationship itself, an idea about the
astonishing possibility for transformation contained within —
what Rogers (1961a, p. 33; emphasis added) came to call — "*a
certain type of relationship.*"

Rogers and Management

Without question, Carl Rogers is one of the most important
American psychologists of the twentieth century. His life's work
spanned seven decades. A prolific writer, Rogers published six-
teen books and over two hundred articles and scientific studies
from the late twenties, when he began as a therapist, until his
death in 1987. In 1972, Rogers became the only person ever
to receive the two highest awards of the American Psychological Association, one for "distinguished scientific contribution"
and the other for "distinguished professional contribution." A
1982 survey of practitioners published in the *American Psychologist* ranked Rogers first among the "ten most influential psy-
chotherapists" in the history of psychotherapy, ahead of Freud

and B. F. Skinner. In another 1982 article, a study in the *Journal of Counseling Psychology* concluded that Rogers was preeminent among a group of major clinicians who "have stood the test of time and are still influencing the field." Deeply personal, his moving and lucid writings have been translated into over *sixty* foreign languages (quoted in Kirschenbaum and Henderson, 1989a, pp. xii and xiii).

The influence of Rogers has not been limited to the field of clinical psychology, however. His thinking has helped transform virtually all the "helping professions": social work, pastoral counseling, education, hospital administration, industrial and labor relations, leadership training, and organizational development. Ever widening the scope of his thought, Rogers successively described his core interest as "nondirective" counseling, "client-centered" therapy, and finally, in the broadest sense, an an existentially grounded "person-centered" psychology.

His impact on the field of management and organizational development is as momentous as that of Abraham Maslow, with whom Rogers founded the "third force" of humanistic psychology, after the "first force" of psychoanalysis and the "second force" of behaviorism. Neither psychoanalysis nor behaviorism, because of their ideological commitment to strict determinism, acknowledged a primary status for consciousness or the creative will of the knowing human subject, the individual. Nor did they fully appreciate the meaning of human relations or the vital need of individuals for community and union, that is, for giving and receiving love. Like Maslow, Rogers eventually went one step beyond humanism to embrace the existential point of view of such thinkers as Rollo May and Gordon Allport. "I would like, if I may, to place myself in this group," Rogers (1961b, p. 87) told the symposium on existential psychology at the 1959 convention of the American Psychological Association.

Through his association with Fritz Roethlisberger, Rogers was also indirectly linked to the Hawthorne research that inaugurated the study of consciousness and human relations — that is, *freedom and community* — in organizations. "When I discovered Carl Rogers and his nondirective approach after I had developed independently a similar approach in the Hawthorne researches," writes Roethlisberger (1977, p. 313), "I thought he had stated the two-person therapeutic or helping encounter much better than I had. . . . There is little question that during [the forties and fifties] human relations almost became identified with the counseling approach." Rogers and Roethlisberger coauthored the classic article "Barriers and Gateways to Communication," published in the August 1952 issue of *Harvard Business Review* and reprinted many times since. Two textbooks on improving organizational communication, based on Rogers' thinking about human relations, were written by faculty of the Harvard Business School (Turner and Lombard, 1969; Athos and Gabarro, 1978) and adopted as required reading for many MBA students.

Rogers was also a prominent member of the "president's labs" (French and Bell, 1990, p. 41) in the early years of the National Training Laboratories, working closely with many company presidents and CEOs to enhance the quality of work life. He spent much of the seventies and eighties facilitating trust and openness in a wide variety of collective settings, from small encounter groups to large intercultural and even international organizations.

One of Rogers's greatest learnings about human relations was that *to listen truly* to another person, not as a technique of "impression management" but as an empathic way of being, is to promote the possibility of spiritual birth and fuller self-realization — a kind of healing of the human soul. With this subtle idea, Rogers was approaching a transpersonal realm beyond humanism, even though he was reluctant to make his spiritual feelings an explicit part of his psychology for fear of having them confused with the religious dogmatism that he had rejected in his youth (Thorne, 1992).

"It is no exaggeration to say," writes Peter Vaill (1985, p. 565) of *active listening*, "that there is no single ability that is any more important for a professional to possess." In the organizational context, to listen actively is to shift from a management-centered to a person-centered philosophy of work life, valuing individual human dignity as much as productivity and profits. "Productive workplaces are those where people learn and grow as they cooperate to improve an organization's performance," says Marvin Weisbord, whose future search conferences bring "whole systems" of people together in the same room to listen actively to each other. "The 'bottom line,' in this way of looking at things, is dignity, meaning and community in work" (Weisbord, 1987, p. xiv). Instead of "experts" solving problems *for* people, everybody searches together to improve an entire system of people and technology, a holistic "sociotechnical system." From even a Taylorite perspective, the costs to productivity of poor listening are astonishingly high. According to Ray and Myers (quoted in Russell and Evans, 1992, p. 143; emphasis added), "For the lack of listening, *billions of dollars* of losses accumulate: retyped letters, rescheduled appointments, rerouted shipments, breakdowns in labor management relations, misunderstood sales presentations, and job interviews that never really get off the ground."

However, in Rogers's view, to listen actively is not a Taylorite technique to improve productivity, even though such improvement may occur as a consequence. In the deepest sense, to listen actively is to move from directive management to nondirective management, from exercising supervisory power *over* employees to releasing the force of creative power *within* employees, from a high degree of domination to a high degree of mutuality. It is to prize the imaginative inner life, the subjective frame of reference, the profoundly felt experiences and perceptions of all people regardless of their rank in the hierarchy. Spiritually speaking, it is to have faith in the human being's capacity for looking within to discover creative solutions to organizational problems, for following one's own direction, for being one's own authority. The heart of Carl Rogers's contribution to the helping professions is that to listen truly to another is to facilitate the psychological growth of a person in the never-completed process of becoming a fully-functioning human being, of accepting and being oneself, the creator or author of one's own life, both inside and outside the organization.

Rogers always worried that his great idea might be misconstrued. That his fear was justified is, unfortunately, evident from a close reading of the April 1993 issue of *Supervisory Sense,* a pamphlet published by the American Management Association

(AMA). Entitled "The Pitfalls of Poor Listening" and full of examples of the harmful effects of poor listening on productivity, this issue sincerely advises managers to practice active listening with employees. Not mastering this "listening competency" (p. 14), warns the AMA, may "ruin your prestige as a capable manager," and even worse, "senior management may see this as incompetence on your part and your employees will be dissatisfied since you are not taking control" (p. 11) of communication in the workplace. "The manager who is a good listener will impress workers," the AMA predicts, "by demonstrating his or her interest in their needs and concerns and desire to hear what they have to say" (pp. 20–21). One can almost hear Rogers asking ruefully: Is the purpose of active listening to retain managerial prestige? To take control? To impress workers with your openness? No wonder that Rogers "hoped the name Rogerian would go down the drain" (Rowan, 1988, p. 71).

The Great Hypothesis of Rogers

What, exactly, was Rogers trying to say? "I can state the overall hypothesis in one sentence," he writes. "If I can provide a *certain type of relationship,* the other person will discover *within* himself the capacity to use that relationship for growth, and *change* and *personal development* will occur" (1961a, p. 33; emphasis added). This hypothesis, as he always called it, was refined and tested by Rogers in almost every conceivable form of human relationship — in the consulting room, at home, at school, at work, and everywhere else in daily living. For a person's creative potential to be released, Rogers found, it is not the helper's authority, knowledge, technique, or interpretations that matter. It is the relationship itself that cures. Paradoxically, it is relationship that allows individuality to emerge, that spawns the self-acceptance necessary for discovering — or better, recovering or uncovering — one's creative potential. Only by willing to be oneself within relationship, by accepting one's own difference and having it accepted by another, can one discover the creativity and strength to change.

While modest about his therapeutic prowess, Rogers outraged psychiatrists and psychoanalysts by asserting that the professional qualifications and training of the helper have no direct connection to the healing process. What matters is communicating that the client is accepted and affirmed, without judgment or evaluation, in becoming and being a person, entirely different from all other people, including the therapist. Cognitive understanding of the client's past (insight) or diagnosis of the client's problem is not transforming by itself. What matters, Rogers never tired of repeating, is the quality of the relationship, a deep sharing between helper and client that offers the possibility of spiritual rebirth. "I rejoice," states Rogers in the preface to *Client-Centered Therapy* (quoted in Kirschenbaum and Henderson, 1989a, p. 170), "at the privilege of being a midwife to a new personality — as I stand by with awe at the emergence of a self, a person, as I see a birth process in which I have had an important and facilitating part."

Otto Rank and the Birth of Client-Centered Therapy

Carl Rogers spent a lifetime testing his hypothesis about the healing effect of experiencing separation and union in one and the same relationship. But how did he develop this momentous idea? What are its roots? As Rogers always acknowledged, the thought of Otto Rank influenced him more than any other at the beginning of his career, when he was still doing therapy in the old-fashioned directive way. Rollo May (1960, p. 42) and Irvin Yalom (1980a, p. 293), the two leading modern existential psychologists, both credit Otto Rank, once Freud's closest disciple, as the most important precursor of existential psychotherapy.

In the twenties and thirties, the field of American psychotherapy was dominated by individuals who stressed the use of "techniques" to maintain control of the interview and direct patients toward therapist-chosen objectives, such as the adoption of socially approved goals. Following the medical model, the emphasis was on diagnosing and fixing a "problem" of the patient, who had an illness that needed to be "treated," and thus the name patient. Few therapists were concerned with the patient's subjective experience, which was considered irrelevant for medical treatment. And almost no one paid attention to the here-and-now interpersonal relationship inside the consulting room.

From 1928 through 1939, Rogers served as a therapist at the Society for Prevention of Cruelty to Children, in Rochester, New York. This was his first professional position after studying psychology at Columbia University, where he had been drawn to adopt "a rigorous scientific approach allied to a coldly objective statistical methodology" (Thorne, 1992, p. 7). Not entirely satisfied with being trained just in research, Rogers was also exposed during his Columbia years to clinicians practicing Freudian psychoanalysis. "If Rogers favored any one deep, therapeutic approach when he came to Rochester, it was '*interpretive therapy*,' the major goal of which is to help the child or parent achieve insight into his own behavior and motives, past and present" (Kirschenbaum, 1979, p. 86; emphasis added).

On his staff at the Rochester clinic were a number of social workers trained at the University of Pennsylvania's School of Social Work, in Philadelphia, where Otto Rank had been lecturing since 1926, after being banished from Freud's inner circle for publishing *The Trauma of Birth* (1924). In this book, Rank overturned the fundamental tenets of the psychoanalytic movement by proposing that the child's pre-Oedipal relationship to its mother was the prototype of the therapeutic relationship between analyst and patient. He delivered the manuscript of *The Trauma of Birth* to his patron as a birthday present in May 1923, with a personal dedication. At first half-receptive to Rank's new idea, Freud accepted the dedication with an ambiguous quote from Horace: *Non omnis moriar* ("I shall not completely die") (Lieberman, 1985, p. 202). Soon thereafter, however, he turned strongly against the book. *The Trauma of Birth* gave Freud a "shock of alarm," according to Ernest Jones (1957, p. 59), "lest the whole of his life's work on the etiology of the neurosis be dissolved." By elevating the role of mother over that of father, Rank was undermining the *causal* significance of the Oedipus complex.

In June 1936, intrigued by social workers who were telling him that relationship therapy, not interpretive therapy, was the emphasis of the Philadelphia school, Rogers invited Rank to Rochester to conduct a three-day seminar on his new, post-Freudian practice of therapy (Evans, 1975, p. 28). No longer calling himself a psychoanalyst, Rank was by 1936 a "world-renowned psychologist whose major works could be read in English, French and German" (Lieberman, 1985, p. 355). In 1935, Rank had spoken at Harvard at the invitation of Henry Murray, then the preeminent American student of "personology."

What did Rogers learn during this brief June 1936 seminar? No one can be certain, but one month after visiting Rochester, Rank published two books: *Will Therapy: An Analysis of the Therapeutic Process in Terms of Relationship* ([1936] 1978a) and *Truth and Reality: A Life History of the Human Will* ([1936] 1978b). Originally delivered as a series of lectures at the Philadelphia School, these writings criticized Freud (who was then still living) for reducing the creative impulse to a mere vicissitude of the sex drive, for failing to recognize what Rank was calling the creative will. Human consciousness, he insisted, cannot be fully comprehended or explained by the "causality" of the natural or social sciences. Not a derivative of biology, consciousness "is only to be understood phenomenologically," Rank told his Philadelphia students. "One might say that in the psychical sphere there are no facts, but only interpretations of facts" (Rank, in press). It is "only in the individual act of will," said Rank, that "we have the unique phenomenon of spontaneity, the establishing of a new primary cause" ([1936] 1978a, p. 44). And with the emergence of consciousness — especially self-consciousness, that is, the full awareness of self — the human being begins "a new series of causes."

In speaking of *The Trauma of Birth*, Rank ([1936] 1978b, p. 2) says he had referred to "the creation of the individual himself, not merely physically, but also [spiritually] in the sense of the 'rebirth experience,' which I understand . . . as the actual creative act of the human being." A creature born out of a biological mother, out of matter, "the human being becomes at once creator and creature or actually moves from creature to creator, in the ideal case, creator of himself, his own personality." According to Rank (pp. 11–12), the development of conscious-

206 In Search of Meaning

ness and "the never completed birth of individuality [seem] somehow to correspond to a continued result of births, rebirths and new birth, which reach from the birth of the child from the mother, beyond the birth of the individual from the mass, to the birth of creative work from the individual and finally to the birth of knowledge from the work." The essence of life and consciousness is ceaseless change. Freud's rigidly deterministic theory, which reduced all experience to a disguised permutation of sexuality, corresponded "to a longing after a firm hold, after something constant, at rest, in the flight of psychic events" (p. 10). As a result, says Rank ([1936] 1978a, pp. 113), "the real I, or self with its own power, the will, is left out." The aim of his new post-Freudian therapy, he says, is "self-development." Simply put, this means that "the person is to develop himself into that which he is" (p. 20).

Neurosis is not a failure in sexuality but a failure in creativity, a refusal to affirm oneself as an individual, to accept the strange and unfathomable existence forced on us at birth by fate. "It is self-willed, a sort of creation that can find expression only in this negative, destructive way" (Rank, in press). Although a "creative achievement," the neurosis is an expression of negative will, the product of a person who denies himself or herself because of excessive guilt for separation and individuation, because of excessive anxiety over the sheer consciousness of living, that is, sheer difference itself.

A biologist of the mind, Freud always insisted that the sexual difference between male and female was "biological bedrock." While not disputing the force of biology or the sex difference, Rank peered below biological bedrock to confront the ontological, or better the *pre*-ontological, mystery of being itself: that is, the ineffable difference between nonexistence and existence. Neither biology nor psychoanalysis has one word to say about the beginning of life or the end of life, about what it means to be conscious during this brief interval, an infinitesimal moment of light between two eternities of darkness.

"The mere fact of difference, in other words, the *existence* of our own will as opposite, unlike, is the basis for the [self-] condemnation which manifests itself as inferiority or guilt feeling," says Rank ([1936] 1978a, p. 56; emphasis added). In the existential sense, therefore, guilt "is simply a consequence of consciousness, or more correctly, it is the self-consciousness of the individual as of one willing consciously" ([1936] 1978b, p. 32). Rank never minimizes the enormous significance of the anatomical difference between the sexes. This difference, however, is the *second* most important difference the child confronts. "First comes the perception of difference from others as a consequence of becoming conscious of self . . . then interpretation of this difference as inferiority . . . finally association of this psychological conflict with the biological sexual problem, the difference of the sexes" ([1936] 1978a, p. 55).

"Neurosis," according to Rank, "is a facing on the part of the individual of the metaphysical problem of human existence, only he faces them not in a constructive way as does the artist, philosopher or scientist, but destructively" ([1936] 1978a, p. 127). Reframing the economic metaphor so central to Freud's drive theory, Rank concludes that the neurotic "bribes" life itself—for which we all have to "pay" with death. Because of extreme guilt and anxiety, the neurotic hurls a big No at living: "he refuses the loan [life] in order thus to escape the payment of the debt [death]. Continuously striving to ward off dying, the neurotic only hastens death "from which he seeks to buy himself free by daily partial self-destruction" (p. 126).

The core of the suffering person, according to Rank, is angst, or anxiety. The human being is born afraid, a shivering bundle of anxiety cast adrift in an uncaring cosmos. "*Angst* seems to be erected as a dividing line between the I and the world, and vanishes only when both have become one, as parts of a greater whole" ([1936] 1978a, p. 198)—in, for example, love or art. The emotion of anxiety divides into two currents, running in opposite directions: one toward separation and individuation and the other toward union and collectivity. The outbreak of neurosis typically comes from the streaming together of these two fears, which Rank also calls the fear of living and the fear of dying. A crisis "seems to break out at a certain age when the life fear which has restricted the ego development meets with the death fear as it increases with growth and maturity.

The individual then feels himself driven forward by regret for wasted life and the desire to retrieve it. But this forward driving fear is now death fear, the fear of dying without having lived, which, even so, is held in check by fear of life" (pp. 188–189). The fear of life is the fear of separation and individuation. The fear of death is the fear of union and merger, in essence, the loss of individuality. Both separation and union, however, are desired as well as feared since the will to separate correlates with the creative impulse and the will to unite with the need for love. To respond obsessively to just one need — by choosing to separate totally or to merge totally — is to have the other fear thrown back at oneself. In a prose style that wraps around itself, like a double helix, as if to protect its author from the very anxiety it illuminates, Rank ([1936] 1978a, p. 124) writes:

> The fear in birth, which we have designated as fear of life, seems to me actually the fear of having to live as an isolated individual, and not the reverse, the fear of loss of individuality (death fear). That would mean, however, that primary fear corresponds to a fear of separation from the whole, therefore a fear of individuation, on account of which I would like to call it fear of life, although it may appear later as fear of the loss of this dearly bought individuality as fear of death, of being dissolved again into the whole. Between these two fear possibilities, these poles of fear, the individual is thrown back and forth all his life.

According to Rank, it does not seem possible to eradicate these two ultimate anxieties, which appear to be an existential burden carried out of the womb by every new arrival on the planet. Sometimes it is fear of life — the fear of becoming and being oneself, separate and different from everyone else — that has the upper hand. At other times, it is fear of death — the fear of merging into the other, into the collective, and losing one's "dearly bought individuality" — that predominates. The eternal conflict between the wish for and fear of separation and the wish for and fear of union has no final solution. It must be solved and re-solved continuously throughout life, at every developmental stage, "from birth, via childhood and puberty to maturity and downward through old age to death" ([1936] 1978a, p. 134), which is simultaneously the final separation *and* the final union. "It can only be a matter of balance between the two, which, however, is not attained once and for all but must be created anew and ever anew" (p. 91).

No one has expressed the conflict between the will to separate and the will to unite better than Ernest Becker, whose *The Denial of Death* (1973, pp. 152–153) captures the essence of Rank with electrifying passion:

> On the one hand, the creature is impelled by a powerful desire to identify with the cosmic forces, to merge himself with the rest of nature. On the other hand, he wants to be unique, to stand out as something different and apart. . . .
>
> You can see that man wants the impossible: He wants to lose his isolation and keep it at the same time. He can't stand the sense of separateness, and yet he can't allow the complete suffocation of his vitality. He wants to expand by merging with the powerful beyond that transcends him, yet he wants while merging with it to remain individual and aloof.

The lifelong oscillation between the two poles of fear can be made more bearable, according to Rank, in a relationship with another person who accepts one's uniqueness and difference and allows for the emergence of the creative impulse— without *too much* guilt or anxiety for separating from the other. Like the double function of fear, the creative impulse itself seems to divide into two currents: "will and guilt," says Rank ([1936] 1978b, p. 31), "are the two complementary sides of one and the same phenomenon."

Although a necessary part of growth, separation and in-

dividuation have an emotional price: "the more we individualize ourselves — that is, remove and isolate ourselves from others —
the stronger is the formation of guilt-feeling which originates
from this individualization, and which again in turn unites us
emotionally with others" (Rank, in press). But the human being who has failed to separate and individuate also feels guilt — a
kind of thrown-back responsibility — for remaining embedded
in the other, submerged in the womb of the collective. This is
guilt for self-betrayal: for refusing the burden of consciousness,
of individuality, for denying the vital need for growth. Yet those
who experience and express the creative impulse to the fullest
extent possible — the artists — also feel a deep guilt for taking on
the greatest burden, creating a whole world in their own image, for rivaling the creative force of the cosmos itself, for "negotiating" as mere mortals "with the problem of the Beyond" (Rank,
[1932] 1989, p. 49).

Rank's view that creatively "negotiating" with the cosmos
leaves *guilt* in its wake is found nowhere else in the psychoanalytic literature. In *Truth and Reality* ([1936] 1978b, p. 67; emphasis added), he writes: "The creative type must constantly
make good his continuous will expression and will accomplishment and he pays for this guilt toward others and himself with
work which he must give to the others and which justifies himself to himself. Therefore he is productive, he accomplishes something because he has real guilt to pay for, not *imaginary* guilt
like the neurotic, who only behaves *as if* he were guilty but whose
consciousness of guilt is only an expression of his will denial,
not of creative accomplishment which makes one *truly* guilty."

By the act of creating, the artist strives toward spiritual
freedom, to make himself independent of the compulsions of
sex and death, of the will of mother nature — reaching toward
the fantasy of *causa-sui:* pure independence (Becker, 1973). However, the project to create oneself, to be one's own parent, so
to speak, is confronted with the existential limits mandated by
biology because death and bodily destruction await us all, artist or neurotic, hero or coward. Rank never forgot the impossibility of the *causa-sui* project, even while exploring its dynamics
as a spur to the creative urge and artistic illusion. He analyzes

the dialectic between freedom and fate, will and guilt, most acutely in his greatest work, *Art and Artist* ([1932] 1989, pp. 328–329): "[M]an's acceptance of his dependence on nature is more honest, while freedom-ideology, beyond a certain point, presumes the negation of that dependence and is therefore, also in a deeper sense, dishonest. This fundamental dishonesty towards nature then comes out as consciousness of guilt, which we see active in every process of art . . . the more strongly man feels his freedom and independence, the more intense on the other hand is the consciousness of guilt, which appears in the individual partly restrictive, partly creative."

As a harmonizing factor between the will to separate and the will to unite, says Rank (in press), guilt seems to be the emotion that cements the I to the Thou, externally, as well as the active and social components of the person, internally:

> I think the guilt feeling occupies a special position among the emotions, as a boundary phenomenon between the pronounced painful affects that separate and the more pleasurable feelings that unite. It is related to the painful separating affects of anxiety and hate. But in its relation to gratitude and devotion, which may extend to self-sacrifice, it belongs to the strongest uniting feelings we know. As the guilt-feeling occupies the boundary line between the painful and pleasurable, between the severing and uniting feelings, it is also the most important representative of the relation between the inner and outer, the I and the Thou, the Self and the World.

Against Freud's assertions that only the analyst's interpretations cure and that the analyst must maintain strict neutrality, Rank constructed "a philosophy of helping": the relationship between client and therapist is itself therapeutic, not the therapist's insight into, or "causal" understanding of, the client's infantile past or presenting problem ([1936] 1978a, p. 2). It is not what the client learns from the therapist's interpretations that is healing. It is, rather, what Martin Buber calls the I-Thou relationship. "All real living is meeting," says Buber (quoted in Friedman, 1985, p. 2), and "by the graciousness of its comings and the solemn sadness of its goings, [the I-Thou relationship] teaches us to meet others and to hold our ground when we meet them."

Each therapeutic hour, according to Rank, is a partial living and dying, a microcosmic experience of separation and union. If one can accept oneself in this fragment of time, without too much anxiety or guilt, then living more fully outside the allotted hour may also be possible. But the problem of human suffering, according to Rank, cannot be solved "in and by the individual himself, but only in relation to a second person, who justifies our will, makes it good, since he voluntarily submits himself to it" ([1936] 1978a, p. 56), in other words, accepts us as we are. Rank maintained that Freud's technique does not do this because it interprets all expressions of will in the therapeutic hour as resistance to the authority of the therapist, who stands in the center of the analysis in spite of his so-called passivity or neutrality.

The "whole psychoanalytic approach is centered around the therapist," Rank complained in a 1935 lecture in New York. "Real therapy has to be *centered around the client,* his difficulties, his needs, his activities" (Rank, in press). Therefore, the therapist is not to play the role of authority, according to Rank, but is an "assistant ego" who provides a helping relationship in which the neurotic — an *"artiste manqué,"* a kind of failed artist — can affirm and rediscover his own positive will, become his own therapist, accept responsibility for his own individuality and difference, and say yes to the often painful obligation of living as well as the dreaded obligation of dying.

According to Rank ([1936] 1978a, pp. 27 and 65), experience (in other words, living itself) is nothing but "emotional surrender to the present." The problem of experience is not how to understand or speak about the past, which has already been interpreted and reinterpreted a thousandfold in memory, but how to live in the present: consciousness, thinking, feeling, and willing are always in the present. "This, then, is the New, which the patient has never experienced before." An emotional experience in the here-and-now relationship with an empathic therapist is more important for healing than interpretations that claim to uncover the repressed "truth" about infancy or make the unconscious conscious.

Although Rank does not use the words *empathy* or *empathic understanding* in his writings, he defined love to his Philadelphia students as an extraordinary form of emotional attunement that allows one to merge into another in order to reemerge as an individual, enriched spiritually in the process. Love, he told them, "unites our ego with the other, with the Thou, with men, with the world, and so does away with fear":

> What is unique in love is that—beyond the fact of uniting—it rebounds on the ego. Not only, I love the other as my ego, as part of my ego, but the other also makes my ego worthy of love. The love of the Thou thus places a value on one's own ego. *Love abolishes egoism, it merges the self in the other to find it again enriched in one's own ego.* This unique projection and introjection of feeling rests on the fact that one can really only love the one who accepts our own self as it is, indeed will not have it otherwise than it is, and whose self we accept as it is [Rank, in press].

"I Became Infected with Rankian Ideas"

Exactly what went on during Carl Rogers's three-day seminar in Rochester with Otto Rank in June 1936? Unfortunately, no record of this seminar exists. Rank himself mentions it only twice, in correspondence with a friend and student, Jessie Taft, without naming Rogers. "Yesterday," wrote Rank on June 10, 1936, "I gave a general lecture somewhat like for the students in Philadelphia"; a few days later, in another letter, he wrote, "Rochester was interesting and successful, but I am tired" (quoted in Taft, 1968, pp. 215 and 216).

And what about Rogers? What could have been the seminar's impact on him? In an interview decades later, while not

referring to the seminar itself, Rogers spoke in almost revela-
tory terms to his biographer of the experience of encountering
Rank's post-Freudian thinking: "I became infected with Rankian
ideas and began to realize the possibilities of the individual being self-directing. . . . I was clearly fascinated by Rankian ideas
but didn't quite adopt his emphases for myself until I left Rochester. But the core idea did develop. I came to believe in the
individual's capacity. I value the dignity and rights of the individual sufficiently that I do not want to impose my way upon
him. These two aspects of the core idea haven't changed since
that time" (quoted in Kirschenbaum, 1979, p. 95). Asked in
the mid-seventies, "Were you influenced by Rank?" Rogers answered: "Yes, I was [by] his ideas of the relationship and focusing more on the immediate present. . . . There's no doubt that
my 'therapy' was influenced by his thinking" (quoted in Evans,
1975, pp. 28–29).

It is impossible now, almost sixty years later, to recon-
struct what Rank said or did during the 1936 seminar with
Rogers. It is likely that during much of the time Rank spoke
spontaneously. He writes ([1936] 1978a, p. 105) that his technique "in every case, yes in every individual hour of the same
case, is different. . . . My technique consists essentially in having no technique." The first practitioner of therapy as a performing art, Rank improvised a new theory for each client, while
always honoring the client's unique expression of the dynamic
interplay between life fear and death fear, separation and union,
creativity and inhibition, courage and despair, will and guilt.

Surely there were many question-and-answer sessions during the seminar, but one wonders whether Rogers spoke at length
with Rank, privately or publicly. How much of Rank, often
a tangled writer, did Rogers actually read? Nobody knows. "One
searches Rogers' writings in vain for even a single quotation
from Rank or even for more than three consecutive sentences
on Rank's thinking" (Kirschenbaum, 1979, p. 92). Yet Rogers
evidently was so moved by the seminar with Rank in 1936, and
later by the lucid writings of Jessie Taft, who became the leading American student of Rank, that his view of the helping
profession changed radically.

In the simplest sense, what was Rank's message to the helping professions? Invited to deliver a lecture in 1938 at the University of Minnesota, Otto Rank summarized his post-Freudian approach:

> From my own experience, I learned that the therapeutic process is basically an *emotional experience* — which takes place *independently* of the theoretical concepts of the analyst, a statement, that is borne out by the fact that therapeutic results have been attained and achieved by various methods of psychotherapy, based on different theories. Furthermore, the emphasis on the emotional experience — instead of on the intellectual enlightenment of the patient — brings two essential principles of my dynamic therapy into focus. Firstly, the emphasis is shifted from the past to the *present,* in which *all* emotional experience takes place; secondly, the therapeutic process allows the patient a much more *active* role than being merely an object upon whom the therapist operates. . . .
> All living psychology is relationship psychology. . . . What we learned from the analysis and understanding of this therapeutic relationship seems to have a bearing on other forms and types of relationships — such as exist between parent and child, teacher and pupil, husband and wife, in friendship, and so forth. That is to say, in all those relationships there seems to be a therapeutic element, if we conceive of that term in the broadest sense of the word. Simply speaking, this is the definition of relationship: one individual is helping the other to develop and grow, without infringing too much on the other's personality [Rank, in press].

In October 1939, Otto Rank died suddenly in New York, at age fifty-five — one month after Freud's death in London, at age eighty-three. Freud had conceived of all human beings as alike, reducible to the same unconscious sexual desires, to "drive." Although he never minimized the power of sexuality, Rank was too absorbed in aesthetic problems, especially the problems of creativity and inhibition of will, to reduce the incalculable variety of human beings to one common denominator. Shortly before he died, Rank asked poignantly, "Will people ever learn that there is no other equality possible than the equal right of every individual to become and be himself, which actually means to accept his own difference and have it accepted by others" ([1941] 1958, p. 267)?

In 1939, the great hypothesis of Carl Rogers was still gestating. According to Rogers, "It would seem quite absurd to suppose that one could name a day on which client-centered therapy was born. Yet I feel it is possible to name that day and it was December 11, 1940" (quoted in Kirschenbaum, 1979, p. 112). On that day at the University of Minnesota, at exactly the same place where Rank had spoken in 1938, Rogers presented his paper "Newer Concepts in Psychotherapy."

Publicly crediting "the thinking of Otto Rank" and his students, Rogers told his Minnesota audience that in recent years he had been developing a different approach. First, he said, "the aim of this newer therapy is not to solve one particular problem, but to assist the individual to *grow*." Unlike traditional approaches, the approach does not *do* anything to the individual; instead of "treating" the person as an illness might be treated by a medical doctor, the newer therapy releases the creative potential from *within*. "In the second place, this newer therapy places greater stress upon the *emotional* elements, the feeling aspects of the situation than upon the *intellectual* aspects. . . . In the third place, this newer therapy places greater stress upon the immediate situation than upon the individual's past. . . . Finally, this approach lays stress upon the *therapeutic relationship* itself as a growth experience" (quoted in Kirschenbaum, 1979, p. 113; emphasis added).

Somehow the ideas of Otto Rank had germinated in the mind of Carl Rogers, whether directly as a result of the 1936 seminar or indirectly through Rank's students. Within a short time, Rogers began writing *Counseling and Psychotherapy: Newer*

Concepts in Practice, which was published in 1942. "It was in this book," observes Brian Thorne (1992, p. 13), who worked closely with Rogers in the last decade of his life, "that the term 'client' first appeared."

Echoing Rank's old-world philosophy of life in *Art and Artist,* or "the volitional affirmation of the obligatory" ([1932] 1989, p. 64), Rogers came to define the fully functioning person as one who deliberately and creatively says yes to the "must." Such a person, concludes Rogers, in words that are almost identical to Rank's, "voluntarily chooses and wills that which is also absolutely determined" (Kirschenbaum and Henderson, 1989a, p. 418).

Rank and Management

The last twenty years have seen a burgeoning renewal of interest in the philosophical and therapeutic ideas of Otto Rank. Brutally attacked by orthodox analysts for abandoning Freud's teachings, Rank "will probably turn out in the end to have been the best mind that psychoanalysis contributed to intellectual history" (Jones, 1960, p. 219).

The Rankian revival began in 1973 with Ernest Becker's Pulitzer Prize–winning *The Denial of Death* (1973), a brilliant merger of Rank's post-Freudian writings with the thought of Kierkegaard. Fritz Perls, one of the developers of Gestalt therapy, was also deeply influenced by Rank, going so far as to describe Rank's writings on art and creativity as "beyond praise" in his foundational work, *Gestalt Therapy* (Perls, Hefferline, and Goodman, 1951, p. 395).

It was not until 1981, however, with the publication of Robert Denhardt's *In the Shadow of Organization* (see Kramer, 1989) that management scholars began to pay attention to Rank, whose *Psychology and the Soul* ([1930] 1961), a cultural history of the belief in immortality, was quoted extensively by Denhardt. At about the same time, Tom Peters and Robert Waterman were writing *In Search of Excellence* and used Becker's *Denial of Death* as "a major supporting theoretical position" (Peters and Waterman, 1982, p. xxi) for their psychology of management, although they knew nothing about Rank and overlooked Becker's subversive critique of the very organizational culture they were promoting. A deeper appreciation of both Becker and Rank came with *Paradoxes of Group Life* (1987), a rich study by Kenwyn Smith and David Berg of the ever-shifting conflict between paralysis and movement — stuckness and creativity — in groups. "One thing I hope my confrontation with Rank will do," writes Becker (1973, p. xii) "is to send the reader directly to his books. There is no substitute for reading Rank. . . . [H]e is a mine for years of insights and pondering."

Interpretation Versus Relationship

By suggesting that the prototype of the analytic situation is the *mother*-child relationship, Rank was radically shifting the psychoanalytic view of therapeutic action. He had made a momentous discovery, a discovery that dawned on him only gradually. He was moving from interpretation therapy to relationship therapy. As soon as it became clear to Rank that the patient's present emotional experience with the analyst is more important than "insight" into the Oedipus complex, he instantly realized that the therapist does not cure by "after-educating" the patient with interpretations, as Freud maintained. Instead, the therapist *himself* or *herself* is the cure. Interpretation of the past, on the other hand, allows both therapist and patient to escape the emotionally charged present, the experience of *two creative wills encountering and transforming each other* in the therapeutic setting. Even interpretation of the present is scarcely valid or reliable while it is being enacted. "It is not a question of whose interpretation is correct," said Rank in a 1930 lecture, "because there is no such thing as *the* interpretation or only *one* psychological truth." According to him (Rank, in press), "Psychology does not deal primarily with facts as science does but only with the individual's attitude toward facts. In other words, the objects of psychology are *interpretations* — and there are as many of them as there are individuals and, even more than that, also the individual's different situations, which have to be interpreted *differently* in every single manifestation."

By creating a symbolic womb in the analytic situation, the therapist is to assist the patient in being reborn spiritually as an autonomous self, a new individual, separate and different from all other human beings, without suffering too greatly for separating from the therapist during the end phase of therapy. Thus, says Rank ([1936] 1978a, p. 106), "my theory of the birth trauma [is] a universal symbol of the I's discovery of itself and of its separation from the momentary assistant I, originally the mother, now the therapist."

Freedom and Community: The Part-Whole Problem

One of the greatest learnings of Otto Rank was that the individual and society are not antagonistic, as Freud always insisted, but complementary. There is an eternal oscillation between the need for individuation and the need for attachment, the will to separate and the will to unite, independence and dependence, aloneness and intimacy. Both are essential. Managing this dialectic, which Rank called the part-whole problem, is the principal task of the human being in the process of becoming a fully functioning person, in the process of "the never completed birth of individuality" (Rank, [1936] 1978b, p. 11). One must solve and constantly re-solve the part-whole problem throughout life.

What does this mean in the organizational context? Rank was not a management theorist, but his concept of life fear and death fear is an extraordinarily powerful way to frame some of the most intractable and unhealthy solutions to the part-whole problem in the workplace. For the obsessive-compulsive — the alcoholic or workaholic, for example — "the miscarriage of this solution [means that] the part is not a substitute for the whole but always the whole itself, because with him the partial always assumes the dimension of the whole, and therewith of finality. With him, accordingly, it is always a matter of life and death, an avoidance of life that leads him to the threshold of death and a fear of death that keeps him from life" (Rank, ([1936] 1978b, p. 140).

Soon after his exhilarating 1936 meeting with Rank, Rogers began to formulate the three "core conditions" that he felt were necessary for spiritual healing. Deceptively simple to state but remarkably difficult to practice, these three conditions offer clues as to how managers could become therapeutic helpers, not just authorities, to their employees: their clients.

What were Rogers's three core conditions, as transposed to the organizational setting? First, and most importantly, the manager-helper must be *congruent,* fully present in the here and now, with no pretense of emotional distance, no professional facade. "It is only as he is, in this relationship, a unified person, with his experienced feeling, his awareness of his feelings, and his expression of those feelings all congruent, that he is most able to facilitate therapy" writes Rogers (quoted in Kirschenbaum, 1979, p. 196). Often misunderstood as simply a passive reflection of the client's emotions, Rogers's approach demands a wholesome self-assertiveness of the helper's own creative will, own individuality, own difference. Obviously, this does not mean that helpers burden clients with their problems or blurt out all their feelings impulsively. For Rogers, however, fully accepting a client never means denying the helper's own individuality, being overly permissive, or becoming weak and ineffectual. According to Rogers, "The therapist [or manager] encounters his client directly, meeting him person to person. He is *being* himself, not denying himself" (Kirschenbaum and Henderson, 1989b, p. 12).

Second, the manager-helper must communicate *unconditional positive regard* for the uniqueness of the other person. Rogers defines this as "caring for the client as a separate person, with permission to have his own feelings, his own experience" (quoted in Kirschenbaum, 1979, p. 199). The perceptions of the client are not distortions of a reality that only the helper has the vision to see clearly. Without excluding the possibility of unconscious factors affecting the perceptions of both parties, the helper accepts the client's phenomenology as reflecting the constantly fluctuating conditions of the moment, whether or not they agree with the helper's view. "Each person is an island unto himself, in a very real sense, and he can only build bridges to other islands if he is first of all willing to be himself and permitted to be himself," writes Rogers. "So I find that when I can accept another person . . . then I am assisting him to become a person" (Kirschenbaum and Henderson, 1989a, p. 22). There are no objective psychological facts for Rogers, only subjective interpretations of phenomena. And the client, not the helper, is the expert on the meaning of these phenomena as they apply to his or her experience. There is, in short, no single reality. Fully accepting the client's frame of reference, therefore, requires extraordinarily active listening.

Third, the manager-helper must express genuine *empathic understanding* for the client. Empathic understanding is a form of nonpossessive love that the ancient Greeks called *agape* — to distinguish it from *eros,* a grasping possessive love that insists on its own desires being met. As Rogers (1980, p. 143) explains:

> The way of being with another person which is termed empathic has several facets. It means entering the private perceptual world of the other and becoming thoroughly at home in it. It involves being sensitive, moment to moment, to the changing felt meanings which flow in this other person, to the fear or rage or tenderness or confusion or whatever, that he/she is experiencing. It means temporarily living in his/her life, moving about it delicately without making judgments, sensing meanings of which he/she is scarcely aware, but not trying to uncover feelings of which the person is totally unaware, since this would be too threatening.

However, Rogers has also made it clear that empathy, or *agape,* does not mean losing oneself in the other. Maintaining the separateness of the helper is essential for permitting the separateness of the client. Only by being separate can empathy be offered. "When I can freely feel this strength of being a separate person, then I find I can let myself go much more deeply in understanding and accepting [the client] because I am not fearful of losing myself" notes Rogers (Kirschenbaum and Henderson, 1989a, p. 121). The key to healing is the emotional experience of being *in* relationship, fully separate yet somehow simultaneously connected with another.

Beyond these three core conditions, the technique of the manager-helper is irrelevant, according to Rogers. Of course no mortal can always be completely congruent, accepting, and empathic. Therefore, Rogers visualized the core conditions, which are met to a lesser or greater degree, as located on a continuum. Moreover, the art of the manager-helper, Rogers believed, consists entirely in moving farther and farther along the continuum, getting better and better at *being* or *performing* these conditions, not just espousing them. Rogers, who was never convinced that he fully met his own conditions, thought it fortunate that "imperfect human beings can be of therapeutic assistance to other imperfect human beings" (1959, p. 215).

In all organizations, in the family, at school or work, a person's basic conflict is to be a self with others, to maintain a separate identity while simultaneously participating in the group, to deal creatively with the dilemma of being one among many, utterly different from everyone else yet still affiliated with the whole human system. According to Rank, reports Karpf (1953, p. 74), the development of the psychologically healthy person proceeds in a back-and-forth pattern "in terms of relationship and separation by a succession of emotional attachments and dependencies on the one hand and independence-seeking separations and detachments on the other hand, with the creation of personality and the emergence of individuality as constantly evolving and expanding goals. From the primal attachment and separation at birth to the final detachment and separation at death, this process of binding and freeing continues, throughout the entire course of human life."

It is to Carl Rogers and, before him, Otto Rank that managers owe the great idea of offering a certain type of relationship to employees as a way of helping them find a vital balance between the part and the whole, difference and likeness, the self and the organization — in short, between freedom and community. This healing through meetings has the potential of allowing a person to merge into the whole in order to reemerge enriched and spiritually reborn in his or her singular individuality. And, perhaps not surprisingly, it was a deep sharing between Carl Rogers and Otto Rank that gave birth to the idea of creating a fresh solution to an existential problem that must be solved and re-solved continuously throughout life, both inside and outside the organization. Like living itself, managing people is a performing art that "is not attained once and for all but must be created anew and ever anew" (Rank, [1936] 1978a, p. 91).

8

Acknowledging the Dark Side
of Organizational Life

Howard S. Schwartz

Over a period of twenty years, I spent a great deal of time in the town of Mamou, which is located in the Cajun area of south-western Louisiana. As nearly everyone knows, the Cajun people have a culture that emphasizes the fun that can be had in life. Cuisine, music, storytelling — put these together with an attitude of carefree abandon and one comes up with a spirit that the Cajuns express by saying, "Laissez les bons temps rouler!" (Let the good times roll!)

Beneath the fun-loving exterior, however, there is another side to Cajun life. The close observer finds that the gaiety and abandon are often forced. There is a manic quality to them. The Cajuns feel as if they *need* to be happy-go-lucky. Delve beneath the surface and you will find a depression and despondency that stand in stark contrast to the surface manifestations. Moreover, since depression cannot be admitted in a culture that makes a point of being carefree, it must be suffered alone. This, of course, makes it worse, and the cycle goes on. The upshot is that, in this locale known so well for its love of fun, the rates of mental illness, alcoholism, drug addiction, and finally, suicide are phenomenal.

What is of interest in the context of this book is that these phenomena are not publicly discussed in Cajun discourse. They are known and discussed privately, but only among intimates and always with an air that what is being talked about is some-

224

thing that should not be discussed. So it is that when someone commits suicide in the town of Mamou, the *Mamou Acadian Press* says in that person's obituary that he or she died of either "a short illness" (the suicide act) or "a long illness" (by which, I suppose, is meant depression, or perhaps life itself). The facts are known, so to speak, beneath the level of performance that others view as Cajun culture. They are part of the dark side of Cajun culture.

We may think of the dark side as that part of a culture that is experienced by participants as what should not be a part of the culture, as the side that causes them anxiety, as the shameful side. Jungians refer to this as the shadow side. It is the part of life that is not acknowledged, that individuals attempt to bar from their conscious awareness.

Organizations have a dark side, too. As observers of organizations, as consultants or practitioners of organizational development, we all know this. We also know that we do not talk about it much, and certainly we do not discuss it when we are writing for publication. It is, after all, sympathetically understood as a topic that should not be written about. So why should we not leave well enough alone? Why should we concern ourselves with matters that are unpleasant? Why not simply confine ourselves to what we may call the light side of organizations? To the parts of organizational life that are unobjectionable, that do not evoke unpleasant emotions?

The point I wish to make in this chapter is that, if we are to understand and work with organizations, it is not enough to confine ourselves to the light side, because that side cannot be understood without reference to the dark side. The two constitute a system: two aspects of the same reality, which must be comprehended as a totality. I would like to illustrate this by returning to the Cajun example.

The Theory of the Organization Ideal

Recall the happy-go-lucky attitude of members of the Cajun culture has a forced character. If we were to look only at the light side, this forced quality would not make sense to us. Now recall the despondency and depression in Cajun culture that contrasts sharply with the light side. To suppose that we could understand the fun side of Cajun culture without considering the dark side would be to suppose that there is not one Cajun culture but two separate cultures. How are we to understand the two in relation to each other?

In trying to understand Cajun culture, I found that I could make some sense of it by considering Cajun history. Refusing to swear allegiance to the British Crown, the people who would become the Cajuns were ejected from their homeland in Nova Scotia (Acadia) and deposited more or less randomly along the east coast of the United States. When they learned that there were French people living in Louisiana, many of them made that their destination. When they got there, they found that the good land had already been taken and that they would have to settle for the outlying swamps and bayous, which many people thought were uninhabitable.

The Cajuns never talk among themselves about their forced exile. It does not appear to be part of their conscious experience. Nonetheless, it is easy to conceive that a sense of powerlessness and terror remains with them from this experience in the form of a depression. If we make that assumption, we can understand that their carefree culture, far from arising in isolation from the depressed underside, can best be understood as an attempt to deny that dark side and is therefore incomprehensible without reference to it. Moreover, we can also understand how the depression comes to be worse in comparison with the carefree life that the Cajuns need to take so seriously. In other words, what we have come to see in this example is that, far from being isolated from one another and comprehensible independently, the light and dark sides exist as mirror images of each other, neither being comprehensible except in terms of their relationship.

Elsewhere (Schwartz, 1990b), I have developed a theory that helps explain how the light side and dark side give meaning to each other. According to this theory, organizational participants project a fantasy of perfection onto the organization. This fantasy is a special case of what Freud called the ego ideal. The ego ideal represents being the center of a loving world, returning to the state of fusion with the mother that represents our earliest mental life. When this fantasy takes the form of an organization, I call it the organization ideal.

The organization ideal is a conception of organizational life and, specifically, of the organizational experience of the individual, as being free of anxiety and of its causes. According to Rollo May (1950), anxiety is the experience of being in the face of nonbeing. The organization ideal represents the denial of the difference between the individual and the organization and therefore a denial that the organization represents nonbeing with regard to the being of the individual.

Within the organization ideal, individuals correspond perfectly and without remainder to their organizational roles. They do their jobs spontaneously and out of desire, not as the result of either external or internal pressure. Moreover, an organization of this sort is conceived to be in perfect concordance with its external environment. The organization's environment is not an independent existence in its own right but merely, so to speak, the participant's mother at further remove. Its whole meaning is to nurture the participant through nurturing the organization of which he or she is a member. It therefore cannot make demands or impose threat or constraint.

The organization ideal is, of course, the light side of organizational life. However, the relationship it has with the dark side is also evident. To see this, we need to observe that the organization ideal, like any ego ideal, never happens. The existential reality of human life is that the individual simply is, as a unique individual, separate and distinct from the rest of the world. This is not a matter of happenstance; it is just what it means to be a unique individual. Specifically, we always experience ourselves as standing out from the organization, and it is the anxiety of this standing outness that drives the fantasy of the organization ideal at all times and again and again.

Returning to the Cajun example, we can see that it is precisely the anxiety of the dark side that drives the enactment of the light side and gives it life. Thus, the view of organizations that emerges is that of a denial, what Ernest Becker (1973) has called a *vital lie*.

An organization is a performance, a drama of perfection in which individuals are perfectly suited to their organization roles. Within this drama, they do what the organization needs doing out of desire, not coercion or obligation. In reality, however, the individuals who enact these roles are driven by the anxiety of powerlessness, limitation, and isolation that the human condition represents and whose denial constitutes and gives meaning to the performance of the organization ideal. Again, then, neither of these two sides may be understood in isolation from the other.

But the dark side also has a moral dimension. The meaning of the performance, the joint project of each participant in the organization, is fusion with the organization ideal and, through that, fusion with others. The organization ideal therefore represents the imaginary play of eros, or love. However, the participants' difference from their roles in the drama calls the drama into question, reveals it as a performance, wrecking it for themselves and threatening it for their loved others. The participants experience it with a feeling of their own unlovability and unacceptability, as moral failures. Thus, in contrast to the perfection of the organization ideal, the limitation, the separation, the finitude, the imperfection of the participants' actual lives are experienced with shame. The shame arises from their experience that, as imperfect and limited, they do not belong in the organization ideal. Taken together, all these processes and experiences constitute the dark side.

Returning to the question of why we should study the dark side, we can now give two related answers. First, without knowing about the dark side, we lose sight of the fact that the drama that organizational participants put on is a drama—that they are playing roles. Within that drama, as in all drama, they *are* their roles. In point of fact, however, individuals are *enacting* these roles. And they are doing so for reasons that are not contained within the roles they are playing. This fact is forced into the dark side. If we consider only the light side, we cannot know it. Second, we need to study the dark side because without it we do not know what drives individuals to do their jobs, to enact their organization roles. In other words, we cannot know about organizational motivation. In regard to both work motivation and dramaturgy, then, ignorance of the dark side leads to a loss of understanding. As I will show, this loss of understanding must have consequences. I wish first to deal with motivation.

Motivation and Hierarchy

When I speak about motivation in organizations, I am not concerned with whether or not a person will commit a specific act, which is the focus of what is called motivation theory. Rather, I am concerned with the motive of the action in the sense of its underlying meaning. This is not a concern with specific actions but rather with a unity that structures many separate actions to produce a more or less coherent life. When I look at the people I know in organizational life in terms of the underlying meaning that structures their lives, one thing that stands out very clearly is the desire for promotion, for rising in the hierarchy, for getting ahead.

In traditional organizational psychology, the value of rising in the hierarchy is explained in terms of the higher rewards that are expected when one is promoted, and this is certainly part of the picture. But this traditional orientation is not capable of dealing with what, to me, is the most striking thing about the desire for promotion, and that is its compulsive and absolute character. As Jackall (1988) puts it concerning the managers he observed, for them, getting ahead is a "moral imperative."

This is certainly in accord with my observations. Many of the people I know in organizational life are absolutely consumed with rising in the hierarchy. They will sacrifice anything for it, no matter how otherwise valuable what they are sacrificing may be. Many of them will sacrifice their family lives, their friendships, work that they love, attachments to places where they live, and anything else. This is not consistent with a rational pursuit of rewards because, rationally, the possible rewards would all have values attached to them, values that would often be expected to outweigh the promise of alternatives. Indeed, if rising in the hierarchy were a matter of obtaining valued rewards, the higher one rose in the hierarchy, the more rewards one would have obtained and the less giving up these rewards in the hope of obtaining different rewards, even if at a higher level, would make sense. However, close observers of executives report that this is not the case (see, for example, Jennings, 1967). Rather, the higher one rises in the hierarchy, the more important further promotion becomes.

What does not make sense in terms of expectancy theory is easily explained from the standpoint of the ego ideal. As we have seen, the organization may be taken for the ego ideal, a process that is the result of projection by the individual and fostered by the organization's own dramaturgy (Klein and Ritti, 1984). Of course, we never realize the ego ideal, and the organization is never the organization ideal. We need a way of maintaining a belief in the organization ideal, while at the same time our experience does not correspond to being the center of a loving world. One way of doing this is by supposing that those who truly are the organization, those in higher positions than we are, are the ego ideal while we, at our level, are not there yet. Thus, the route to the ego ideal is through promotion.

Now, to be sure, our image of promotion never lives up to our fantasy about it. We had thought that we would no longer be subject to forces that are outside our control, that we would, instead, be the force that controls others. As it turns out, however, we are still subject to forces outside our control; they are just bigger. Moreover, the fact that we have control over others turns out to be less salient to our sense of well-being than the forces acting upon us. We find out that our control over others is often only nominal and deeply problematic. From the standpoint of the ego ideal, however, this is no problem since it can be resolved by further promotion. Thus, the vertical dimension of the organization becomes the route to the ego ideal that, like the horizon, is never attained but always stands before us and beckons us toward it.

Viewed in this way, promotion appears to many of us and to many organizational participants as offering unlimited rewards, as opposed to the limited value of any finite rewards that have already been obtained. Indeed, at its core, the idea of promotion offers the end of limitation itself. Under the circumstances, it is not surprising that individuals would give up anything to obtain it; everything they already have is merely finite. Their fantasy of what they will have when they are promoted is, well, fantastic.

The compulsive character of getting ahead refers to the fact that what drives it is precisely the anxiety whose absence the ego ideal represents. Taking the ego ideal seriously, as we know, drives the anxiety into the dark side, where one cannot understand or evaluate it. It exists for one only as a nonspecific drive that presses for satisfaction, a wish that comes to be represented by the ego ideal in the form of promotion.

The fact that the higher one gets, the stronger the compulsion becomes is accounted for by the fact that the whole mythology of the organization ideal is built around the idea that the higher one gets, the more at peace one should be. Thus, as one rises higher, the contrast between the peace one is supposed to experience and the anxiety that does not abate becomes more intense; this contrast has to be resolved in the only way one knows, and has left, to resolve it: further promotion. What is apparent in all of this is, again, the way the ego ideal and the anxiety of the dark side live off each other and keep each other active. The horror of remaining in one place is amplified by the idea that promotion would resolve one's anxiety, while the intensity of the wish for the resolution of that anxiety is driven by the anxiety of the dark side itself. Again, these two mirror images of each other can be distinguished but not separated.

We can see some of this dynamic played out in the account of one of Studs Terkel's (1972) interviewees, a former corporate president named Larry Ross.

As a kid, living through the Depression, you always heard about the tycoons, the men of power, the men of industry. And you kind of dream that. Gee, these are supermen. These are the guys that have no feeling, aren't subject to human emotions, the insecurities that everyone has.

But

> You get in the corporate structure, you find they
> all button their pants the same way everybody else
> does. They all got the same fears [1972, p. 407].

And

> As he struggles in this jungle, every position he's
> in, he's terribly lonely. He can't confide and talk
> with the guy working under him. He can't confide
> and talk to the man he's working for. To give vent
> to his feelings, his fears, and his insecurities, he'd
> expose himself. This goes all the way up the line
> until he gets to be president. The president really
> doesn't have anybody to talk to, because the vice
> presidents are waiting for him to die or make a
> mistake, and get knocked off so they can get his
> job. . . .
>   You have the tremendous infighting of man
> against man for survival and clawing to the top.
> Progress [p. 408].

Which ultimately led to this:

> I left that world because suddenly the power and
> the status were empty. I'd been there, and when
> I got there it was nothing. Suddenly you have a
> feeling of little boys playing at business. Suddenly
> you have a feeling — so what? . . . I've been to the
> mountaintop. [Laughs.] It isn't worth it [p. 412].

When Larry Ross quit, a confrontation with the dark side
that he had avoided, his own limitations and finitude, evidently
followed:

> It was very difficult, the transition of retiring from
> the status position, where there's people on the
> phone all day trying to talk to you. Suddenly no-

body calls you. This is a psychological . . . [Halts; a long pause.] I don't want to get into that [pp. 412-413].

Indeed, I suggest that it was only this confrontation with the dark side that enabled Larry Ross to grow and make a new life for himself based upon an acceptance of his limitations. This is what Maslow (1970) means by self-actualization (Schwartz, 1983). As is often the case, this transformation involved finding a value in one's experience that could be of use to others. Thus, Ross became a consultant to top management on the basis of the fact that he knew what they were going through and could provide someone for them to talk to when they (as earlier he) could not talk to anyone else.

What we see here is that the sense of limitation, separation, finitude, and mortality, which is part of the dark side, remained with Larry Ross and drove his pursuit up the hierarchy. Further, the vision of perfection that promotion represented led him to suppress his anxiety and drive it into the dark side. Again, we see the interplay between the wish and the anxiety and the fact that one cannot be understood without the other. Finally, a confrontation with the dark side enabled Ross to grow into a more differentiated and integrated human being who could find a meaning for his life in the full consciousness of his limitations.

The Dark Side and
the Performance of the Organization

The fantasy of the organization ideal structures the organization's performance. To employ the motivational power of the organization ideal, the organization consciously and unconsciously attempts to portray a picture of itself as perfect and of its participants as perfectly matched to the organization. It demands that participants redefine their identity in terms of the organization (Shorris, 1981). It requires the presentation of self to adhere to a norm of a perfect concordance between individual motivation and organizational necessity. In a sense, the organization may be seen as just this process of dramatization (Goffman, 1959).

The trouble with this is that the organization only fulfills this motivational function at the expense of an accurate perception of reality. This drama works, or gives participants the hope of the ego ideal, only if they do not understand that the organization is a drama. They have to take it as real, spontaneous, unself-conscious, if it is to fulfill its psychological purpose. However, this is inconsistent with participants' experience of themselves as the actors in this performance and with their roles as creating the drama. Thus, for the drama to have meaning, the participants must somehow remove from organizational discourse what they know about its performed character. Yet this places the basic facts about the performers of the organization — as opposed to the roles that they play — into the dark side, where the facts cannot be known. The organization thus becomes blind to its own reality. This can pose a number of problems. For example, the real motivations of the performers of the organizational drama may become inconsistent with the meaning of the organization.

A delightful book by Michael Lewis (1989) illustrates this phenomenon. Lewis's first experience with the organization ideal of the investment banking business came when he was interviewed at Princeton for a job as an analyst with Lehman Brothers.

[Interviewer]: You know we interview hundreds of people for each position. You're up against a lot of economics majors who know their stuff. Why do you want to be an investment banker?

[Lewis]: (Obviously, the honest answer was that I didn't know. That was unacceptable. After a waffle or two, I gave him what I figured he wanted to hear): Well, really, when you get right down to it, I want to make money.

[Interviewer]: That's not a good reason. You work long hours in this job, and you have to be motivated by more than money. It's true, our compensation is in line with our contribution. But frankly,

we try to discourage people from our business who
are too interested in money. That's all [1989, p. 29].

Later, Lewis came to understand his experience:

Even if analysts were not paid as well as the older
investment bankers, I had thought they were meant
to be at least a tiny bit greedy. Why did the square
young man from Lehman take offense at the suggestion? A friend who eventually won a job with
Lehman Brothers later explained. "It's taboo," he
said. "When they ask you why you want to be an
investment banker, you're supposed to talk about
the challenges, and the thrill of doing deals, and
the excitement of working with such high-caliber
people, but never, ever mention money" [p. 30].

And:

I did not learn much from my stack of Wall Street
rejection letters except that investment bankers were
not in the market for either honesty or my services
(not that the two were otherwise related). Set questions were posed to which set answers were expected.
A successful undergraduate interview sounded like
a monastic chant. . . . My Lehman interview was
representative not just of my own experience but
of thousands of interviews conducted by a dozen investment banks on several dozen college campuses
from about 1981 onward [p. 30].

Forcing interviewees to dissemble if they were to get jobs
ironically led to the investment banking firms' hiring only people who were willing to dissemble in order to pursue their own
selfish interests. And this is something that the firms precluded
themselves from knowing. Tied to a grandiose image of themselves, hiring only individuals who would reproduce that grandiose image, the organizations lost the very culture they were

trying to preserve. Rather than hiring investment bankers, with
the whole complex range of motivations, convictions, and ways
of relating to others that constitute the capacity to do that work
successfully, the firms hired individuals whose only motivation
was their own advancement, who had no convictions that would
have stood in the way of their dissembling, and who were unrelated to anything. Rather than being investment banks, they
became dramatizations of their fantasies of investment banks.

 Lewis, who managed to dissemble well enough to get a
job at Salomon Brothers, observes what happened as a result:

> In retrospect it is clear to me that my arrival at
> Salomon marked the beginning of the end of that
> hollowed institution. . . . [T]hat they let me — and
> other drifters like me — in the door at all was an
> early warning signal. . . . They were losing touch
> with their identity. They had once been shrewd
> traders of horseflesh. Now they were taking in all
> the wrong kinds of people. Even my more commer-
> cially minded peers — no, especially my more com-
> mercially minded peers . . . — did not plan to de-
> vote their lives to Salomon Brothers. And neither
> did I.
>
> Nothing bound us to the firm but what had
> enticed many of us to apply: money and a strange
> belief that no other jobs in the world were worth
> doing. Not exactly the stuff of deep and abiding
> loyalties. Inside of three years 75 percent of us
> would be gone (compared with previous years when
> after three years, on average, 85 percent of the class
> was still with the firm). After this large infusion of
> strangers intent on keeping their distance the firm
> went into convulsions, just as when any body in-
> gests large quantities of an alien substance.
>
> We were a paradox. We had been hired to
> deal in a market, to be more shrewd than the next
> guy, to be, in short, traders. Ask any astute trader
> and he'll tell you that his best work cuts against the

conventional wisdom. Good traders tend to do the unexpected. We, as a group, were painfully predictable. By coming to Salomon Brothers, we were doing only what every sane money-hungry person would do. If we were unable to buck convention in our lives, would we be likely to buck convention in the market? After all, the job market is a market [1989, pp. 38–39].

The organization ideal is a presentation, an image of organizational life free of anxiety. However, it only makes sense because of the anxiety connected with our own separate existence. To say that no organization ever gets to be the organization ideal is to say that we all retain a level of anxiety. But notice that this anxiety, whose denial is the very meaning of the organization ideal, becomes anomalous. We cannot acknowledge it within the drama of the organization because that would seem to be a sign that we are out of place in the organization ideal, that we do not belong. We must therefore experience it with shame, as part of our dark side.

That is not the end of the matter, however. As Karen Horney (1950) notes, we can either attribute the cause of our shame to ourselves or project the cause outward, experiencing it as humiliation. If this were to happen, in the context of our belief that promotion is, at least for others, the route to the ego ideal, we could come to experience our existential limitations as caused by others, as a conspiracy to keep us limited and powerless. Consider the case of the glass ceiling.

In an article in the *Wall Street Journal,* Trost (1990, pp. B1, B2) observes that women managers he interviewed did not quit jobs because of their families but because they felt blocked in their advancement. Moreover, women were much more likely to feel they were blocked than were men. There is no doubt that women often face discrimination in the workplace, arguably the residue of traditional forms of the division of labor. Yet when we consider the apparent phenomenology of their distress, another possibility presents itself.

First of all, consider the imagery of the glass ceiling. The image here is one of a state of perfection that a person believes she can see but that, despite any visible barriers, she cannot get to. Notice that this image fits perfectly with the organization ideal, which is a fantasy of perfection that a person locates at high levels of the organization and that the organization demands as a performance. Someone who bought into this picture and accepted it would be surprised to find out that at whatever level she had reached in the organization, her subjective experience would not match the perfection she expected to find. From this, she could easily conclude that she was not being allowed to rise to the level where the real goodness was, that she was being blocked, thwarted, and kept from participation in the bliss that she still believed to be there.

This is the kind of language the women Trost writes about use to describe their condition. They say they did not find "job satisfaction," "respect," "really meaningful work," and so on. In other words, they were not finding the subjective dimension of their work to be what they expected.

This view is given credence by one of Trost's (1990, p. B2) interview subjects: "'The reasons I left had nothing to do with family,' says Gloria Webster, who used to be a financial analyst for a multi-national chemical corporation. In her 14 years there, Ms. Webster says, she won regular promotions, yet could never break into management. Though she had supporters and good training opportunities, she says she finally 'hit what I felt was my glass ceiling,' feeling blocked as a woman by 'people who didn't want me to succeed in any way.'"

The critical phrase here is "could never break into management." What strikes me as odd about this is that, on the one hand, virtually anybody above the rock bottom of the organization can think of himself or herself as management. I know, for example, many first-line supervisors who think of themselves in this way. Webster, with fourteen years of regular promotions in a staff function could surely think of herself as management.

On the other hand, as Jackall (1988) points out, consistent with the theory of the organization ideal, managers always experience themselves as on the margin and never able to feel sure of their status. He calls this the probationary character of

management. Of course, managers experience this probationary feeling without being able to talk about it or otherwise allow it to be known by others. Indeed, the performance of their
organizational roles is built around denying it. To the outside
observer, they may easily appear to have a sangfroid that the
observer lacks. It is perhaps this sangfroid that Webster is thinking of when she talks about being "management." What she has
not seen, of course, is the dark side. If she had, she would have
known (as Larry Ross could have told her) that in corporate
life, especially at high levels, nobody wants you to succeed—
not so much because you are a woman but because you are
competition.

Trost (1990) concludes the article by saying that organizations must deal with women's dissatisfaction through explicit
policies to further their promotion. From the standpoint of dark-
side psychology, this is a dubious strategy, since there is no reason to believe that any finite rate of promotion is going to make
much difference. On the contrary, the higher someone gets
within this psychodynamic, the more miserable and enraged she
is likely to be because the greater the gap between the bliss she
is supposed to feel and her own emptiness. Moreover, increasing the promotion rate of women just because they are women
creates problems of equity that will be no less real for the fact
that they, too, are liable to be found in the organization's dark
side.

The Projection of the Dark Side

The capacity to blame others for one's own experiences of limitation and finitude suggests that one's own dark side is being
projected onto others, where it can be freely and righteously
condemned. In this case, one and the other members of one's
group are free to nourish themselves with the fantasy of the ego
ideal, gaining a sense of identity through the process.

If we reflect upon what has been said about the psychological significance of hierarchy, we may observe that this is a
familiar process in organizational phenomenology. Thus, Sennett and Cobb, in their monumental study, *The Hidden Injuries*

of Class (1972), observe how lower participants in organizations bear the brunt of shame as a result of their placement in the social structure. It is likely that the experiences of job dissatisfaction, stress, alienation, and so on, which organizational psychology has traditionally associated with low position in the hierarchy and which it has attempted to alleviate (see, for example, McGregor, 1960), are largely the results of this projection and condemnation. What such psychologies lose sight of is that the motivation to avoid such condemnation by rising in the hierarchy has been a major element in the psychological structure of organizations as we have known them. This, of course, simply adds to what we have seen about the dark side of hierarchy.

This raises an interesting question about the future course of organizations. In recent years, perhaps at least in part as a result of the moral desert that the psychology of hierarchy has created within them, the effectiveness of hierarchical organizations has come into serious question (see, for example, Peters and Waterman, 1982). The contemporary trend in organizations is certainly to reduce the hierarchical dimension and flatten their structure. The question that this raises is What happens to the dark side?

If the dark side is not acknowledged as being within oneself, it must be projected outward. If the abolition of hierarchy precludes its being projected onto lower participants in the organization, the possibility develops that it will be projected outside the organization. Then the function of the organization will be to condemn and attack parts of its own environment, under the guise of a crusade against badness.

The process I have described is certainly a familiar one in political affairs. For example, Jerrold Post (1986a, 1986b) has observed how terrorist groups divide the world into "us and them," good and evil, and achieve a sense of consolidated identity for their members by attacking the evil that they see in the world outside them. Indeed, the group defines its own goodness by its attack upon this badness.

It is easy to see this mechanism at work in a group like ACT-UP or Earth First!, whose reason for existence is political. It is harder to imagine how a business organization could adopt this orientation. One may speculate, however, that as such organizations develop, their conscious business strategy may come to be based on the deployment of moral revulsion against those who do not buy their products and those who would regulate their activities. Again, internally, those employees who do not put themselves entirely at the disposal of the organization could come to be seen as "foreign bodies," so to speak, and threatened with condemnation or expulsion. Totalitarianism would not be too strong a term for this development. At any rate, the reasoning reveals a potential dark side to the adoption of overtly political stances and imagery by organizations such as The Body Shop and Benneton.

What makes this incipient movement even more disturbing is the way it seems to fit into other trends within society. As Post (1986b, p. 29; emphasis added) observes: "This labeling process . . . bolsters the tendency to look outward for the source of problems and to strike out to get rid of their sources. *This rhetoric of polarization is psychologically attractive to the alienated and troubled adolescent/youth as well as to individuals with borderline personality structures.*"

It takes little imagination to conceive that such organizations may become very attractive, not to fringe elements but to the very mainstream of today's youth. Certainly one does not want to condemn an organization for doing good. However, this psychology defines doing good as destroying evil, and that is not always the same thing, especially if the putative victim is innocent or even no more guilty than anyone else.

Toward Acknowledging the Dark Side

It may be useful to observe here, as I have suggested concerning Larry Ross, that Maslow understood that reconciling oneself with one's dark side is a necessary element in the process of self-actualization:

> [Self-actualizing people] can accept their own human nature in the stoic style, with all its shortcomings, with all its discrepancies from the ideal image

without feeling real concern. It would convey the
wrong impression to say that they are self-satisfied.
What we must say rather is that they can take the
frailties and sins, weaknesses, and evils of human
nature in the same unquestioning spirit with which
one accepts the characteristics of nature. One does
not complain about water because it is wet, or about
rocks because they are hard, or about trees because
they are green [1970, pp. 155–156].

And:

Be it observed that this amounts to saying in another
form . . . that the self-actualized person sees reality more clearly; our subjects see human nature as
it *is* and not as they would prefer it to be [p. 156].

The capacity to accept human reality for what it is, in
oneself as well as others, makes for the possibility of an identification with others that is more real and therefore more profound than that of mutual idealization in the ego ideal. It in-
fuses all our activities because it represents a fundamental change
in the way we experience ourselves and others.

Certainly this capacity for identification contributes to
what Maslow (1970, p. 179) has called "the resolution of dichoto-
mies in self-actualization," of which he says: "The dichotomy
between selfishness and unselfishness disappears altogether in
healthy people because in principle every act is *both* selfish and
unselfish. . . . Duty cannot be contrasted with pleasure nor work
with play when duty *is* pleasure, when work *is* play, and the
person doing his duty and being virtuous is simultaneously seeking his pleasure and being happy." The implications of this for
the psychology of work motivation are easy to imagine.

The current tendency toward the politicization of organizational life, looked at in its most positive light, represents
a search for a basis for morality in our lives. These days, the
desperation behind this search has become almost palpable. Our
times offer us, it seems to me, two options for defining its metric.

First is the externalization of the dark side and the pursuit of morality through its destruction. Second is the integration of the dark side and the experience of identification.

My argument here is that the suppression of the dark side leads not only to a loss of intellectual leverage but also to a loss of personal, organizational, and even social vitality. This suggests that bringing light to the dark side, painful though it may be, is likely to be less painful and more productive in the long run than leaving it in the dark.

9

The Four Questions of Life: Their Effect on Human Motivation and Organizational Behavior

Frederick I. Herzberg

Existential questions evolve from the existential pause in human development, not the pause of animals listening or choosing a path in the woods but of human beings reflecting on their own capability: If I am so damn smart, why am I so damn helpless? To answer, they invent tools, grow crops, develop pesticides. In other words, they "determine into" the system of the physical universe.

Human work is a product of the human determination to create a different world. At the empirical level, human work is an attempt to harness the system of natural laws for our own purposes through the development and application of technology. However, science can only help us invent more glasses to see the boundaries of the physical system better. We develop bigger and bigger encyclopedias, but they are still bounded by hard covers. Even primitive humans could see that if they had all knowledge and were able to harness the system perfectly, they would still be bounded by a system that they did not choose. If the answer to the musical question, Is that all there is? is yes, we refuse to accept it. We are also determined to create a mystery system.

Mystery systems exist in all human cultures, created to answer four scientifically unanswerable questions: (1) Why me? (2) Whom do I turn to? (3) What should I do? and (4) Who am I? This chapter briefly contrasts the different answers to these existential questions offered by mystery systems of the West (Hellenism, Judaism, Christianity, and Islam) versus mystery systems of the East (Taoism, Hinduism, and Buddhism). Some effects of these answers on human motivation and organizational behavior in East and West are also suggested.

Why Me?

Why me? is the first unanswerable question asked by human beings, and it has been asked throughout human history.

Primitive Man and Primitive Organization

When a primitive man comes home from a hunt and discovers that his house has been blown down by a strong wind, what is the second thing he says? (We know what the first is: !&!!%.) He does not just sit back and say to himself that this was a meaningless event in a meaningless world. He asks something to the effect of Why me?

Man cannot accept meaninglessness, so he asks the question, Why? Since his family cannot answer, the primitive man turns to the shaman (a group authority), who tells him: "I know why your house blew down. You failed to propitiate the great god, Thor." The primitive man is relieved; he has an answer to why his house blew down. It is not important that he has the right answer. As long as there is some kind of existential explanation, then what happened to him is no longer meaningless, and therefore he is no longer meaningless.

Now we bring a meteorologist into the picture, and he says to the man whose house was blown down: "Thor had nothing to do with it. Your house was destroyed and will again be destroyed because you built it in the wrong place." The meteorologist shows our primitive man homes built in a protective cove on the other side of the hill that have never been blown down. Do the shaman and primitive man welcome the new explanation with open arms? No. The primitive man becomes confused and angry, while his shaman forms a vigilante committee to hang the meteorologist.

Is our primitive friend dumb? No. If he had accepted the meteorologist's explanation, then every significant encounter in his life would have required a completely different compartmentalized explanation; and that runs counter to another very real need, namely, the human need for unified explanations. This need for psychological ecology is just as real as the need for biological ecology.

Life, after all, is made up of a lot of bewildering encounters. All scientists can do is tell you what is happening and how it is happening. The primitive man's house blew down; the meteorologist gave him an explanation. But suppose the primitive man's wife runs away, his daughter dies, and his tools are stolen? The meteorologist has no explanation for these events. The man would have to talk to a marriage counselor, to a physician, and to a police officer to get comparable "scientific" explanations. Yet that isn't necessary, or existentially satisfying, because the shaman has the answer to Why me? and Whom do I turn to? for all these events. The house blew down (Thor), wife ran away (Thor), daughter died (Thor), tools stolen (Thor). He gives a one-stop, one-premium homeowner's policy for all of the bewildering encounters in life. He gives a semblance of unity, a personal mystery system.

A mystery system is an empirically unverifiable explanation promulgated by an institution to maintain its own organizational integrity and believed in by its constituency to maintain a semblance of the unity of their existence.

First Principle of Organizational Behavior

Is the shaman dumb? No, he couldn't create an explanation like Thor and be a stupid man. Out of the shaman's explanation grows an entire organization, with all its helpers, shrines, and payrolls. The need for the original explanation is no longer so important to the shaman because he is now in charge of an organization that has taken on life of its own. And here we have one of the first principles of organizational behavior: The primary obligation of the leaders of any organization is to maintain the integrity of the organization.

Answers of the Mystery Systems

The three major mystery systems of the East—Taoism, Hinduism, and Buddhism—answer the Why me? question this way: Your pain is existentially unimportant. See these bewildering events as insignificant in terms of the aeons of time that the universe has seen. You are only part of this immense and mysterious whole.

Taoism, a religion and philosophy of China, reputed to have been founded by Lao-tzu (604–517 B.C.), teaches that human pain comes as a result of being out of harmony with Tao, the way the universe functions. Hinduism, a complex body of beliefs and practices largely confined to the Indian subcontinent, holds that Brahman, the supreme world soul, forms the innermost essence of all life. All individual souls pass from body to body in a round of rebirths until they become pure enough to be united with Brahman, when the soul is liberated from individual existence and pain. Most Hindus worship Siva, the destroyer, who replies to Why me? with the answer: To make room for the new. Buddhism, the teaching ascribed to Gautama Buddha (563–438 B.C.), holds that suffering is inherent in life and comes from the folly of individual desires.

In contrast, the major mystery systems of the West—Hellenism, Judaism, Christianity, and Islam—all agree that human pain is significant, but Hellenism and Judaism had difficulty answering the Why me? question. If individuals matter, as Western mystery systems hold, then why do the worthy and the innocent suffer? Hellenism—or Greek thought—explained that man is the tragic victim of a pantheon of gods and fates. The individual can turn to the gods for help, but they are unreliable: man must rely on his wits. To do this, the Hellenes developed scientific methods for obtaining knowledge, but the rules of silence do not permit ultimate Why? questions, only questions of What? (bewildering event happened) and How? (it happened). The Jews were perplexed by human pain. They could turn to Almighty God with the question, but God did not have to answer. The book of Job shows that the Jews who wrote the Old Testament concluded that the Why me? question is unanswerable. So have the modern survivors of the Holocaust.

Christianity, on the other hand, was able to answer Why me? with the concept of original sin. All humankind is guilty of Adam's disobedience. No one is innocent, and so no one deserves to escape suffering. Since a human being cannot bear meaningless events, the explanation "You are guilty" can bring great relief. Islam, which means submission, also answers Why me? questions simply: The will of Allah.

Earning Loyalty

Organizations earn loyalty from their members when they help unify beliefs that fit into the underlying mystery systems of their cultures. The Eastern systems tend to agree that individual human pain is unimportant in the overall scheme of the universe and that the individual should strive to lose his ego as part of a larger whole—to become like Buddha, an egoless wonder.

The manager of an organization in Taiwan, Singapore, or Japan, when asked Why me?—for example, Why do I have to retire so early?—can frequently answer, You are part of this company and that policy is good for the company. The small *i* egos supported by mystery systems of the East tend to give loyalty to organizations that emphasize dependence and to struggle for self-denial. This means that organizational loyalty is not so difficult to achieve in the East. For the Japanese to say, "What is good for Sony is good for Japan" is considered very proper. Yet, when onetime U.S. Secretary of Defense Charles E. Wilson observed that "what's good for General Motors is good for the country," he was vilified.

Western mystery systems agree that individual human pain is important, but they have disagreed on the answers to Why me? Hellenism answers: I am tragic. Judaism answers:

I am perplexed. Both conclude: I am worthy. In contrast, Christianity concludes: I am guilty; Islam concludes: I must submit. Schizophrenia of these conflicting capital *I* identities is much more difficult to manage than an inferiority complex.

Whom Do I Turn To?

Whom do I turn to? is the second unanswerable question asked by human beings. Echoing many authors in this book, this question poses the problem of existential loneliness. That loneliness dynamic underlies most of the pain that human beings suffer in this world. Does a tree in an unknown forest exist? The answer to that question is yes. Does it exist with meaning? The answer is no. To have meaning is to receive attention from a being capable of self-awareness. Only humans—and presumably God—have that capacity. That is philosophically having your cake and eating it too. The tree exists, but it has no meaning. Does an individual living unknown exist? The answer is yes, like that tree. Does that individual have meaning? The answer is no. As we live our lives, parts of us fall like that tree. If no one knows or cares, we still exist, but not meaningfully.

Answers of the Mystery Systems

In the mysteries of the East, the deity is not interested in me as an individual, so I must turn to the group—family, government, and business organizations. The Eastern mysteries normalize the inferiority complex—I am insignificant—a disease that makes it very easy for organizations to manage people.

Because Brahman has no human attributes, to answer the question Whom do I turn to? Hinduism allows the worship of a multitude of gods as stepping stones to understanding Brahman. To answer the same question, Buddhists turn inward and escape into Nirvana (extinction of desire). Taoism is also a cold concept that does not answer the existential question Whom do I turn to? So the Chinese turned to a pantheon of household gods for comfort, and to the family itself. The teachings of Confucius (551–479 B.C.) attempted to answer the question without reference to a mystery system at the top. The central answers of Confucianism are *chu,* or loyalty, and *ko,* or filial piety. Japanese Confucianism emphasized *chu* as a support for feudal lord-vassal relations.

In the West, Jews and Muslims turned to Almighty God, and Christianity to a compassionate Christ. During modern times, however, the West has exported Christianity to underdeveloped countries and has tended to live by the scientific method of Hellenism, which has fractionated the egos of modern man. Whom do I turn to? If I am in a hospital with twenty specialists working on me, am I comforted? No. The demigods of medicine only pull me apart because each deals only with part of my anatomy or psyche. I am better off believing in a transcendental God, even if I cannot prove his existence, than being pulled apart psychologically.

Humans have a need to know and a need not to know. It is much better for mental health to patch up a unity of beliefs than to be empirically correct but fragmented.

The Caring Dynamic in Organizations

Organizations can find no ultimate answer to the pain in life. No solution for Why me? questions. The best we hope for is to minimize our pain. Nor can we find ultimate satisfaction in caring and being cared for, as a solution to Whom do I turn to? We cannot experience as much relief from a pat on the back as a dog can because underlying all human relationships are reservations and expectations for the ultimate. A dog has fewer reservations because he has no concept of the ultimate. He cannot experience human happiness, but his animal relief from being cared for is tremendous. Because we have been taught to despise and yet overvalue the animal side of our nature, we have learned to mask our need for animal comfort with all kinds of symbols, slogans, and demands for reciprocity.

The new emphasis by organizations on people assets is an example of the worst kind of reciprocity in all aspects of caring. Historically, management's approach to its workers has been that of animal trainers. Many of the people problems in orga-

nizations result from attempts to manipulate humans' animal
needs as a means of getting more work out of them.

Should managers expect workers to be grateful for a good
job environment? No! Caring for the animal needs of workers
does not make managers better human beings. It simply makes
them more compassionate animals. Paternalism was hated precisely because of this inversion of expectations. An animal does
not expect or deserve a reward for its compassion. Caring is
a natural animal reaction; even chimpanzees care for wounded
members of their tribe. We see today in our school curricula
a decline in the study of the humanities and a rise in the study
of technological crafts. This has spilled over into human relations. We feel we can rise to humanity through technology, but
more technology has meant more depersonalization.

Our institutions have created depersonalized organizations to deal with the problem of depersonalization. The organizations have created professional carers rather than compassionate carers. *P* caring stands for professions, paid, and so often,
pretentious. It is practiced by all the *P* professions: priests and
pastors, physicians, professors, psychologists, politicians, police
officers, prostitutes, and the press and lawyers. Lawyers definitely belong on the *P* carer list, and I am sure there is something typically lawyerish in their managing to have a name that
does not begin with the appropriate letter *P*. The *P* carers have
learned the technology of "stroking" antiseptically, with the organizational and "profession" procedures screening out any genuine human contact and with it any genuine comfort for the
sufferer. The *P* carers, in turn, generate their own creatures:
more laws, bureaucratic regulations, and psychological red tape,
which only lead to less understanding on the part of the individual and add the pressure of bewilderment to all the other
pressures.

Modern human beings are having to turn more and more
to such *P* carers. We are expected to pay for all caring in money,
favors, or at least groveling gratitude. I object to the lack of
simple compassion that results when the professional rules of
the organization absolve the *P* carer from responsible human
involvement. The bureaucracy injects itself more and more into

the intimate life of the individual. For every move one makes, one must "negotiate" some contract, a contract not designed to solve one's problem, to relieve one's suffering, but to preserve the integrity of some organization and to absolve that organization of the responsibility for ethical behavior.

To administer the technology of all these contracts, we are educating more and more narrow specialists to whom the individual must apply for help for relief from pain. If one cannot speak the correct technological jargon of the P carer assigned to one, one is accused of failure to communicate.

Today we are taking more training in communications. We have to learn to communicate on the job with our boss, with our co-workers, with our subordinates. At home we have to learn to communicate with our spouses, with our children. Why can't we get through to each other? Why all this need for communications training, for human relations technology? Because we are demanding reciprocity in areas of our lives where we have no right to expect reciprocity, and we are not demanding justice in those areas where we do have the right to expect it. Human relations technology fails because it demands quid pro quo for decent treatment. We have to be able to interact on the human level without the "contract" and stop asking to be paid back for caring. Otherwise, if we want a breath of fresh air, we cannot simply step outside; we must go to a national park and face more crowding and bureaucratic regulation. If we want sun all over our bodies, we must join a nudist organization and adhere to its regulation. If we want sex, we must read the manual and sign the "contract" ensuring satisfactory performance.

Such contractual arrangements bring relief to organizations but not to the individuals involved. The result for individuals is that we rely more and more on the cold flesh of technology, which furthers our desperation and creates more addiction to that cold flesh and less confidence in our ability to find human satisfactions in life.

Our cultural evolution has outrun our biological and psychological evolution. The result is that all our adaptations today are pathologic: adaptations that allow us to read the fine print of all the contracts that are supposed to relieve us of the pain in life but which drive us farther toward insanity. We are devoting more of our energies to sustaining our pathologies because we fear that if we do not read all the fine print, we will be destroyed psychologically or even biologically. This obsession with trivia leaves little room for our aspirations to rise to humanity.

In their communications with workers, both as individuals and in the group's structures, managers must recognize that the demands they will hear will be cries of pain. They must alleviate that pain insofar as possible but also recognize that no matter what they do or how much they spend, those cries of pain will still be there. There is no final solution to the animal needs of human beings. People will always find something that hurts, especially if they hate their jobs. Managers should not expect, however, that because they have shown that they care by minimizing workers' pain that workers owe them something in return. Managers have no "right" to expect gratitude or other kinds of reciprocity for the animal compassion of caring for the animal need to be comforted.

How do managers minimize the animal pains we all suffer? By having compassion, making the workers' environment (including their interpersonal relationship) as comfortable as possible. But managers should not try to motivate a human being by taking advantage of his or her animal needs. They try it every time they give a person a decent wage, provide him or her with an adequate working environment, and in return expect that person to repay them with increased production and higher-quality work. When they satisfy a human being's animal needs there can be no quid pro quo.

What Should I Do?

Belief in participative management receives support from the mystery systems of the East — Taoism, Hinduism, and Buddhism — which promise pain reduction through avoidance of human conflicts. Their heaven is the death of ego. They have provided for participation primarily through processes for coping with the pain of self. The major Western mystery systems — Hellenism, Judaism, Christianity, and Islam — have been concerned with self-actualizing participation.

All of these systems have endured because to some degree they have met three criteria:

Mystery, inspiring interest and awe
Protection from rational analysis
Ability to provide for a method of participation in the mystery system — an answer to another existential question: What should I do? or How should I participate in the system?

Mystery Systems of the East

Taoism, the ancient religion of China, focuses on a mysterious first principle of the universe — Tao, "the Way" — which satisfies the first criterion for a lasting mystery system. All existence and change in the universe spring mysteriously from this first principle. Contradictions in Tao are protected from rational analysis by the secondary principle of the unity and harmony of opposites. All things spring from a combination of the positive, bright, masculine *yang* principle with the negative, dark, feminine *yin* principle. Taoism instructs human beings to participate in the mystery by conforming to Tao through unassertive action. The teachings of Confucius later elaborated on the cardinal virtues of loyalty and filial piety.

Hinduism, the ancient religion of India, also tends to view all forms and thoughts as aspects of the one eternal being and truth — Brahman. It is protected from rational analysis by the endless numbers and complicity of all of its sacred aspects and also by the doctrine of reincarnation. (Respect for all aspects of life is reinforced if one believes that in the next life one may be a cow or even an insect.) The Hindu participates through the "way of works" (doing good), the "way of knowledge," or the "way of devotion" as a means of release from the round of rebirths and union with the one great eternal being and truth, a state of Nirvana (extinction of the individual desire). However, the caste system reinforced by this religion, reaching from untouchable at the bottom to Brahmins at the top, became so rigid that it killed the hopes and motivations of individuals in this life.

As for Buddhism, Gautama Buddha focuses on the mysterious human ability to escape into Nirvana in this life. Nirvana in Buddhism is not a negative state. It is, rather, an awakening to a new reality that defies the usual logic and rationality of thinking. The state is one of nonthinking and expanded awareness. The state of Nirvana is protected from rational analysis by rituals designed to put the mind at rest — to give up all mental struggles. The Buddhist participates by mental and moral purification — a major method of which is meditation similar to that practiced by Buddha and one also favored by Hindu yogis.

The goal of participation in the Eastern mystery systems is always to lose individual desire and come into harmony with the environment; the goal is never to "mold it nearer to the heart's desire," as in the West. There are now transcendental meditation groups in the United States that try to use their techniques to reduce the number of casualties in foreign wars, a predictable Western inversion of methods of participation in an Eastern mystery: trying to change others rather than oneself.

Mystery Systems of the West

The Greeks (or Hellenes) saw mystery in the natural order of events. When Aristotle saw the beauty and simplicity in his method of classification, he elevated it to a metaphysical mystery, as Pythagoras before him had made a mystery of mathematics. The Hellenic mystery system presupposed that inherent in the universe is a rationale, a logic that is discoverable. This assumption led to the mystery system of science. Einstein said: "I shall never believe that God plays dice with the world," even though his dream to develop a unified field theory was frustrated. Every new discovery in science leads to more questions; hence, ultimate answers are protected and are beyond analysis. The appeal of science is its mystery, and the way to participate in this mystery is through the discovery of natural law. It meets all the criteria for a lasting mystery system:

Mysteries of the natural universe
Protection from rational analysis (Human beings can never find out everything about the universe; progression and regression are infinite.)

Ability to provide for a method of participation (One should seek knowledge through scientific method.)

To get reliable, empirical knowledge, humankind has developed scientific methods for determining which knowledge is reliable and which is not. The first, and still the most pervasive, method of gathering reliable knowledge is experience: observation. All organisms have some kind of sensory mechanisms that enable them to process incoming information into reliable knowledge. But, of course, individual observations often prove to be wrong. A second method of developing reliable knowledge is classification. Things tend to classify themselves in certain ways. Look-alike is one common classification method, although we have to be careful — whales look like fish, but they are mammals. Still another method is co-relationship, which has evolved into what we call the statistical method today. Just as classification is a more powerful method than simple observation (freeing one from having to observe every detail of every event), so the statistical method is more powerful than classification. However, its focus on relationships can be dangerous because relationships do not necessarily mean cause and effect. Finally, we invented the most powerful method for getting reliable knowledge: experimentation. This method consists of techniques to minimize the number of spurious cause-and-effect relationships and allows us to select those over which we have a measure of control. The danger here lies in ignoring causes that cannot be controlled, which are frequently the most significant.

Historically, humans started out with scientific method at its most primitive level: observation. Then they reverted to the method of authority because they needed to answer Why me? questions. But *why* questions are not permitted in science. Science is the study of *what;* religion is the study of *why.* Science assumes that the world is governed by natural laws and that human beings are capable of discovering those laws. Religion assumes that the world is governed by supernatural laws and that these laws can be revealed by God or his authorities.

These different assumptions lead to very different methodologies for gaining knowledge: seeing is believing versus receiving is believing. Trying to give religious answers to scientific questions leads to physical illness and mishap. And trying to give scientific answers to existential questions leads to fragmentation and insanity. To remain sane, the Western mind has been forced to segment the scientific methods favored by Hellenism from unifying methods of authority favored by Judaism, Christianity, and Islam.

Judaism centers on the concept of a transcendental deity, which satisfies the first criterion of a lasting mystery system. Transcendental means extending beyond the limits of capable human experience. In other words, the Jews made their God so mysterious that he-she is beyond human comprehension. Their God was protected from rational analysis by the first commandment: (1) no other gods, (2) no graven images, and (3) no misuse of God's name.

Why not, like the Greeks and Romans, have a whole pantheon of gods? Because, as one tribe fights the other in battle, each praying to its own god, the losers begin to lose faith. If there is only one God, he cannot be tested. Without comparison, there is no rational analysis. The Jews went even further: they blocked off sensory observation (no graven images), and they made God's name sacrosanct. It was not to be spoken or written. As a result, Judaism never developed a theology. How could it attempt to explain the unexplainable?

To meet the third criterion — participation — architects of Judaism had several alternatives open to them. Sacrifice was one of the more popular forms of participation in the pagan religions of the time. However, sacrifice is meant for a rich society. Lambs are expensive, and only overpopulated societies sacrifice people. The Jews were neither rich nor overpopulated. They were nomadic tribes. What they really needed was cohesiveness. So Moses gave the Jews the Decalogue, a set of laws governing human behavior. That became their cohesive force and the means for participating in their religion. Moses' laws are generalized statements of ethics and morality open to a myriad of interpretations. The questions What does it mean? and How and when do you abide by it? have occupied formal and informal Jewish scholars for centuries. How should I partici-

pate in the Judaic mystery system? I should develop the meaning of the law, applying it to every aspect of human life. This
development still goes on today. Since God in scriptures prescribed how the rituals, not the law, were to be implemented,
there were few lasting precedents. Therefore, although the Decalogue provides the standards with which Jews satisfy the need
for unity in their lives, it also allows them the variability so necessary to the individual. The Judaic mystery system idealized the
goal of social justice. Its strength lay in its affirmation of life
and the validity of seeking knowledge to live a better, more ethical life. But it did not answer the *why* of pain and death.

The public relations practice of hyphenating to give an
appearance of unity is nowhere more inappropriate than in the
term *Judeo-Christian*. There could hardly be two more different
systems, if you consider their essence (not the numerous sects
that have sprung up). The Jewish belief in the Messiah, the
anointed one, was tied to a belief in a Messianic Age, an age
when participation in the Jewish mystery system, the living of
the Decalogue on earth, would be fulfilled. But no matter how
much the prophets preached, life was getting worse, more unethical, not better, at the time of Christ. How did the Christian
explain this? Man was trying to create something — a Messianic
Age — that could not be done on earth. Why not? Because man
is imperfect, so the concept of original sin became very important. Why me? was answered. All humankind was guilty of
Adam's sin of disobedience, seeking knowledge of what humans
had been commanded not to know, the sin of pride (discovery).

But if there was not to be a Messianic Age on earth, why
did Christ come? To make imperfect humans whole again, to
expiate for original sin by sacrificing himself on the cross. The
criteria for a lasting mystery system were met:

> Christ was hidden in the mystery of the Trinity and the
> Kingdom of Heaven, both beyond human empirical
> comprehension.
> Christ was the Son of God, who died for our sins and was
> resurrected from the dead — a personality and an event

that defy rational analysis. Answers were not of this world; thus, no event in this world would challenge the mystery. Christ could comfort one's pains and ensure one's salvation and resurrection after death. This was a great strength, especially to a slave population from which Christianity drew its first converts. But what was the weakness of Christianity as a mystery system? Christianity's answer to What should I do? was I should seek salvation in the Kingdom of Heaven. This was such a problem to early Christians that it resulted in mass suicides. Early converts were by and large slaves. If one persuades people who are in the depths of misery and despair that the answer to their pain is in the Kingdom of Heaven, then certainly they will try to get there as soon as possible. This became such a problem that the church had to condemn suicide in its dogmas.

How should Christians seek salvation? Avoid sin. However, Christians were caught in a bind. Everything they tried to do as perfected human beings could be viewed as a sin of pride. Should one become a Mother Teresa, a rationalist like Descartes, or a self-flagellating monastic? St. Augustine and later Calvin in the concept of predestination decided that there was no way for Christians to earn salvation; they could only be elected to it by God's grace. Christians never developed a unique method of participation because they were caught in the double bind that sin is necessarily produced out of attempts to avoid sin. Great acts of humanity and great brutalities were committed in the name of Christianity. The ritual of absolution seemed the only way out, and Christians became addicted to forgiveness. Many focused on proselytizing as a mechanism for fulfilling the command, "Love thy neighbor as thyself." But, as Freud explains, proselytizing is a symptom of the defense mechanism called projection — projecting your needs onto the other person: You must need what I need. Islam solved this problem by combining Judaic and Christian methods of participation, that is, studying the law (the Koran) *and* proselytizing for converts.

Adversarial Participation

How should I participate? The standard answer of most organizations is: You should do it our way. The Eastern ego will
tend to accept this organizational answer because the focus of
its participation is to seek harmony. Management in countries
like Japan can encourage ritualized exercises and meditation
to reduce stress levels in individuals and allow them temporary
escapes that are reinforced by their mystery systems. Management in the East can send out a consistent participation message, primarily: We did it our way. It relies on methods of consensus that can dissolve contradictions through emotion because
of the small *i* emphasis in the Eastern mystery systems.

Western capital *I* egos will not accept "Do it our way" as
an answer without rational proof; and any appearance of injustice will rankle. Western mystery systems lead to adversarial participation messages: Let me convert you to my way with
authority (God is on my side) and scientific method (here are
my data). The authority of the individual sings out, I'll do it
my way, while management counters, You must be a team
player.

Such inconsistent social messages place employees in a
double bind and reinforce a split mind, unless managers recognize the existential need to leave some room for "I'll do it my
way." Without the possibility of individual variability, workers
cannot find meaning in the content of their participation, and
motivation to work will diminish.

Who Am I?

To survive, organizations have to manage within the values of
the religious mysteries predominant in their cultures. The mystery systems of the East — Taoism, Hinduism, and Buddhism —
all emphasize the subjugation of the individual ego to a larger
whole. In other words, the Eastern answer to the existential question Who am I? tends to be: You are meaningful only as part
of a larger universe. It emphasizes an expanded group ego: Tao,
Brahman, Nirvana. Eastern mystery systems reinforce a small

i ego goal — and with it an inferiority complex that is very easy
for organizations to manage.

In contrast, the predominant mystery systems of the West —
Hellenism, Judaism, Christianity, and Islam — all agree on the
elevation and development of the individual ego as a larger and
more important self with a capital *I*. Their answer to the existential question Who am I? is: You are meaningful as a unique
individual. But the Western mysteries are split on what that
means. Adversarial religions have reinforced the Western disease of the split mind, the double bind — a disease that is very
difficult to manage.

Inferiority Complex of the East

All mystery systems overgeneralize some of their values. The
Eastern mystery systems have overgeneralized the goal of static
or circular harmony at the expense of growth and justice. Chinese Communists felt that they had to get rid of the old values
of Taoism and Confucianism in order to achieve growth. However, they continued to reinforce their citizens' inferiority complex, which had been normalized by the old systems of belief.
The "nonassertive conformity" to Tao and Confucian "filial piety"
to parents were simply transferred. The ego goal of "i am in
harmony with Tao" became "i am in harmony with Mao."

The ego goal of Hinduism has been "I am in harmony
with Brahman (all soul)." The modern government of India has
outlawed many of the debilitating practices of the ancient Hindu
caste system in an attempt to achieve greater growth and justice,
but the country continues to be ruled by families of the highest
caste. The inferiority complex of those in the lower castes is much
more profound than that of the so-called lower classes in the
West. They will defend themselves against the adversarial Muslims in their midst, and on their borders, but their tendency
is to bow to the authority of higher castes.

Buddhists of India, China, Japan, and other countries
of the East have emphasized inner harmony by coping with displaced hostilities that inevitably flow out of the inferiority complex. The Buddhist ego goal is "i am in harmony with Nirvana"

(extinction of individual desire). The ritual exercises of yoga among the Hindus and tai chi among the Chinese have served much the same purpose as Buddhist meditation.

The "laws" of hostility dictate that frustration must be expressed. Either it will be expressed directly against those in our environment who are frustrating us, or it will be displaced onto innocent parties, or it will be turned inward on ourselves. The mystery systems of the East forbid direct expression of hostility against the authorities. Since justice is not a central value in the East, organizations can allow frustrations to be displaced downward in the hierarchy—to the lower castes, to women, or to minorities—much more than this can be allowed in the West. However, such displacement must be limited or social order is disrupted. It can be turned inward, but this leads to self-destructive depression unless regular coping mechanisms are developed. Through such coping mechanisms as ritual exercise and meditation the Eastern mystery systems have answered the problem of displaced hostility. The ritual exercises that precede and interrupt the labor of Japanese workers serve not only to ease cramped muscles but also to cope with the workers' displaced hostility.

Americans tend to believe that Japanese who begin work with the company song and calisthenics are satisfied with the way their companies treat them, even if they have boring jobs. However, a 1981 "critical incidents" study of a variety of jobs in Japan conducted by Y. Kobayashi and I. Igarashi of Tohoku University shows that events that make Japanese workers feel very good on the job are almost never related to hygienic factors of treatment (company policy, supervision, interpersonal relations with peers and supervisors, working conditions, or security). Instead, events that make them feel very good involve motivator factors (their own achievements, recognition, interesting work, responsibility, advancement, and growth)—the same factors that bring job satisfaction to workers in the West (and that I discuss in my books, *Motivation to Work,* 1959; *Work and the Nature of Man,* 1966; and *The Managerial Choice,* 1982). Kobayashi and Igarashi (1981, p. 82) conclude: "These results were not consistent with the view implied in discussions with Japanese management that Japanese find their job satisfaction in inter-

personal relationships or in unification with organization."
The "feel good" factors are the same in Japan as in the
United States because human nature is inherently the same in
both East and West, regardless of mystery systems. Seeking oblivion in group harmony cannot bring long-term motivation and
happiness, only the short-term hygiene of pain avoidance. Different mystery systems explain many different behaviors in organizations, but the universality of "feel good" factors explains the
deeper nature of all human beings. All humans need to *do* something they can learn from. This need for achievement and growth
supersedes any cultural and religious compunction in the long
term.

Split Mind of the West

The mystery systems of the West have overgeneralized the adversarial goal of individual justice at the expense of harmony.
Supporting adversarial values of individual competition, freedom, and proselytizing salesmanship have emphasized not only
the boundaries between individuals but also the schizophrenic
contradictions within individual psyches.

The Greeks elevated individual pursuit of excellence (*arete*)
to a mystery system. The goal of the individual ego was to be
able to say, "I am first" among my competitors. In the Olympic
Games of Ancient Greece there were no prizes for second place
in running, jumping, javelin, or bow and arrow events. Notice
that these were all individual efforts. "The team" was not important in Greek games and combat until development of the
Spartan phalanx began to require more cooperation in warfare.
Since sport and warfare analogies are applied to participation
in business in both East and West, it is useful to remember that
our schizophrenic "How to," "I did it my way; but I'm a team
player," are based on our underlying Hellenic mystery system.

The Judaic mystery system elevated the concept of freedom from enslavement, which has been a powerful guideline
to the value systems in the West. A rallying cry of many Western
social and political revolutions has been: Let my people go! The
ego goal behind this cry has been, I am free—to say no to the
pharaoh, a Caesar, or other earthly authorities. This meant op-

portunity to think, study, argue for one's opinion, and seek justice. Freedom did not mean oblivion, loss of desire, or escape from pain, as it did to Taoists, Hindus, and Buddhists.

The Christian mystery system elevated the concept of salvation of individual souls from death. The ego goal of Christianity has been: I am saved. But conflicting arguments on how to find salvation have led to religious debate, each side insisting: You must need what I need. Islam elevated submission to the will of Allah as revealed in the Koran. However, individual interpretations of the will of Allah are in conflict. The adversarial ego goals — "I am free to say no" but "You must need what I need" — became incorporated into Western existential values, along with "I did it my way; but I'm a team player" and also "God is my authority, but I rely on scientific method." The mystery systems of the West support a unique ego identity, but a fragmented one.

Western mystery systems permit direct expression of hostility against frustrating authority figures much more than do those of the East. If those in authority do not permit overt expression, hostility will tend to be expressed passively through lack of cooperation or even sabotage. When we cannot figure out who is in charge (who's to blame), we will sometimes displace hostility onto those who cannot hit back — but this will be strongly disapproved by Western justice values. If we are forced to turn our hostility inward, we become very depressed — a disease we have not learned to cope with as well as have people of the East. However, we are borrowing many of their methods of meditation and ritual exercise as our depression deepens. The West's copycat syndrome of turning to the East for the secrets of motivating workers is a symptom of psychological depression in the West. In such a period, do we go in copycat directions or do we examine the malaise and discover our own direction? We have no choice but to go in our own direction. East/West ego projections of the universe are too different.

Ego Projections

While the goal of Eastern mystery systems is to deny the individual ego, the effect of mystery systems of the West is to split it. The Eastern systems view nature as sacred. A natural wonder like Mount Everest is to be revered. Art emphasizes landscapes, with human figures given little more importance than animals and plants. Ritual is maximized in every aspect of life to displace hostility and reduce the painful number of individual choices in exercise, work, recreation, and social routines. Finally, death itself is seen as part of the endless harmonious cycles of nature, a process to be accepted—and even sought—when one can no longer fulfill one's part.

In contrast, the Western systems view nature as challenging. Everest is to be conquered simply because it is there. Art has emphasized portraits of human beings in sculpture and stone, with the rest of nature playing a secondary role. Since the Western systems view freedom as the opportunity to develop individual abilities and tastes, rituals are minimized to allow more individual choice. Death is seen as a defeat to be fought at all costs, with artificial hearts for individual bodies and salvation for individual souls. To control individual egos, however, Western mystery systems also have to introduce conflicting messages of teamwork, obedience, and guilt. Surviving amid these conflicting messages has required individuals in the West to struggle for effectiveness in ambiguity, a source of both anxiety and creativity.

Eastern cultures, like human cultures everywhere, have always had to rely on the creative abilities of individuals, but their overemphasis on harmony goals has tended to overcontrol and discourage creativity much more than in the West and to make workers less effective when they encounter the loneliness and ambiguity of independent thought. To get the creativity they now seek, and to continue to grow, Japanese organizations and those of other Eastern cultures are going to have to give individuals more psychological space for experiment, not more managerial boot camps where they learn patience in pursuing meaningless tasks. Authorities are going to have to learn to absorb more direct hostility from subordinates as women and minorities inevitably become less willing to accept displaced hostility and demand more justice. The elaborate rituals of exercise, meditation, etiquette, and military tradition will continue to help displace hostility and to achieve harmony, but not creativity. However, Eastern cultures' overriding goal of harmony will continue to make it easier for them to adopt and adapt ideas generated in the West than it is for our adversarial system to adopt and adapt theirs.

The often-conflicting Western goals of individual happiness (through growth and justice) are based on a real individual nervous system that is more difficult to manage than a manufactured "group mind" but can generate growth as a group mind cannot. The Western problem is overgeneralization of adversarial demands for justice, which heightens debilitating anxieties. To achieve greater harmony, it will be necessary to reduce expectations of absolute equity without giving up the ideal of justice. Only a child expects parents to spend excessive amounts of time dividing the ice cream into mathematically equitable portions. But to manage well, Western organizational policies will have to operate within Western answers to existential questions while encouraging greater effectiveness despite the ambiguity of our conflicting messages.

Expanding my own motivation-hygiene theory of human nature to the existential level, the first two questions, Why me? and Whom do I turn to? follow hygiene dynamics—the need to avoid pain. The third question, What should I do? follows motivator dynamics—the need to seek achievement and growth. The fourth question, Who am I? attempts to unify motivator and hygiene ego identities.

Because of different mystery systems, Eastern answers do not work well in Western organizations and vice versa. But organizations everywhere must take into account the two very different dynamics of human nature. In the West, the do's and don'ts of providing meaning to human existence at work must take the capital *I* into consideration, without encouraging egotism.

• Why me? Don't answer that individual pains and perceptions of injustice are unimportant in terms of the "team effort." Do absorb some direct hostility and give time for individual attention. We tend to assume that individual pains are covered by the legalities, so we overlook them. Special problems require compassion, not due process.

- Whom do I turn to? Don't answer with a company song and ritualized meetings. Do offer individual relationships behind open-door policies and support groups. One-on-one communication will work best. In all organizations, richness of meaning tends to be destroyed by the agenda.
- What should I do? Don't answer that team participation comes first. Do answer that members of the organization should participate as individuals who take responsibility for a good or service, including service to other members of the team. Participation will be more fruitful. The individual who serves must be at least as happy as the individual who is served.
- Who am I? Don't answer that the individual ego is unimportant. Do answer that the individual ego is unique and needs opportunity to grow to be more effective and happy in ambiguous situations. Adversary relationships and anxiety are reduced in those who develop unique expertise and know who they are, in and out of the organization.

With great difficulty and occasional pathology we in the United States have been able to enhance the doctrine of social pluralism. It has been assumed that this tolerant doctrine has elevated the individual. However, we have too long confused the sanctity of the healthy individual ego (who learns to grow without hurting others) with that of the pathologically selfish egotist (who demands that all others must revolve around him). George Meredith, in his novel *The Egoist,* describes such a character perfectly in the person of Sir Willoughby Patterne, who can function only like the central willow pattern on a plate of china, around which all other people are forced to circle harmoniously. The weakness of our mystery systems in the West has been that we can often see no justice unless we are treated as the central ego pattern on the plate. It takes real growth and maturity — not conversion to Eastern mystery systems — to see that as the feast of life progresses, each ego must often play a supporting role.

Part Four

Two Stories
of the Search
for Meaning
in Organizations

10

Organizational Culture and Its Discontents: Life in a Spiritual Community

Burkard Sievers

The fact that the organizational culture literature almost completely lacks reference to Sigmund Freud and his *Civilization and Its Discontents* ([1930] 1957b) may just reflect the reconnotation that psychoanalysis has undergone in the process of its English translation (Bettelheim, 1983). Because Freud in the original German version (*Das Unbehagen in der Kultur,* 1930) explicitly refers to culture and the discomfort and uneasiness it brings with it on the broader societal level, it is appropriate by analogy to look at organizations and the uneasiness with which their members (and clients) are confronted.

Although Freud's main emphasis is on culture and cultural development at the more general level of society, he explicitly refers to the community of the city (of Rome) (Freud, ([1930] 1957b, p. 14). It, therefore, can be assumed that the "soul" of an institution/organization like the soul life of an individual maintains its past as a constituent element of its presence. Like society in general, organizations can thus be perceived as arenas in which the life struggle between "eros and death, the drive for life and the drive for destruction" ([1930] 1957b, p. 97), plays an important role through the organizational culture and its development. As for the individual, organizations also have a limited capacity for happiness: to quite an extent they are predestined to experience misfortune and suffering. As Freud (p. 25) elucidates, this suffering results from three different sources: from the transience of the human body (and the inevitability of individual death), from the potential destructivity through external forces, and from the relationship with other people. Freud (pp. 128–129) further leaves no doubt that the creation and maintenance of a larger human community always contradicts the idea of happiness of its members. "The processes of individual and cultural development meet with hostility and mutually challenge each other's ground." Like the "above-I" (superego) in the case of the individual, organizations can be understood as having a cultural "above-I," an organizational idea that raises its demands (Freud, [1930] 1957b, p. 131; see Schwartz, 1990a).

Contrary to the almost exclusive emphasis on the pursuit of effective task accomplishment and permanent growth in predominant organization and economic theories, organizations, from such an extended understanding of human existence and the struggle for life, appear to be much more ambiguous. On the one hand, organizations allow the accomplishment of goals that go beyond individual capacity and competence; through the identification with something that is greater than oneself, they mediate a sense of identity, potency, and grandeur (Becker, 1973). On the other hand, however, they postulate the renunciation of drives and desires and demand conformity to the norms and discipline of the larger community.

Although it may be true for every organization, the culturally mediated uneasiness and discontent will be extreme if the organization is based on a lifetime or even an "eternal" membership of its staff and/or clients. Despite the fact that people in organizations in general and those at the top of industrial enterprises in particular tend to identify with the institution and to derive their own individual immortality from the fictitious collective one, members of ecclesiastical organizations are embedded in a cultural time horizon from eternity to eternity; the way they are able to cope with cultural discontent during this life is immediately related to their life after death. And often the expected easiness, comfort, and context of eternal life in heaven may even cause or contribute to the discontent with the narrower organizational culture in this world.

It seems that religious or ecclesiastical organizations increase the possible experience of ambiguity to an enormous extent in comparison to other organizations in general and to work enterprises in particular. Contrary to the latter, in which one's work and its related experience more often than ever may be accompanied by imaginations of purgatory or even hell, the former are explicitly oriented toward heaven as the empire of the blessed and eternal blissful happiness. In promising the fulfillment of religious needs (primarily in a life after death), these organizations nevertheless, at least latently, contribute to the reactivation of feelings of infantile helplessness and the strong desire for a father, on which, according to Freud ([1930] 1957b, p. 18), these needs are based. Although these organizations predominantly aim to reduce the suffering in the world through works of charity, they often enough tend to sustain a helplessness toward the suffering that results from the relationship among its members (and/or its clients).

Whereas organizations in general are supposed to be only successful in a creative sense if they incorporate a "spirit of enterprise," religious organizations have to be built on spirituality in a much broader sense. Spirituality as man's collective attempt and capacity to relate human life and existence meaningfully to the universe and the cosmos thus necessarily must refer to God as the world's creator and the guarantor of human life. Regardless of whether a particular ecclesiastical organization favors sexual procreation among its members or excludes it via the vow of chastity, this spirituality irrenounceably includes a vision of how men and women are supposed to cope with their sexuality and how it may be related to their eternal existence.

In this chapter, an attempt is made to understand the possible psychosocial dynamics of a home for "fallen girls" run by sisters of the Order of the Good Shepherd. The exploration of some of the root metaphors, guiding rites, myths, and symbols leads to various working hypotheses that can be further explored in consultation or action research. It will also be shown that the basic inequality from which the organization derives its

meaning—in other words, that of "holy sisters" and "fallen
girls"—serves, from a psychoanalytic and systemic perspective,
as a surrogate for and defense against the underlying equality
or similarity of the predominant pattern of object relatedness:
regardless of whether the actors are "nuns" or "girls," the women
in this institution relate to "the man" through partial object relations. Whereas in its particular case the inequality among
members and inmates is culturally primarily managed through
a religious spiritualization of sexuality, it becomes evident that
the cultural management of equality/inequality among people
in (social) organizations is more often than ever not only artificial, or sometimes even fictitious, but is also the main source
of the discontent, uneasiness, and discomfort experienced in organizational cultures.

Although the following case vignette leads into a social
reality that for most contemporaries may appear unfamiliar, it
nevertheless mirrors fundamental human concerns; regardless
of their specific "answer" or "solution," these concerns must
be dealt with in almost every organization and its culture,
in terms of the meaning that its members relate to their work,
lives, and death and how the organizational task, boundaries,
differences, resources, and so on are supposed to be perceived
and managed.

From Organizational Culture
to Organizational Symbolism

The (re)discovery of culture was the central issue in the discussion of organizational theory during the last decade. The debate on organizational culture (for example, Alvesson, 1990;
Frost and others, 1985; Schein, 1985; Turner, 1990) can be seen
as a kind of counterreaction to previous attempts at describing
and shaping organizations in a rational and objective way. In
place of the issue of optimization of organizational configura-
tion, structures, and processes, the question arises as to whether
and how the organizational culture of enterprises can be shaped
in such a way as to turn them to competitive advantage "in [the]
search of excellence" (Peters and Waterman, 1982). The prom-

ises made in this process, above all by Peters and Waterman, are usually similar in character to statements made by the church. The organizational culture of a successful enterprise must be such that the enterprise not only guarantees the income of its employees but also relieves them of having to question the meaning of life. Enterprises, especially multinationals, are not infrequently styled as guarantors of immortality (Sievers, 1990a, 1990b, 1990c, 1994).

Parallel and in contrast to this marketing of the concept of organizational culture, a significant reorientation of the scientific discussion has been going on. The approach adopted by Berger and Luckmann (1966) to the social construction of reality, themes, and issues that had hitherto been associated with ethnology, theology, psychoanalysis, or epistemological sociology found its way into the discussion of organizational theory. Thus is account taken of the fact that only parts of an organization are visible and that the behavior of its members and its fundamental orientations tend to evade the daily discourse (Adams and Hill Ingersoll, 1990, p. 15). The newly forming self-image of these organization- and management-oriented social scientists is occasionally referred to as *organizational symbolism* (Pondy and others, 1983; Turner, 1990, 1992; see also Gagliardi, 1990); besides the cultural dimension, central attention is focused on the study of myths and emotions as well as the aesthetics of organizational reality (Strati, 1992). Beyond dealing with metaphors, symbols, allegories, or myths in themselves, reference is also made to the basic values, ideas, and beliefs of an organization (Gahmberg, 1990, p. 155). Proceeding along with this is a significant shift of basic metaphors underlying the theoretical perspectives on organization. Besides the cultural metaphoric references to psychic prison (Morgan, 1986, p. 199), theater (Mangham and Overington, 1987; Sievers, 1992) or, more recently, chaos takes the place of the imagery of machines or organisms. In this sense, sexuality also can be understood as a metaphor in dealing with gender in organizations.

Special significance is attached to the concept of myths, a significance that is increasingly supplanting so-called unshakable findings and objective truths in this constantly changing process of understanding organizations. Though occasionally in this process a rather rationalist position is taken that it is the other, the barbarian, who subscribes to myths, another understanding of myths is gradually gaining ground in two senses. On the one hand, if dealt with as a body of objective cognitions, myths continue to contain unconscious individual and social assumptions, fictions, fantasies, and illusions. On the other hand, these myths seek to answer fundamental questions that are as old as humankind. With special reference to organizational myths (Westerlund and Sjöstrand, 1981), current myths are mostly the result of long-standing (sometimes centuries old) formations that like archaeological or geological formations are characterized by superimpositions and faults. Quite often, original myths are supplanted by surrogate or derived ones that contribute to letting the original spirit of the enterprise fall into oblivion or to reducing it to a caricature of the original (Sievers, 1990b, p. 220). Images that were originally held to be valid in the organization are—as occasionally old paintings are—painted over in the course of time (Adams and Hill Ingersoll, 1990, p. 22; Zeri, 1987). McWhinney and Batista (1988) have shown in the case of the Walt Disney Corporation how, through the process of *remythologization*—that is, the reconstruction of the founding myths—access to the original creative potential that had been hidden for such a long time when the primary corporate culture had been distorted by the spirit of the outmoded or deceased founder was reestablished.

Although in the view of several authors the task of organizational cultural analysis is to unearth the hidden issues of context, purpose, and value (Smircich, 1983, p. 355), I have observed that psychoanalytical cultural critique as established by Freud (1930) (see Erdheim, 1986) has found very little response in the course of this debate (see, for example, Schwartz, 1990a, 1990b; Gabriel, 1983, 1986, 1991). My own work has, above all, been influenced by the British tradition of institutional analysis as it has been evolving over the past thirty years or more within the context of the Tavistock Institute and the Tavistock Clinic in London.

A Case in Institutional Analysis

Arising from one of the working conferences that we have been holding in Germany in the British tradition of institutional analysis is the following case study, which illustrates some of the psychosocial entanglements that in a concrete context could unleash and perpetuate "the organizational culture and its discontents." The immediate cause for this was a role analysis (Auer-Hunzinger and Sievers, 1991; Reed, 1976; Weigand and Sievers, 1985) with one of the seminar participants, a young female psychologist employed in a girls' home run by the Sisterhood of Our Lady of the Good Shepherd. While our task during the seminar was mainly directed at helping this psychologist actively organize her role in this home, the following attempt at an institutional analysis transcends the boundaries of the immediate empirical material. It does not represent a concrete institution of this sisterhood; rather, it is based on my subjective attempt as an external, a man and an organizational analyst, to understand the possible psychosocial dynamics of this institution without having worked as a consultant with it. As already noted, this attempt is not only a subjective one; it is more of a general attempt to provide material for working hypotheses whose examination, modification, and amplification are left to those who, irrespective of their roles, work in one of these homes or in similar institutions.

On the basis of the material acquired from the role consultation and my own associations and thoughts, the psychosocial dynamic of the home appears quite entangled. In a nonclinical sense, it points to the pathology of the organization (Türk, 1976, 1980; Steiner, 1990; Dejours, 1990).

On the one side are the "morally endangered or fallen" girls and women, as they are called in the objectives of the religious order, which was founded in the first half of the nineteenth century and traces its origins from Saint Jean Eudes, who died in France in 1680. These are girls who are "addicted" to sex, that is, girls who have earned a living from sex and who in the process are unconsciously acting out the sexual conflicts in their families of origin (Drewermann, 1991, p. 283). They represent an attitude toward sexuality marked by dependency, immaturity, and violence but one in which real bonding with "the man" cannot take place. Although these girls have been penetrated by men, an interpenetration in a mature sense has not occurred. The inability of these girls to bond also means that they are unable to keep "the man" inside themselves; the real physical and psychic man to whom they have "given themselves" is more a representation of men in general; the "wedding," "the marriage," and the realization of a common future life could not take place. The "phallus of the man" appears to have remained the father's; it could not be introjected (Sievers, 1989).

At the same time, these girls have, as Jocaste's daughters (Olivier, 1989, p. 59, 1991; compare Reinke, 1987), remained in the shadow of their mothers, no "satisfactory" objects for them, alienated from their own bodies. It seems reasonable to suggest that these girls are at the same time acting out the tragedy of their parents, that is, of fathers who were not able to take possession of the phallus of their own fathers, and of mothers whose female genealogy has been interrupted in a concretely individual way as well as in a cultural-historical context (Irigaray, 1991, p. 135). The families of origin of these girls are presumably based less on parental (husband/wife) relationships than on surrogate (father/daughter, mother/son, brother/sister) relationships, which further suggests that their own mothers were not allowed to be and could not be women but only girls.

On the other side, facing these "fallen girls" are the Sisters of the Good Shepherd. They are the "brides of Christ," who with their vows and their final entry into the nunnery, enter into their marriage with the Son of God as virgins (Theobald, 1990). They are therefore wives of the bridegroom in the tradition of the German marriage laws that were valid into the nineteenth century (Borneman, 1978, p. 1490). At the individual level, they replicate in this way the theological metaphor according to which the church itself is understood as the bride of Christ. However, there is something peculiar about this engagement. While according to traditional marriage law, marriage was sealed by the act of sexual intercourse—"the wedding represented a later ceremony by which the marriage was celebrated" (Borneman, p. 1490)—this is spiritualized in the case of nuns; the actual marriage is postponed to life after death, after the resurrection of the dead into eternity in heaven (McDannell and Lang, 1990, p. 228). Intercourse with the Savior is not sexual; according to the mythology of the Catholic church, it remains not only spiritual but also oral; the nuns internalize the body of the Lord by eating it. In contrast to the majority of monks (who are priests), this also means that the blood of the Lord is denied to the nuns. Similar to several other Christian myths of this kind, especially that of the virgin birth (Schaberg, 1989; Kohn-Roelin, 1989), this engagement makes references at the same time to early matriarchal images; it suggests associations of sororal polygyny, in which several sisters have intercourse with a single man (Borneman, 1979, p. 208). Although nuns are or were physically capable of conception during a greater part of their lives and are or were reminded of this constantly by their own blood, they cannot as a rule live out this part of womanhood. They have to split it off. They live it partially in secret friendships with men. But neither do they dare talk openly about these friendships nor do these men dare take physical shape; even private "particular friendships" among nuns are forbidden (Drewermann, 1989, p. 187; Curb, 1986, p. 22). What has to be prevented at all costs is a child being born out of a relationship with a man. This would not only expose the sexual relationship (Martin, 1990, p. 348) but (as opposed to the case of monks) would also mean an end to the nun's membership in the order. Because of the vow of chastity and celibacy, these male friendships either have to remain platonic or the nuns have to personalize the illegality of their relations with men as a sin or even reflect on or conceal a breach of contract regarding their vows to the order.

Several authors have argued that these institutions, especially those that belong to the charitable wings of the church with life membership, generally seek to "compensate for the shortcomings of real parents" and provide "protection against narcissistic insults" (Schmidbauer, 1991, pp. 52, 79; compare Mentzos, 1988, p. 79). Further, it seems reasonable to suggest that the individual biographical dispositions upon which the entry of these nuns into the religious order was based (just as in the case of the fallen girls) can be traced to the families of origin and the experiences of sex and sexuality there (Moser, 1976, 1990, p. 5). Just as the "early Christian call for chastity [also] has to be related to the social situation of those times . . . to the constraints of ancient family structure and to the factual position of the woman" (Flasch, 1991; quoted in Pagels's review, 1991), one can also say that the saving of souls, as the fourth vow and the objective of the religious order in terms of its superego function (Schmidbauer, 1991, p. 52; Schwartz, 1990a), is based more or less on the individual nun's wish for atonement and rectification. To the extent that one can assume that the call to sisterhood in this order is based on the unconscious identification with a fallen or morally endangered girl belonging to the generation of one's parents or grandparents (Hellinger, 1991) and that a girl, in her identification with a related girl, feels called to become or remain a sister, her identification as a woman is potentially eliminated. This is increasingly impeded upon entry into the religious order because she appears before the mother superior — whose spiritual motherhood is moreover deeply rooted in patriarchy — as a novice, as a younger sister, above all as her daughter (Gebara, 1989).

The regression and immaturity that potentially accompany this call and choice of profession should not, however, lead us to the conclusion that nuns in general and those of the Good Shepherd in particular are "condemned" to remain immature and asexual girls for life. As much as I am convinced that the homes of the Good Shepherd are part of but not exclusively what Foucault (1976, pp. 385, 393) describes as a dungeon network in which "society's penal system ensures that the physical body is actually taken into custody and placed under constant observation" (see Riley, 1990), I also believe that sisters can succeed in becoming mature women. At the same time it is important to remember that human maturity is no constant condition. Just as adulthood is rooted in one's infancy (Klein, 1959), maturity is only a potential condition, that is newly acquired regarding the psychosocial dynamics of institutions and relationships (Winnicott, 1950).

In the context of the home and the activities of the sisters, this means that the latent or manifest constellation of the family of origin, which a sister unconsciously tries to escape by entering the religious order, can be reactivated in the course of her daily work and within the home and order's systemic context. The girls in this home embody and live a disturbed relationship to sexuality that the individual sister may have experienced or felt unconsciously within herself and/or in her family and that made her decide to take the vow of chastity, of eternal virginity. However, to assert that the nuns have renounced all sexuality and have become plain neuters is as naive as the attempt to deny the sexuality of a virgin. Mature nuns can claim to have sexuality that they experience in themselves and others. They have sexual dreams, fantasies, and desires and are able to discover for themselves ways of dealing with them other than continuously accusing themselves of sin or suppressing this aspect of their humanity.

The obvious age difference between the nuns and the girls and also their different views of the world make it possible to ignore similarities or even what they have in common. This seems to apply above all to their man-woman relationship patterns. Man is perceived only as a partial object by both groups. To the former he is represented in the soul and to the latter in the phallus (Segal, 1972, p. 396; Laplanche and Pontalis, 1973, p. 371). Although neither of them can let a whole man take form, the major difference consists of the fact that this heterosexual partial-object relation is proof of the nuns' completeness and the girls' incompleteness. The respective splitting of the man or men carried out by nuns and girls can hardly be seen as something they share in common (Drewermann, 1991, p. 280). It is acted out as a cleavage in the systemic context of the home; it presumably constitutes the basis of existence of such a home.

Sexuality in dealing with the wards of an institution is generally problematic (Burrell, 1984; Hassard and Porter, 1990; Mills and Tancred, 1992; Spiegel, 1990; White, 1987). In our case, it seems hardly possible for nuns and girls to talk about and work together on sexuality in a mature pedagogical way, let alone live it with each other in a mutually acceptable manner.

In Search of Meaning

The denial of sexuality becomes more important than its realization. And this leads again to new dynamics: these girls who have obviously "failed" in dealing with sexuality (they would otherwise not have been placed in the home) have to be denied doing it their own way; such a denial could well be regarded as the principal pedagogical or healing method that the home can provide. At a time when the traditional idea of such a home is increasingly being questioned — that is, making repentants out of sinners as a first step and then making rehabilitated Christians out of repentants — these girls are being made to renounce their passions. They have to atone for the sexuality they have previously acted out despite their increasing lack of belief in the sacrament of atonement. The presumably successful objective of such an educational process appears to consist more in the creation of girls who substitute the abstinence demanded of them during their residence with an oath of temporary asexuality. The ideal inmate is the female neuter, the nonwoman, who must still be preserved as an ideal type even when she has a child to care for. Like the Holy Virgin Mary, she has to assume the role of a mother without ever being a woman. In the face of this institutionally required asexuality and the condemnation of abortion in the Catholic church, the fact that some of these girls have to come to terms with one or more abortions must be ignored.

The prohibition of active sexuality (especially in the form of heterosexual intercourse) on the part of these girls as a central aspect of the pedagogy of correction and conversion (Treiber, 1990, p. 166) is reminiscent of the church's ritual of baptism, which incidentally is repeated like a second baptism in the process of vow taking: Do you renounce Satan? It is the image of the archangel Michael who finally defeats the dragon (Grubel, 1990), Satan, and makes him a fallen angel (Blass-Simmen, 1991, p. 19) that resonates and is repeated in the dichotomy of consecrated, chosen virgins and fallen girls. While Satan forever remains the fallen angel and the ruler of hell till the end of time, the relationship between the nuns and the girls contains an element of hope for the nuns that the girls have the opportunity of returning to the lap (!) of the church to become once again the children of God and to attain eternal life.

The difficulty of dealing with gender and sexuality in a potentially mature way in such a home appears to me to be supported and reinforced not least by the patron saint after whom the home was named: Saint Gabriel. While Jesus, the heavenly bridegroom and son of God, is clearly a man and has been portrayed as such in the two-thousand-year-old iconography of the Catholic church, the archangel Gabriel is, like all angels, sexless. He is a spiritual being in contrast to the often maidenlike or androgynous portrayal of Him. His spiritual significance "is the rebirth of the divine spirit in the earthly being. Gabriel announces the second, eternal rebirth of Man, the one who acknowledges himself as being of heavenly origin" (Bauer, Dümotz, and Golowin, 1980, p. 213). His name means "God is almighty." According to the legends, Gabriel led Adam and Eve out of Paradise, he was sent along with Michael by Allah to collect the dust out of which Adam was created, he is the one who suckled the infant Abraham with the little finger of his right hand, he foretold the birth of John the Baptist, and he is present at the annunciation of Mary. The latent sexual metaphorism surrounding the angel Gabriel finally reaches its summit in the portrayal of him as a hunter "who drives the precious unicorn to the virgin" (Biedermann, 1989, p. 113; Schmidt and Schmidt, 1982, p. 46). Just like other angels, Gabriel is a partial object, sometimes iconographically portrayed in the form of a winged head, which has symbolized the incorporeal nature of angels since the twelfth century.

The partial-object character repeats itself much more clearly in the name given to the order or the name by which it is commonly referred to by omission or through lack of knowledge of the first part: (Our Lady of) the Good Shepherd('s Love). Although the portrayal of Christ as the good shepherd can be found in primitive Christian art and as a mythological representation transcends the New Testament and even goes beyond Jewish mythology in the image of Mercury/Hermes (Schmidt and Schmidt, 1982, p. 17), in the above context this image is clearly marked by its resuscitation in the second half of the seventeenth century. The reactivation of the good shepherd, just as the worship of the holy heart of Jesus, can be traced to Jean Eudes, who though acknowledged as one of the revivers of religious life in France and as a protagonist of the people's mission was certainly not free of the misogyny of that time (Riley, 1990, p. 44). Similar to other female orders founded at around the same time (Holy Heart of Jesus, Divine Prophecy, Precious Blood, and the like), this religious order differs significantly from its larger predecessors, such as the Benedictines, Dominicans, Franciscans, or Ursulans, not only in its church reformatory and social demands. With the partial-object reference to Christ, the possibility of identifying with the founder of the order as a complete person was relegated to the background (contrary to the importance of this given by the traditional orders, especially in the symbolic representation of a Saint Benedict or a Saint Ursula, for example).

What is worth contemplating is not so much the question of what circumstances led to the founding of the Good Shepherd order and later the sister congregation of Angers within the context of Salpêtrière in seventeenth-century Paris, an event that definitely appears worthy of a remythologizing in terms of reworking original myths. Much more important is the peculiar aura of antiquatedness that seems to cling to the image of the good shepherd in reference to this home today. The good shepherd is "a symbol of care for the helpless" (Biedermann, 1989, p. 197). He feeds his flock on green pastures; he knows his sheep and even searches for the lost ones. On the day of judgment he will separate the sheep from the goats (Breuk, 1966, pp. 36–51). Besides the regressive and sexual symbolism this image contains ("Thy rod and thy staff, they comfort me!"), it serves at the same time—in the form of pastorhood—as a means of legitimizing not only the institutional ecclesiastical power of the bishop but also that of the head of the monastery or the monastic authorities (Regis, 1932, p. 45).

The question I pose to myself is whether the symbol of the good shepherd is not something hypocritical in a reformatory home for girls. I can imagine this good shepherd standing somewhere at the portals of this institution in the form of a sculpture or at least an enamel plaque on the door to symbolize to any entrants in whose sphere of influence they find themselves. It is made irrevocably clear to the inmates, the girls, who the shepherd is and who the sheep are. Even though no one can officially use the expression "fallen girls" with impunity these days, this contributes to sustaining the defamatory picture. The nuns and perhaps those employed can also identify themselves as shepherds; the sheep are the others. Such a separation of shepherds from sheep may well also encourage the narcissist-omnipotent attitude on the part of the nuns and employees that only they themselves are good shepherds. This is a temptation easily invited by this symbol for there is mention neither of help-ers nor of dogs. Finally, the use of the male connotation sup-ports the expectation that this role, be it as a warden or pastoral director, ultimately requires a man.

What needs to be done is for these pictures of the good shepherd and the archangel Gabriel to be sorted out again and their dysfunctionality recognized in order to keep them, to a limited extent, where they belong: in the nuns' chapel. They could, I think, do a lot more there than just be a source of de-votion and edification; namely, they could be an aid to the nuns' spirituality, which contributes to working in this world without losing sight of the other. The alternative function that these pic-tures seem to have for the girls is akin to that of pornography. It seems to me that these holy icons are being used in this home in the way that pornographic pictures of women are used by men to activate their unfulfilled desires about women and sex-ual intercourse with them as partial objects. They make the nuns believe that without having to enter into an actual relationship with the girls an "intercourse," or working relationship, is pos-sible with them. They hide the fact that a mature relationship between the nuns and the girls has to include the reality of sexuality — its tragic aspects as well as its dangers of self-destruc-tion, apart from its possibly inherent lust and enrichment.

With reference to the approach to sex and gender in such a home and its inherent potential for separation and alienation, the employed personnel are also undoubtedly involved and affected by it. They, however — with reference to the psychoso-cial dynamics of such an institution — appear to be playing no more than supernumerary or odd-job roles. I do not mean this in a general sense and by no means in a pejorative one. What I mean is that the dynamics that exist between the nuns and the girls fundamentally and historically predate those that exist between the girls and the employees. In my view, the secular employees fulfill more of an auxiliary function because the reason for employing them can be traced to the fact that the nuns of this order had been confronted with the alternative of closing down the various homes — one of their main sources of income and resources — as a result of difficulties in recruiting younger nuns. The fact that these employees could play an additionally important role in rehabilitating and reintegrating the girls to lead meaningful lives may have been realized in the meanwhile and taken more seriously; it was not, presumably, a consideration when the changes were instigated. It also appears to me that demands are being made on these employees to respect and perpetuate the existing structure of psychosocial dynamics instead of transforming it, because changing it would require understanding and elucidating the structure to the degree that I have tried to do here. At the moment, however, this is precisely what seems to be impossible for these employees.

One reason for this lies in the way the employees deal with their own sexuality; I can foresee the potential personal and social implications. I can imagine that, as in the case of the nuns, corresponding latent personal-biographical dispositions may either have unconsciously influenced the choice of employment or have been activated by the relationship existing between the nuns and the girls. The latent character of these dispositions results in conflicts that remove and suppress the employees' own sexuality from and in their daily work. My assumption is that their experience of possible disturbances in their own sexuality leads them to conduct themselves in a relatively asexual manner when working. At best, this results in an institutionalized mimicry, a throttling of sexuality and eroticism at work and a more or less disturbed expression in one's leisure time, in friendships or marriages. At worst, one becomes a neuter, a partial subject or object of oneself.

Implications for Organizations

As explained in this chapter, the psychosocial entanglements of people with the organization on the one hand and of the nuns, inmates, and employees among themselves on the other hand are neither an isolated occurrence nor something peculiar to institutions under the influence of the church or religion. What has emerged from this analysis is more of a generalized picture of the phenomenon of human interrelationships in organizations regardless of whether they are business enterprises or nonprofit organizations (Sievers, 1994).

At the same time, social institutions are predestined for these entanglements for two main reasons. In contrast to other work relationships or membership in an organization, membership in a social institution is marked by its totality (in Goffmann's [1973] sense of total institutions) and a higher degree of existential concern. First, these institutions "usurp" people either temporarily or for life, as in the case of prisons or psychiatric institutions. Second, they are often based on a profound integration of their members' individual commitment, dependency, disability, or ailment. The purpose that these institutions pursue and the task to which they commit themselves are often a matter of life and death, of being or not being. As a rule, this total commitment not only is restricted to inmates or clients but also influences those who earn their living or spend their (professional) lives in these institutions.

Insofar as social institutions are often the product of a division of labor that is as hidden as it is subtle in its "keeping" and "administering" of illnesses, disabilities, depression, and death—which are ignored and suppressed in other areas and systems of society—their employees are much too often exposed to special difficulties that drive them to their individual limits and also often place excessive demands on them. I clearly recall the consternation of certain prison officials as they began to realize, within the framework of a long-term organization development project, not only that the prison as a bastion of depression affected their own well-being but also that it was they and not the prisoners who were serving "life sentences." Not until we consultants had grasped the cultural discontent, as Freud ([1930] 1957b) described it (the difficulty or even impossibility of being happy in the social environment), were we able to recognize the discontent in the prison's organizational culture and to work with the prison officials to find ways of managing the boundaries between themselves and their roles rather than only exporting the discontent of the institution to their homes every evening.

The immense difficulty of managing the evident differences (and similarities) that exist between different groups of people and roles and of realizing what feelings of impotence could arise out of the entanglements in social institutions again became clear to me recently in conjunction with a self-help organization for people with AIDS (Sievers, 1993). In the face of the obvious differentiation between those employed and paid by the association and the "others," the fact that there were people classified as HIV-positive and HIV-negative in the association as well as among the employees was relegated completely to the background. Those classified as positive in the association unconsciously exerted such dominance that the basic psychosocial dynamics of envy that resulted could not be permitted. Not only did the "positives" envy the "negatives" because of their presumably higher life expectancy, but to a certain extent those not infected envied those infected and felt inferior and excluded. This envy was exemplarily expressed by an HIV-negative employee who wished he could be terminally ill just once in his life. The potentiality and immediacy of death of those with AIDS in this association cast a dark shadow over the institution (Bowles, 1991), which causes those not infected to feel constantly compelled to take "suppressive actions."

To the extent that in social and other institutions the differences and similarities that people consciously and unconsciously embody are not adequately admitted and managed, discontent, entanglements, and suffering increase within those organizations, as do meaninglessness, frustration, regression, and contempt in the experience of employees and others involved (Lawrence, 1979, 1982). Even though discontent in the organizational culture cannot be totally eliminated, institutions and people are not automatically condemned to hopelessness, however. Culture in general and organizational culture in particular not only represent the impossibility of happiness but at the same time provide a shared context in which people's wishes and beliefs can be symbolized and updated. In the final analysis, the spirit of an enterprise or social institution and its success largely depend on whether a (secular) spirituality can be developed and maintained in a way that enables those affected, individually and collectively, to harmonize life, work, and death.

Developing a spirituality for today would, in the case described above, mean overcoming the apparent particularization of gender relationship and the organizational splitting derived therefrom. The attempt to remythologize must therefore elaborate and transcend the limitations of Jean Eudes's images of woman and man, which are expressions of the seventeenth century and its feudal patriarchy. It may start, for example, from the mythological figure of Saint Gabriel, the patron saint of this institution, whose spiritual significance is regarded as "the rebirth of the divine spirit in the earthly being" (Bauer, Dümotz, and Golowin, 1980, p. 213). To what an extent the reactivation of the divine spirit has to be based on a more matriarchal image of goddess, as offered in contemporary feminine theology, is, however, primarily a matter of the women in this order and their collective capacity to relate their own (and their clients') experience of their lives to the cosmos and the meaning they allow themselves to invest in death and the notion of an eternal spirit.

Meaning at Work

What should by now be obvious is the fact that more often than ever before organizational reality is much more complex and diverse than predominant theories of management and organization make it out to be. In addition to structuring and controlling production and economic processes, organizations are also spaces in which often high numbers of people both individually and collectively spend their entire working lives as a constituent part of their lives. And as these people conceive much broader qualities than those traditionally perceived as the characteristics of rational individuals, organizations, in addition to pursuing their primary tasks, will be perceived as arenas or theaters in which men and women are taking part in and acting out their dramas of life, comedies and tragedies alike. Con-

trary to the predominant conviction that organizations and organizational experience add a further, rather limited dimension
to an individual's life, organizations must be understood as places
in which life occurs and in which human existence is realized
to an enormous extent.

As soon as we are prepared to give up the fictitious construction that work organizations serve primarily to provide the
income and produce the goods that we then consume in what
is supposed to be a private life, both our work and our lives
have to be seen from another, much broader perspective. If we
are able to overcome the limited pragmatic notion of work as
an activity toward which one has to be mobilized via motivation and all kinds of incentives, work in organizations can be
perceived and experienced again as a constituent dimension of
the individual's and humankind's attempt to lead a meaningful
life. Although the linking of work with the payment of money
is reasonable and almost indispensable, there can be no doubt
for most contemporaries that money itself does not provide
meaning.

Meaning, as Elias (1985, p. 54) describes, is a social
category referring to a plurality of interrelated people as its subject. Meaning has a transcendent dimension that surmounts the
obvious. For example, reality beyond the frame of a picture is
the logical precondition for perceiving the special reality of the
picture and its particular message; to understand the meaning
of the picture, we must necessarily relate the picture to something else, at which point its meaning becomes transcendent.
Similarly, the meaning of the work one is doing can only be
actualized if it has a significance in one's life. And the meaning
of one's life does not only go beyond the narrow answers that
the social sciences and psychology in particular are offering
(Rank, 1958); ultimately, meaning can only be grasped if it surmounts this frame. In other words, the meaning of life can only
be referred to from the perspective of death as its end — no matter whether the assumption of a life after death is shared or how
it is interpreted. Thus work can only have meaning in its fundamental sense if it is regarded not just as a dimension of the

employing institution but also as a part of an individual life and our collective lives. Because meaning can only be understood from beyond the frame of life, the meaning of work has to be qualified by the fact of human mortality (Sievers, 1990c).

However, although meaning can thus be seen as the essence of human existence, it is not a commodity. It has to be searched for; it is more an invention than a discovery; more often than ever before it is problematic; it may be lost and need to be rediscovered again. The quest for meaning is not an easy venture. It includes becoming aware of the relatedness of our own inner world, our dreams, hopes, and anxieties, with the outside reality and its social construction. It also involves acknowledging more and more our own dependency on what is being reconfirmed every time we buy into it. Part of this dependency will also be discovered in the personal helplessness and emptiness that prevent each of us from regarding as a lie what otherwise is commonly taken as a truth. There can be no doubt that "truth is not discovered by proofs but by exploration, it is always experimental" (Weil, 1970, p. 135).

In our attempt to grasp the spirit of an enterprise, we have to reintegrate in both our practice and our theories an awareness that includes the knowledge that we are neither the first nor the last nor even the only individuals who live on this earth but that we are a part of humankind, related to our predecessors, contemporaries, successors, and the cosmos. In this attempt, we may well be reminded that the ancient notion of wisdom may have a more important meaning than just something put into the wheelchairs of the elderly.

In trying to understand what wisdom can be about, I found a statement by Joseph Campbell very valuable. In *Myths to Live By* (1973), he writes that every human attempt at institutionalization must take two basic considerations into account: the inevitability of individual death and the survival of the social order. This twofold realization may offer us a meaningful image of what wisdom can be about. Bringing wisdom back into our institutions in general and into our work enterprises in particular would therefore mean maintaining the dialectical realization that every member is inevitably mortal and that the institution itself is supposed to survive and is therefore immortal. In contrast to the ongoing attempts to diabolize immortality and mortality — that is, to split them — wisdom then can be regarded as the symbolization of immortality and mortality. Consequently, to the extent that an enterprise is capable of managing wisdom in such a sense through its mature members, its leaders are, potentially, agents of wisdom. If a corporate culture contains and symbolizes such a wisdom, the leaders of the enterprise can be regarded as mortal agents of immortality.

11

Not from These Parts:
A Tale of Organizational Turmoil

Narayan Pant

I wanted to look at organizational existences but wasn't quite sure how to start. I was trained as an academic of sorts, sent forth to teach what I know of how organizations follow strategies. Such training gave me a truckload of rules about ways to look at organizational phenomena and told me how to label what I saw and how to extract truths from my labeling that might be corroborated by colleagues. Existences in organizations, too, almost by definition, follow sets of rules about what to see, how to label and interpret. Unfortunately, sets of rules rarely come with rules about how to look at themselves, how to look at the issue of rules in any existence. The usual communications between organizations and academics who study them involve addressing the one using the rules of the other, an enterprise of uncertain value in the existence of either.

The following story describes what happened over a few days in a small bank in the southeastern United States. The tale touches on the delicate fabric of trust and good faith that makes such institutions possible. It does so by focusing on a seemingly absurd and coincidental series of events that befall an otherwise healthy institution. At one level, the story derives its plot from Albert Camus's *The Plague*. It suggests that ordinary human beings are carriers of an insidious germ much like the plague bacillus. This germ lies dormant until some quirk of circumstance causes symptoms of the infestation to appear in large groups of people. Some attempts to place this story in the larger context of other such infestations appear at the end of the tale.

Not from These Parts

And indeed, as he listened to the cries of joy rising from the town, Rieux remembered that such joy is always imperiled. He knew what those jubilant crowds did not know but could have learned from books: that the plague bacillus never dies or disappears for good; that it can lie dormant for years and years in furniture and linen chests; that it bides its time in bedrooms, cellars, trunks and bookshelves; and that perhaps the day would come when, for the bane and the enlightenment of men, it roused up its rats again and sent them forth to die in a happy
· city [Camus, 1947].

Yelena Moshansky stared at the man rummaging through the wire trash basket at the other end of the square. She glanced at her watch and tried to calculate how long it would take him to reach the basket that stood some five feet away from her. She didn't think the bank would open before he got to it. Yelena was sixty-seven years old, but she wasn't afraid of the solitary derelict. Ordinarily, she would have paid him no attention; he and his kind were a common enough sight. Only today, in light of what she was about to do, she hoped that the man would not remember her waiting for the Neighborhood Savings and Loan to open and then waylay her when she emerged.

At the time Yelena Moshansky stood waiting for the bank to open, Ben Seward and other employees of the same bank had already been at work for about an hour. They worked a regular nine-to-five shift like other people who worked in offices. The only difference was that they had to deal with customers, who kept them from doing any real work, between ten and four. Ben's current job had him sifting through all mail addressed to the general manager of operations, Jim Bailey. It wasn't the most fascinating of jobs, but it kept Ben occupied for the first hour of the day. It also permitted him to nurture dreams of one day coming across that crucial piece of information that would have Bailey forever in his debt.

Stewart Griggs wandered over to where Ben sat making neat piles of paper, some that Bailey would sign, others that he would peruse, and still others that he wouldn't see. Stewart was widely thought to have gotten his job solely because his father happened to own the largest source of employment in town. All people got their jobs because they knew somebody, of course, but Stewart was special in that he couldn't consistently find buttons on his calculator. Ben suspected that he had gotten his own job because his father worked at the county surveyor's office. Still, he knew that if he had applied to any of the big banks in Tampa or Orlando, or even Richmond, he'd have had a good shot at them. Ben was qualified. He had a bachelor's degree in business from Florida State, with a respectable grade-point average. He hadn't taken one of those possibly fancier jobs because Neighborhood had surprisingly offered him more money than had any one else.

Ben sat back in his chair and reflected on Stewart's comment about last night's football game between the Miami Dolphins and the Denver Broncos. He wished he could have Stewart's almost cavalier attitude toward his work. Stewart seemed to treat work as a somewhat distasteful interruption of the general flow of civilized conversation. He usually made it a point to discover other people's interests and could make some not totally inane comment on a vast variety of subjects. However, the same Stewart found it difficult to give customers a clear explanation of the difference between the rate of interest and the yield on a deposit. Ben's passion was football, in particular the Miami Dolphins and their legendary coach, Shula. He never really minded that every Tuesday morning Stewart would start a conversation about the previous night's games. Yet it was usually Ben who regretfully had to end the discussion by asking: "Have the doors opened yet?"

"About five minutes ago."

"Well, Jim's going to want these any minute now, so I'd better see to them."

"Don't burn yourself out Ben," and with an almost solici-
tous cluck, Stewart sauntered back to whatever desk he was oc-
cupying that day.

Neighborhood Savings and Loan was a medium-sized savings and loan association in a small town named Moxahachie
in the Florida panhandle. It would have been unexceptional in
every way were it not for the fact that the current management
had installed themselves in a remarkable coup d'état two years
earlier. The current president was originally a finance and management consultant who had encouraged the former management team to convert their unambitious operation from a mutually held bank to one owned by stockholders. They had followed
his advice and subsequently gone to the markets to replenish
their equity base. At that point, the management consultant and
a few friends cornered enough of the bank's new equity to enable them to relieve those managers of their jobs.

The management consultant installed himself as the president of an apparently aggressive, professionally managed bank.
The bank's asset base soared under his direction, and the bank
boasted borrowers who were from as far away as California.
Even the decor of the bank took on a rich leather and velvet
finish that seemed to belong to New York, the place the president came from, rather than Moxahachie.

Professional appearances notwithstanding, two people
effectively ran the bank: the president and Jim Bailey, a Chicago
business graduate. There was another general manager who
managed the administration of the bank. This, according to
critics, meant that she, Eleanor Boyce, ensured that the pay-
checks were issued on time and that supplies of stationery never
ran out. To Eleanor's credit, this did sometimes require advance
planning so that goods and services from Tampa would arrive
in a timely manner. Eleanor also went out on various public
relations jaunts for the bank. The president reasoned that in
their region an attractive white woman in her late thirties could
probably generate more goodwill than an African-American
general manager from Chicago or a Jewish president from New
York. It probably helped that her husband was an assistant to
the Democratic state senator from that region and aspired to
become a senator himself someday.

Jim Bailey usually started his day with the bank president, reviewing imminent decisions. As a policy the bank avoided substantial exposure to any single industry though, of course, this was not always possible. With the new laws, however, assets had spread across state lines and this was causing Jim to look more closely at suffering Texas oil fields than he would have liked. The bank's major local exposure was in the real estate sector, and he could see nothing that caused him immediate concern. The bank had made a large loan for the development of a condominium complex, several units of which had been sold well before completion of the project. The construction was progressing well, and the few cost overruns seemed not to concern the developers.

The bank had made one speculative investment that very few people knew about. It had entered into a joint venture whose principals included Eleanor's husband. Technically, there may have been nothing wrong with the arrangement because no particular favors had been done for anybody and Eleanor herself had stayed out of the negotiations. The joint venture had subsequently entered the development business, backed by a letter of credit from Neighborhood Savings and Loan. The investment itself didn't bother Jim too much because even a total write-off of that one account would not really cripple the bank. It might, however, raise difficult questions about how the bank chose to interpret the law regulating direct investments in real estate by savings and loan associations. Since nobody knew the answers to these potential questions, all concerned had tacitly agreed to avoid any mention of the transaction. All in all, at the conclusion of his morning meeting with the president, Jim didn't feel any sense of unease or anxiety about any aspect of the bank's position.

Jim first became aware of the existence of Yelena Moshansky when he heard the sound of rushing feet outside his door. He opened the door just in time to see Ben Seward scurrying down the staircase to the main office. Jim turned to his secretary and asked her what had prompted the young man's precipitous exit. The secretary, who was intelligent enough to hold down her position without unnecessarily exercising her extremely overweight body, picked up the telephone and dialed the office

manager's extension. The phone was answered after an unusually long interval, and the secretary informed the party at
the other end that her direct superior wished to know what was
going on. Jim knew the office manager, Dan Dalton, well enough
to understand that the pitch of the reply emerging from his secretary's phone was that of a person under substantial strain. So
when the secretary turned around to tell him that a woman was
withdrawing her life's savings from the bank, he took the telephone.

"Dan, Jim Bailey; what's the fuss?"

"Jim, there's a woman here who wants to close out her
account."

"I understand that. What's the problem? Is she a big depositor?"

"Oh no, Jim, she's a pensioner. We're only talking about
$20,000 or so."

"Right, so what's the problem? People close their accounts
with us all the time."

"Jim, she wants to take all her money out in cash. She
says our cashier's check isn't good enough."

"Do we have that much float? Did you explain that large
withdrawals of cash always require advance notice?"

"I tried explaining it to her, but she began to get nasty
and said that if she wanted to take her money out at any time
she ought to be able to. A couple of other customers started chim-
ing in, saying that she was just an old lady and we shouldn't
be harassing her. The thing is, Jim, I know the woman. She's
old Walter Moshansky's widow, usually one of the most sensible people I know. I can't imagine what's got into her. I know
her daughter quite well too; the thing is she lives in Tampa and
I can't get her to talk to her mother on such short notice."

"Dan, Dan, calm down. There's nothing you can do if
people want to throw their money away; it's their money. Did
she say what she wanted it for?"

"Yes, she said she wants to put it in CitiBank across the
square."

"What?"

"That's right, Jim. She said as loud as you please that we

weren't allowing her to take her money out because we didn't want the world to know that we had money problems."

"I'm on my way. Where is she now?"

"I put her in the vault visitors' room, and told her I'd see what I could do. I wanted her where she couldn't spook any more customers."

"You did fine, Dan. Hold on, I'm coming down."

Jim hurled the phone toward his secretary before heading down the stairs as rapidly as his dignity would permit. As he descended the last few steps, he was confronted with a puzzling sight. Little knots of people composed of varying combinations of employees and customers dotted the main floor. Conversations trailed off as he entered the area, and heads turned toward him. He was gratified to note that there must have been something about his demeanor that prompted most of the employees to return to their stations as if a brief period of entertainment had ended. With a nod to those whose desks he passed and a laconic, "Your desk misses you, Seward," Jim negotiated the office floor and entered the office manager's cubicle.

"All right, Dan, let's get this cleared up at once. Give Joe Webster at Citi a call and tell him that there's some cash coming down to him. Tell him we'll need a float from him until we can replenish—usual rates. Send Charlie Huff over with the woman and her money so that nobody gets any funny ideas while she's on her way over there. He can wait while she fills out the papers and bring the cash right back. Is that clear? Good, let's move on this. The people out there need to get back to work."

In little towns like Moxahachie news travels swiftly, and ten minutes later workers in offices and shops around the square stopped whatever they were doing and watched Neighborhood's guard, Charlie Huff, and Yelena Moshansky set out in a procession of two across the square. But the watching people seemed uncertain about what to make of the sight, and Charlie Huff was perhaps the most confused of all. You see Charlie wasn't much of a guard. He was well over fifty, overweight, and a bit disheveled looking in his slate gray uniform and cap. He was the butt of jesters who frequented the square during working hours and the Pig & Whistle after hours. What's more, he didn't usually have much to guard. Whenever large sums of money were transferred either into or out of the bank, the armored car company sent along its own guards. The bank itself wasn't considered a likely holdup risk simply because it wasn't a very important bank. At the moment, however, Charlie felt that he was earning the right to some respect because he was finally doing what he was hired to do, namely, to protect money. Nevertheless, he was doing it as much as a favor to this old lady as he was because it was his job. As a result Charlie didn't work too hard to catch anybody's eye as he walked across the square.

Having been told that he had to bring the same money back from where he was escorting it, Charlie had asked Dan Dalton whether he should take the little money box that came with a cuff that he could put on his wrist. He had thought Dan's response, telling him not to be dramatic, was a trifle brusque, and he had let Dan know that by saying that he was sure that the money would fit in his front pocket. Of course, by the time he reemerged from CitiBank, there was nobody around to observe him because everybody had assumed that the excitement was over.

Ben Seward was in trouble. As he stood in front of Jim Bailey's desk, he reflected on the unfairness of a life that had made him commit an apparently serious error on the same day that he had been caught away from his desk, gawking at some happening like a kid at a fairground display. Compounded with this general sense of unfairness was a rising restlessness at the accusation being leveled at him.

"I'm sorry, Jim," said Ben. "It looked just like a standard memo that I should mark FYI and low priority."

"Didn't you remember my telling you that whenever we receive news of independent appraisals of any of our properties, you should bring it to my attention, immediately?"

"Right, Jim, but the notice said that this was an appraisal of Panhandle Development's properties; that isn't one of our properties, is it?"

"The problem with you, Ben, is you're smart, but that makes you lazy and you don't think. Why do you think the bank

requesting the appraisal sent us notice of it if it didn't have anything to do with us? Remember, you're not only paid to follow
instructions but also to try and make some decisions of your
own."

A shaken Ben Seward left Jim Bailey's office to the sound
of the irate general manager's instructions. Any notices at all
referring to Panhandle Development were to be brought to Jim's
notice immediately, not sometime next week.

Sitting with her son and facing a loan officer in the hall
was Catherine Stefanik. Jim Stefanik was starting college in the
fall, and he and his mother had come to the bank to apply for
a student loan. Both of them couldn't help but catch the last
furious words of Jim's instructions to Ben. They both knew Ben
slightly, Jim from watching him play football for the local high
school and Catherine because she and her husband knew the
Sewards socially. At least they knew Ben well enough to be able
to have a civil conversation with him whenever they met. Poor
boy, thought Catherine. Still, that was the price one had to pay
whenever one went to work for people who weren't from these
parts. They might be the nicest people otherwise, but they just
didn't have the manners that people here were accustomed to.

Catherine had not come along with Jim just because she
thought he'd need her moral support. She had wanted to drop
in on her husband at work and decided that she might as well
see Jim taken care of. Besides she knew one or two people at
the bank, and she was sure that with their help she could get
any potential loan problems ironed out. As she and her son left
the bank and headed toward her husband's office a few blocks
away, she noted that Jim was unusually quiet.

It isn't easy for any young person to come face-to-face
with the dreary aspects of employment, but the tongue lashing
he'd seen Ben Seward receive had caused Jim Stefanik considerable discomfort. At one level, he expected that college would
be exciting. Getting away from home and from parents who
bordered on the suffocatingly protective was a good end in itself. Still, Jim couldn't help asking himself what a high-flying
college education counted for if it only transferred suffocation
from parental hands to those of superiors on the job.

Ray Stefanik, Jim's father and Catherine's husband, ran
the local office of a large mutual fund operation in the southeastern United States. Such brokerage branches staffed by single agents, had sprung up all over in response to changed rules
and regulations governing financial institutions. Running the
office meant handing out application forms to local retirees and
white-collar workers and mailing the completed forms and checks
to the fund's regional office. For this, Ray received a commis-
sion on every package that he sold. He was one of Hanson
Mutual's first agents and one of the first to recognize the potential of such mutual funds to attract private resources. The company had rewarded him for his foresight, and he now received
a base salary in addition to his commissions. In return, once
in a while, Ray handled some transactions that the company
undertook nearby.

Ray greeted his wife and son with none of the impatience
that afflicts some people when their relatives visit them at work.
Family members seem to take on different hues at work, vari-
ously becoming taller, shorter, fatter, dowdier, and dressier than
they appear in their natural habitats. But Ray, being relatively
unencumbered with work and unusually fond of his family, dis-
played an almost genuine heartiness as he saw his wife and son
walk into his office.

"So, did you get however much you wanted?" asked Ray.

Now Ray could have easily paid for his son's college education. In fact, he had resolved that he would eventually pay
off his son's student loan, but Jim didn't need to know that just
yet. The boy could do with practical experience in the discipline
of planning and keeping to a budget. Ray had told him to find
a part-time job and put away some of the money he earned
toward repayment of a student loan. The low interest on student loans compared to what money was earning anywhere else
made it almost criminal to pass them up. Even if Jim didn't need
the money to live on, it would have been worth his while to take
out a loan, reinvest it, and make a tidy profit on the spread.
Ray clearly felt that there was a difference between that possibly unethical course and his own proposed course of action.

"No trouble at all," replied his wife. "The loan officer was quite helpful, and Jim should start getting deposits in his account in September."

"Ben Seward got into trouble while we were at the bank," said Jim, uttering more than a grunt for the first time since leaving the bank.

"That's right; it was quite silly," added Catherine. "I can't imagine that anybody would make such a fuss over a little thing like not being given a memo yesterday. Still, those people are not from these parts, and one must expect them to do strange things once in a while."

"Well," said Ray dismissively, acutely aware that his own secretary had often been on the receiving end of similar reprimands and could hear every word being said. "There's no telling how important Ben's slip was, and sometimes the only way to get young people to remember things of importance is to raise your voice at them."

"Oh, I'm sure it was nothing important. It had to do with some land belonging to some other company, or something like that."

"Panhandle," Jim noted.

"What?" asked Ray.

"It was Panhandle Development. The man told Ben that he wanted to see every paper that had anything to do with Panhandle Development," answered Jim, showing signs of some of his father's fussy attention to details.

"That can't be," replied his father, who justly considered himself an authority on all business transacted in his neck of the woods. "Neighborhood Savings doesn't have anything to do with Panhandle."

"Well, perhaps it was Piper, dear, Piper Development maybe," said Catherine, with instincts born of years of practice at heading off family confrontations in their early stages.

"No, it was Panhandle Development. I know what I heard."

"Well, it doesn't matter anyway." Turning to his wife, Ray said, "I should be home around twelve for lunch."

"It's pork chops and lemon tart today. Try and be on time, or else the chops will get too dry and you won't eat them."

"I will, I will. There's not much happening here today."
Ray Stefanik sat back in his chair after his wife and son
left and thought about what he had heard. Panhandle Development was said to be taking its investors for a bath. The principals had gone into business to develop an attractive new town-
house complex that would eclipse the one presently going up
on the outskirts of town. Panhandle's complex would have everything necessary to attract yuppies who worked in the nearby
city — swimming pool, tennis courts, saunas, exercise rooms, and
more. The one thing the plan needed was a highway near the
complex leading to the city. The state had conveniently agreed
to permit a new highway to be built but refused to pay for all
of it. The state had asked the county to shoulder a large propor-
tion of the costs, and this the county had agreed to do. The new
highway would almost certainly cause the surrounding land to
appreciate considerably in value. Some speculators in the know
had taken advantage of their knowledge and sold a tract of land
adjoining the proposed highway at an inflated price to Panhandle Development. Panhandle nevertheless believed that it had
received a bargain because the new development would sup-
posedly yield several times the original investment.

The problem Panhandle ran into was that the county
treasury tap suddenly ran dry. It now appeared that there would
be little chance the county could complete existing projects, let
alone embark on new ones. There was even talk that the local
police force and hospital might be facing cuts in staffing and
services.

All this came as quite a shock to investors in Panhandle
Development. The entire basis for their investment was the highway that was to run past their land. Now it appeared that for
the development to proceed the developers themselves would
have to raise some of the funds needed to build the highway.
The developers next decided to approach a bank for the money,
putting up the land they owned as collateral. The loan officer
at the bank they went to wasn't accommodating enough to see
the money they had paid for the land as evidence of its true
worth. Then the developers decided to hire an independent ap-
praiser who would tell the bank what the land being offered was
really worth.

Some of this Ray Stefanik knew and some of it he could surmise, but what did come as a surprise to him was that Neighborhood Savings was somehow involved in the whole sorry business. Even the new owners didn't strike him as the sort that would bet the organization on a throw of the dice. In fact, he didn't even think Neighborhood was allowed by state or federal law to own more than a very small amount of real estate.

Well, it didn't matter to him or Hanson Mutual in any way. True, Hanson did sometimes invest in multiples of $100,000 in different savings and loans around the South. This was because it got the best rates when it invested in those amounts and because a prudent portfolio strategy demanded that Hanson put some money into quickly transferable near-cash securities whose principal was safe. In fact, Ray had just recently moved about $300,000 from Neighborhood to Alamo Savings and Loan, according to instructions from his head office. He had been told to make the move because Alamo was offering twenty basis points more than Neighborhood on short-term loans. Perhaps it was just as well.

That reminded him, he had that morning checked on the status of the transfer and discovered that the money had started earning interest as of that day. He had filled out the appropriate form informing headquarters of the status of the investment and mailed it. Ray had also tried to reach Hanson's investment officer in Tampa to tell him that the money had started earning interest, but he hadn't been able to get through.

"Delores, I'm going home for lunch. If Bob Zelnick calls, would you tell him $300,000 is out of Neighborhood and earning at Alamo?"

"Sure, Ray."

"Thanks. I should be back at two, if anybody wants to know."

Delores wished she could go home for lunch, too, although she wasn't sure what would be waiting for her there other than a carton of milk and part of a loaf of bread. Well, another day of hot and sour soup and garlic chicken on rice ordered from Peking Palace down the road.

Afternoons usually went slowly for Delores. Most of the firm's clients usually came in first thing in the morning. Those who could, tended to avoid going out in the hot afternoon sun. And so Delores would start surreptitiously gazing at her watch from about four o'clock on. She needed to be surreptitious because she suspected that Ray sometimes found really important work for her to do when he thought she was openly looking forward to leaving. Usually, he was quite good about her time and didn't make her stay late, but occasionally, particularly when she seemed eager to leave, she would suddenly have to go to the main post office to mail something off or type up an urgent letter. She had learned to look nonchalant even when she was counting the seconds till five o'clock.

Dinnertime, for Delores, meant meeting up with friends at the Pig & Whistle, sitting at the counter with a beer and having some idle conversation. Several of the town's single residents usually congregated at the Pig & Whistle in the evenings. The police chief would come by for his nightly cheeseburger and onion rings and look over the assembly to ensure that none of its number would give Costas, the proprietor, any trouble at closing time. Not that he ever had to contend with any serious troublemakers, just a few young locals who might try to pick a fight with visiting out-of-towners. The exciting thing about dinner for Delores was that she never knew whether she would run into someone new. As it turned out, this particular evening there was just one person Delores didn't know on the diner side of the Pig and Whistle. He was sitting alone and eating a steak dinner. Delores guessed that he was waiting for the local magistrate's court to open at six o'clock.

As she slipped into the chair at her usual table at one end of the diner, Delores found herself near a group of people having an animated discussion of the day's events in the town square. Two of the people worked in offices on the square; one of them, an animated woman, worked for the local travel agency. This woman seemed to have an uncanny ability to ferret out dubious information about town residents, embellishing her tales with details that listeners found hard to verify or disprove. At the moment, she was loudly expressing her belief that Yelena Moshansky's son-in-law, who worked in the bank examiner's office in Tampa, had told Yelena that Neighborhood Savings wasn't safe.

"Now, there's no reason for you to go around saying things like that," said Police Chief Orsi, who was concerned that people around him seemed to be paying too much attention to these words. "And besides, everybody knows that bank money is insured. I mean it's insured by the government, not some two-bit operator."

"All I'm saying is what I heard," replied the woman, "and someone who works for the bank examiner's office ought to know."

In fact, Yelena's son-in-law didn't really work for the state bank examiner or for the Home Loan Bank, which monitored federally chartered savings and loan associations. He was actually a CPA who worked in the municipal treasury in Tampa. If asked, he would probably have replied that as far as he knew all bank deposits below a certain ceiling were insured by either a state or federal insurance fund. That didn't mean that deposits were totally safe, of course; insurance funds could go broke. Still, it was unlikely that either the federal or state government would permit that. All he had said, which Yelena had misinterpreted as a call for action, was that in the present climate the big money center banks seemed less vulnerable than savings and loan associations.

"Would someone please tell me what you're talking about?" asked Delores for the second time.

"Old Mrs. Moshansky took all her money out of Neighborhood Savings this morning — in cash."

"Who's Mrs. Moshansky?"

"You know her, old lady lives in the house next to the Baptist church. Well anyway, her son-in-law told her that the bank wasn't safe and that she should take her money out."

"Really? When did you say she took her money out?"

"Now Delores," cut in Chief Orsi, "there's no need for you to get all excited. There's no reason to believe that the bank's in any trouble at all."

"I don't know about that," Delores replied. "All I know is Ray took all of Hanson's money out of that bank today."

All motion and talk in the diner came to a halt. The only steady sound that could be heard was that of the stranger's knife scraping against the cheap ceramic on which Costas served his food.

"What are you saying?" asked the formerly loud travel agent, her eyes alight at having discovered yet another snippet of proof of the world's perfidy.

"Just what I said," answered Delores, already annoyed with herself for having said something that might or might not have been confidential. Still, Ray hadn't said that she shouldn't mention it, and he always made such a big thing of whatever he didn't want mentioned, so she really didn't think she had done anything wrong. "Ray took $300,000 out of Neighborhood and put it in Alamo in Jacksonville."

In the disjointed babble of conversation that ensued, a triumphant voice could be heard: "Chief, I want to know what you're going to do about this." After all, Orsi was the chief of police, the uniformed representative of all that was fair and just in Moxahachie. It was every citizen's right to demand that the sworn protector of the peace uphold the peace when it was threatened. If any of the concerned citizens in that diner could have been magically transported out of there and asked whether they really believed the bank was going broke, they might have been confused. Surely what they believed was beside the point. Here were two events: Mrs. Moshansky, whose son-in-law was an important and knowledgeable person, took all her money out of the bank; then Ray Stefanik, known to all the county as one of the canniest businessmen to hang up a shingle, took all his fund's money out of the same bank. What could this possibly mean other than that the bank was in trouble?

Perhaps there are some people who find it easier to understand the nature of coincidence than do others. For each of the former, there must be several of the latter, who react as the group in the diner did, by constructing a simple scenario that could account for some important known facts. Of course, there were logical problems with such scenarios. For instance, how many times did banks really go broke; didn't insurance mean that depositors couldn't lose their money? Even if the diners had considered them, they may have thought that logical objections didn't reduce the truthlike sound of their scenario by a single jot. For those whose impressions of bank failures were shaped by Jimmy Stewart's experience in *It's a Wonderful Life,* that banks go broke was as unquestioned as humidity in August.

Again, perhaps some people who understand the nature of coincidence can also resist the weight of others' faith in sharply contrasted realities of black and white. These recalcitrants, destined to be strange and lonely voices on the very fringes of the social order you and I know, are even fewer in number than folks who understand but don't resist. If to understanding and resistance we add the further requirement of an ability to stem the tide of apprehension that builds around these simple constructions of reality, we are left with a very small number indeed. As a consequence, the air in the Pig & Whistle was pregnant with unspoken thoughts, such as outsiders are running Neighborhood Savings — what if they came down here especially to rip us off?

Annoyed with himself for having allowed the conversation to take such an alarming tone, Chief Orsi's voice cut rather brusquely through the intense atmosphere: "All right people, get a hold of yourselves. Look at you going on about something you know nothing about. Still, because you have some real questions that need answering, I tell you what I'm going to do. I'm going to call Mr. Bailey and talk to him. I'm going to tell him there are some serious questions about the bank that need answering and see if I can't get some answers. Now you all go about your business and let this alone for tonight."

Right. Orsi's little speech stood no chance of getting people to stop talking about what they had heard, let alone forget it. Each party to that evening's conversation was already thinking through his or her next steps and the reactions of the people the steps would pass by. Information ownership can provide as much if not more of the light-headedness attributed to more traditional intoxicants, and to be the first owners of information like this — well, the chance might come along only once in a lifetime.

That evening, nearly every telephone in Moxahachie was working overtime. No single person made more than a few calls really, but it was amazing how quickly they added up. The reactions to the calls were as varied as the people who answered them. The commonest reaction suggested that the current informer had the facts wrong or that none of this mattered since depositors were insured anyway. To some, the fact that Chief Orsi would be calling the bank's general manager lent authority to the story; to others, it was met only with disdain. Perhaps the net result of all this was nothing more than a buzz, if you will, on the surface of the collective psyche of the town.

And what of the police chief's call to Jim Bailey? Well, he made the call all right, but rather than the personification of authority and decisiveness seen by the Pig & Whistle crowd, it was a subdued and diffident chief who spoke to Bailey: "It's just a few rumors going around, Mr. Bailey, that I thought you should know about. You understand I know there's nothing for anyone to worry about, but some folks who aren't very well educated were saying these things about the bank."

"What things, Chief?"

"Well, sir, the general idea seemed to be that the bank's in some kind of money trouble. Now you never can tell how these rumors get started. I tried to tell the people there was nothing to it, but they weren't listening. I just thought you should know that."

"I understand, chief, and thank you for bringing it to my attention. And no, I assure you, there is nothing wrong with Neighborhood Savings and Loan. It's in good financial shape. You probably know that we had the bank board people down just last month on their quarterly visit and they gave us a clean bill of health. There's absolutely nothing to these rumors that you heard, and I just wouldn't worry about them at all."

Then why didn't Bailey say he knew how the rumors started? Why didn't he tell me why Mrs. Moshansky's and Ray Stefanik's withdrawals didn't matter, wondered the chief. What was that man trying to hide?

Jim Bailey went to bed that night slightly shocked at the impressionable nature of people who saw an old woman take her life savings out of an institution and naturally assumed that the institution was broke. Didn't they understand the nature of deposit insurance? Didn't they know that the sort of bank failure that resulted in irreparable losses to depositors was a thing of the past?

Many of the people of Moxahachie went to bed slightly disoriented by the possibility that they might be the focus of something significant, however unwanted. Some wished that something, anything, *would* happen if only to break the monotony of their lives. Even a few of those who had their own money in the bank and thought it might be in some danger sort of wished the bank would go under. Now that would truly justify their belief in the verity of catastrophe, the perpetual imminence of doom. This belief required little in the way of real nourishment, but what little it did require was deeply cherished. An event of this magnitude, the total or partial loss of all their savings, would truly be a vindication of their lack of faith.

Anticipation was in the air as people went about their business the next morning. The deli directly opposite the bank was always the first establishment to open, at seven on weekdays and at eight on Saturdays and Sundays. Before the deli officially opened, two workers swabbed the floor, cleaned the counters, and put new liners in the wastebaskets. The first few customers of the day were usually blue-collar workers, men and women on their way to the sawmill on the outskirts of town or city sanitation workers. The proprietor of the deli knew all his early morning customers and what they had for breakfast: usually bacon with eggs on rolls, coffee, and sometimes orange juice. Later-arriving customers preferred bran muffins and toasted raisin bagels. The proprietor usually used the lull between the two waves of customers to lay out his fresh stock of bagels and muffins.

It was during this lull, at around a quarter past eight, that one of the deli workers directed the proprietor's attention to the police cruiser parked outside Neighborhood Savings and Loan. This was odd because if either of the two night-duty officers stopped at the square on her way home, she would usually come into the deli. When he next looked toward the bank, the proprietor noticed that it was the chief of police who stood outside the cruiser, apparently talking to a group of people who had gathered there. He wondered whether the gathering had something to do with the reported trouble at the bank.

The proprietor's wife had informed him the previous evening that Yelena Moshansky's was only the first of several withdrawals from the bank that day. She had heard this from friends

312 In Search of Meaning

at the grocery store. She had rushed home to implore her husband to take their money out of the bank the first thing next morning. He had asked what money she was referring to. The bank owned the mortgages on the deli and their house. The line of credit he used for operating expenses also came from the bank. The bank owned them several times over. In fact, he wasn't sure that it might not be a good thing for them if the bank were to go broke. He was tempted to walk over to the bank and listen to the conversation in progress. But at that moment the first of the "glazed doughnut and coffees" walked into the deli and he was forced to remain where he was.

Had he walked over, the proprietor would have heard Chief Orsi using his sincerest voice to address the dozen people who had gathered outside the bank almost two hours before opening time. "Now you people understand that this is foolishness," Orsi said. "It isn't even the bank that's protecting your money; it's the government. All money in this bank that's in accounts of less than $100,000 is 100 percent insured by the government. Nothing can happen to your money. You know that."

"I know all about that government insurance, Roy Orsi, and there's no point in you telling me otherwise," spoke a well-dressed woman who appeared to be in her early sixties. "A friend of mine in Texas had her money in a bank that went broke, and that's what they told her. 'Don't worry,' they said, 'your money's insured.' Well, she didn't worry then, but she's real worried now. It's been a year since the government took over that bank, and she still hasn't seen all her money yet. I'm too old to be taking that kind of chance."

The chief was now boiling inside, but he maintained a pleasant exterior. Institutions like the bank and people like its president and other senior officers were his main support when the time came for him to run for reelection as police chief. While he wasn't going to break any law for them, he felt it was his duty to somehow help them through any rough spots. The chief, who was no less venal than any of the other people who look out for themselves, had at least some notion of fair play, a notion that included standing up for people that stood up for you.

And so, even though he didn't particularly care for the bank's president or general manager, who obviously didn't belong to Moxahachie, Orsi still felt compelled to help.

Less than an hour later Chief Orsi was sitting in Jim Bailey's office and reporting on his encounters: "I can't understand it, sir. It's as if there's no reasoning with them at all. I tried asking them why they were doing this, who had said what to them about the bank. Like you said, I told them that the money was insured by the government, but they just kept saying they'd feel safer with their money somewhere else."

"Don't blame yourself, Chief. You did what you could. I wouldn't worry about this anyway. We have cash coming in this morning. In fact, it should be in any time now, and that should be able to take care of withdrawals of more people than are standing out there right now."

"Well, I don't know, sir. I just keep thinking that if word gets out about this, you'll have half the town beating a path up to your door and then this thing could really get out of hand."

"I don't think so," cut in Bailey. "Our cash reserves are adequate to meet this crisis, and if by some chance we do run out, well our check's still good anywhere in the state. Once people see that we can cover anybody who comes in, they'll be reassured and this thing will be over."

Well, Orsi had tried to tell him. Bailey was almost as obstinate as the people outside. Who knows why some innocuous events snowball into crises? Heaven knows, you can't blame the people who have the crises dumped in their laps. The real stupidity is to find a crisis staring you in the eye and then to pretend it doesn't exist. Well, maybe the bank was that solid, thought Chief Orsi, but the people of this town certainly weren't going to be reassured at the sight of a dozen people taking their money out of the bank and running. To his way of thinking, that was how panic started. However, there were some things he could do. Until something else turned up, he could have two squad cars stationed outside the bank. The police officers would be of some assistance in crowd control or at least could discourage any vagrants from making off with some panicky depositor's money. This was turning out to be one fine day indeed.

At nine o'clock sharp, Jim Bailey walked down the stairs of the bank to confront a staff in the throes of a full-blown anxiety attack. Through the windows in the front of the bank, everybody inside could see the people gathering outside. The bank employees had sensed no personal animosity as they had shouldered their way through the waiting crowd and walked inside, but the intent written on all the faces staring in couldn't help but disconcert them. Two of the employees apparently couldn't stand the strain and were actually trying to communicate with some of the depositors through the plate-glass windows.

"You probably know," Bailey began, "that some rumors are circulating about the strength of the bank. Some of you already know what I'm going to say because you deal with the reconciliation statements. Some others worked with the regulator's team last month. Anyway, just in case there are any doubts — there is absolutely nothing wrong with the bank. Today is going to be a day like any other, except that a lot of the business you do in the first few minutes is going to involve closing accounts." A murmur of appreciation met Bailey's halfhearted attempt at humor. "I want you to believe that nothing extraordinary has occurred. For some reason the natives are restless, and we will have to attend to them. That is all; you can go about your business now."

"Jim?" asked Stewart in an unreasonably calm voice. "Wouldn't it be a good idea to open the doors early and have the people standing outside taken care of immediately? I mean some of them don't even really believe that they're going to get their money back."

"No," replied Jim in as patient a voice as he could muster. "We're running a bank here, and we really cannot be responsible if people start paying attention to crazy rumors. The bank will open at ten o'clock as usual. Now if there are no more questions, I really do suggest we all get back to work."

Actually, Stewart's idea had been a good one. By getting people in, instead of having them wait on the street where the rest of the world could see them, the bank might well have defused the gathering crisis. Unfortunately, he had phrased his suggestion in terms of the mental condition of their customers. Jim Bailey, a normally astute man, might in other circumstances have been able to separate the meaning of the suggestion from its form. However, he wasn't feeling very friendly toward his customers just then, and the sentiment clouded what little remained of his judgment.

Meanwhile, Ben Seward sat at his desk on the second floor, going through the mail addressed to Jim Bailey. Though it was only yesterday, it already seemed an age since he had been reprimanded for apparently falling down on his job. He would be much more conservative in deciding what messages he would withhold, with the result that today Jim was going to be presented with flyers about real estate deals in Tampa and hot-air balloon rides in Moxahachie, among other things.

After the usual interval, Stewart Griggs sauntered up to Ben's desk and asked him if he'd seen the nationally televised football game the previous evening between the New York Giants and the Chicago Bears. Why not, thought Ben, Stewart did this every Tuesday, and hadn't Bailey said that this was a day like any other? Reflecting on Stewart's question it suddenly occurred to Ben that he tended to see the world in football metaphors and that was because he understood football. Just a few minutes ago he had caught himself thinking that last night's goal-line stand by an aging Giants defense player was one of the finest he'd ever seen. When it came down to it and your back was against your own goal line, character was defined by what you did. The coaches could teach you the plays you should make and could even call in the play, but the result on the field had to come down to who wanted it the most. It was no surprise, then, that Ben believed that if all the bank personnel wanted to pull through badly enough, why then they would.

In a burst of unreasonable anger, Ben looked at the casual Stewart Griggs and thought that it was lightweights like Stewart who were going to cost him his job. "Sorry Stewart, I've got to get back to these. There are a pile of them today."

"No problem, Ben. I'm sure it beats fiddling while the world erupts in flames around you." With that, Stewart wandered over to the window facing the street. "You might find it interesting to note, however, that there's a bit of a line outside our doors. I'm afraid it's beginning to stretch a bit . . . uh oh . . . "

"What, what?" asked Ben.

"Smile folks; you're on camera. Television has arrived."
And so it had. The relentless communicator, the great
equalizer, the protector of the many from the depredations of
the few appeared outside Neighborhood Savings in the form of
a van belonging to a local TV station. A reporter and the van
driver, who apparently doubled as the cameraperson, emerged
from the van and looked first at the line of people outside the
bank and then up at the faces that were staring down at them
from the second floor. At the sight of so many people, the reporter's face broke into a broad smile, and with a friendly wave
she joined the cameraperson as he went over his equipment.

Jim Bailey spoke into the telephone in his office. He was
calling Joe Webster at CitiBank, and of all the calls he had made
that morning this one may have been the most important. "Hello
Joe, this is Jim Bailey at Neighborhood, how are you? . . . Well
things could be quieter around here, Joe, to tell you the truth
and that's part of the reason for my call. . . . You did, huh? . . .
Thanks, Joe; I sure could use a little help right now. Our cash
float's been bolstered this morning, so we figure on being able
to handle most of the crowd that might be coming our way. If
we run out, rather than asking you for a short-term loan, we
thought we might be able to get you to treat our cashier's checks
as cash. Now this would be for a short time only, Joe, probably
into mid-morning or so, until the dust settles. . . . Uh, $100,000?
Joe, figuring on an average deposit of $10,000, that's just ten
people. . . . Well, would you clear it, Joe? If your people could
see their way to giving me up to about half a million, that should
tide us over this thing. . . . All right, Joe, I look forward to hearing from you."

By now the news was probably all over the state, thought
Bailey. Everyone would know that Neighborhood was looking
for quick money. How long could it be before those sharks in
Tampa found out? Any legal advisor would have told Bailey
that he couldn't any longer pretend that he didn't have a serious cash crisis. If the regulator's office heard about this, the bank
could be legally liable for not having informed it of the trouble
earlier. But it wasn't going to happen that way, was it? There
couldn't be more than, what — forty people out there? They could

handle that many; of course they could. After that they'd be cash starved for a few weeks, but business should pick up by Thanksgiving. He'd done the arithmetic, and there was no point in panicking now.

"Yes, what is it?" Jim snapped at his secretary.

"Jim, KTLV-TV is on the line. They want to know when might be a good time for you to speak to them."

Jim tried to control his rage. On the one hand, not speaking to the press gave them the liberty to concoct whatever stories they pleased. On the other hand, if he did speak to them, they just might twist his words as they chose. In either case, the whole event would get unwanted publicity. One thing was sure: he could have done without this added trouble.

"Would you please tell the television people that I'm in a meeting, but if they'll leave a number I'd be happy to call them back."

Two hours later Jim Bailey was still behind his desk and still on the phone. This time, though, the phone call wasn't at his behest. "Yes, Mr. White, everything will be available to your people. Yes sir. . . . There's no cause to do that, sir. As you will see when you get here, this is a well-run operation. . . . Absolutely, it is my judgment that the bank need not be closed. . . . Yes sir, the deposit to loan ratio has undoubtedly fallen, but we can't say by how much. Still, I do believe the end is in sight. . . . Cashier's checks. Yes sir, we explained to them that they're as good as government money. We don't know why they prefer those to leaving their money in the bank, no sir."

The following are extracts from the transcript of a KTLV-TV special report on the mysterious failure of Neighborhood Savings and Loan.

Voice-over: In his comments the chief regulator, Jeremy White, confirmed that Neighborhood was, as of that evening, formally out of business.

White: Every depositor's money is safe. The moment we can establish some order here, every depositor will be able to access his or her account. We will be working very hard to find a new owner for the bank, and until we do, the federal government will act as de facto owner of this institution.

Q: How soon will it be before you establish order?

White: We can't say. It all depends on how clean the books are.

Q: Can you rule out the possibility of criminal conduct of any kind on the part of the management?

White: We are in no position to rule out any possibility right now.

Voice-over: Rumors about the shaky financial position had started circulating in Moxahachie well before Tuesday's spectacular run on the bank. We spoke earlier to some residents of the town and bank depositors about their fears.

Q: Would you tell us your name, sir, and what you do for a living?

Eldon: My name is Eldon Harrison, and I work a wood lathe at the sawmill.

Q: Shouldn't you be at work on a Tuesday morning? Would you tell us what you're doing standing in line outside this bank?

Eldon: Well, I'm waiting to take my money out. I heard the bank isn't safe.

Q: Do you know that your money is insured by the Federal Savings and Loan Insurance Corporation?

Eldon: Yeah, but I heard that if a bank goes broke, it takes a long time before you can get your money back, and I've been saving real hard to make a down payment on a cabin cruiser. I'm not looking for any surprises.

Q: Would you tell us where you heard that it takes a long time to get your money?

Eldon: I can't remember. I just decided I didn't want to take any chances.

Q: Would you tell us your name, sir, and what you do?

Costas: My name is Costas Dimitropoulos, and I own the Pig & Whistle, a restaurant and bar here in Moxahachie.

Q: And did you hear of trouble concerning Neighborhood Savings before it actually struck?

Costas: In my line of business, you hear many things. Who's to say what's true and what's not? People get drunk, they feel lonely, they want to talk. Sometimes they talk about things that trouble them, and sometimes they talk about things they'd like to trouble. Usually I pay no attention to these things. But Neighborhood, well, this is different. This is the place where the whole town has its money, right? Whoever runs the bank should be elected, that's what I say, and not just be someone who comes from New York to run a business. This is not a business; this is people's lives.

Q: And you're saying you heard something concerning the safety of the bank before today?

Costas: Sure, I heard. Everybody heard, right? I just didn't pay any attention because I thought I was a sensible person; I don't get excited, so I ignored it, and now my wife won't speak to me. Sure, I heard.

"My name is Stewart Griggs, and I will be your host for this evening."

I can't remember how many times I've said those words since coming to New York. I work in a little bistro below Houston, just off West Broadway. I came here almost immediately after the events I've described to you above. I don't really need to work as a waiter, or host. My father could take care of me for the rest of my life and probably will as far as I know. No, that's not why I'm here. I just felt that by getting away I might make more sense of what happened, of what I allowed to happen.

You have probably guessed that I was in this from the beginning. I was there when old Mrs. Moshansky decided to pull her money out of the bank. I also saw Jim and Catherine Stefanik's eyes go wide when they heard Ben getting yelled at. I was at the Pig & Whistle the evening its patrons came upon their huge discovery. When Delores made her earthshaking announcement about the Hanson money, I knew the effect it would have. All I needed to do to calm things down would have been to say that the jumbo CDs have a fixed duration, and that after a time, they stop. Of course, I don't know that my saying it would have changed anything, but now we never will know, will we?

Oh, don't worry about the people who worked for Neighborhood Savings. Most of them landed on their feet. Take Ben, for instance. With the mass transfer of deposits from Neighborhood to the local CitiBank, Joe Webster found that he suddenly had to recruit more employees. Who better than people who knew the business, understood the clients, and most importantly, were from those parts.

You see, I have a theory. The reason Neighborhood went belly up wasn't because the management did something wrong but because they weren't from those parts. Oh, the Home Loan Bank and even the district attorney's office kept staring hard and long at the affairs of Jim Bailey and the bank president, but they couldn't really make anything stick to them. There was that business about writing a promissory note to Panhandle Development, in which they had an ownership share, but though they may have stretched the law, they never really broke it. And in any case, if the DA had wanted to make a case out of an abstruse technical issue, there was also the state senator who was unwilling to see his protégé dragged through some unwelcome publicity.

I'm also not prepared to believe that Jim Bailey was any more corrupt than old man Richardson, who'd run Neighborhood earlier. The whole town knew that the last two generations of Richardsons were as crooked as they came and still did nothing about them. Can you believe that? Not minding being taken to the cleaners because the people doing the taking happened to be born a few miles from where you were?

Well, whatever. I suddenly became tired of people from my parts. I thought I needed a change from myself and them. Moxahachie had begun to resemble a town recovering from a three-day carnival. After the local TV stations, the national networks started paying attention, simply because there hadn't been any savings and loan scandals in a while and there was a presidential campaign on. This was an opportunity to lambaste the current administration over their failed economic policies. Then came the reporters writing the feature pieces, and the town lapped them all up. Around the same time, my father began talking about getting me started in local politics, and I thought it was time to take my affairs into my own hands. I left.

One final piece of news that may interest you. At her daughter's behest, Yelena Moshansky entered a rest home for the aged with special needs. The daughter felt that Yelena needed institutional assistance because of some of her new proclivities, which included breeding chickens in her living room. The doctors said that Yelena was regressing to the days of her youth in eastern Poland.

"Good evening, my name is Stewart Griggs, and I'll be your host for this evening."

The Tale and Organizational Existentialism

Why does the preceding tale belong in a book on the implications of existential issues for an understanding of organizations? What do either organizations or the tale have to do with Albert Camus's *The Plague*? In the rest of this chapter, I attempt to provide the outlines of answers to these and similar questions.

I do not propose to address the question of how Albert Camus's stories and ideas relate to existential philosophy. Such a relation would have to be drawn not just with care but with some stretching of the boundaries of that body of philosophy and of Camus's own intentions, given that he declared categorically, "I am not an existentialist. . . . Sartre is an existentialist, and the only book of ideas that I have published, *Le Mythe de Sisyphe*, was directed against the so-called existentialist philosophers" (Camus, 1967, p. 259). However, as noted elsewhere in this book, existentialists themselves are uncertain over where to draw the boundaries to their field, or indeed whether it is a field (Pauchant, 1993).

Commentators have suggested that *The Plague* may be read and taught as literature, philosophy, or even history (Kellman,

1985). None of these approaches explicitly addresses the aspects of *The Plague* that deal with the organization of human beings in collective activity. Yet Camus's ideas have particular implications for students of such collective activity however the activity manifests itself. Speaking only months after the cessation of hostilities in the European theater of the Second World War, Camus said that "the last five years [have] brought out . . . the extreme solidarity of men with one another. Solidarity in crime for some, solidarity in the upsurge of resistance in others. . . . When a Czech was shot, the life of a grocer in the Rue de Beaune was in jeopardy" (1967, p. 260). Writing to Roland Barthes, Camus said that *The Plague* represents a "movement from an attitude of solitary revolt to the recognition of a community whose struggles must be shared. . . . [T]here [is] an evolution . . . towards solidarity and participation [in my world]" (p. 253).

What is this plague, and how does it demonstrate the existence of such solidarity? At the level of the narrative, the plague is an infestation of bubonic plague visited upon the town of Oran on the southern shores of the Mediterranean. Beneath this superficial level, Camus's plague is commonly thought to refer at least in passing to the "infestation" of France by conquering German troops during the Second World War (Brée, 1985, p. 16). It would be a mistake, however, to draw direct parallels between the German occupation and the plague because several structural characteristics of the occupation are absent from the tale (Maquet, 1958, p. 82). In fact, the plague may not be the symbol of an "outer abstract evil" at all but derive rather from the "values implicit in the unconscious attitudes of [its victims]" (Brée, 1961, p. 118).

Camus himself has provided insights into the nature of plague by characterizing its defining feature as monotony. Calamities such as the plague represent extraordinary misfortunes precisely because they persist over long periods of time. And while they persist, they cause their victims to experience "the same thing over and over again (Camus, 1947, p. 134). These calamities are "unflagging adversar[ies] . . . shrewd organizer[s], doing [their] work thoroughly and well" (p. 148).

More insights into the nature of plague emerge from its effects on its victims. Those people to whom their own peace of mind is more important than a human life display symptoms of being infected by the plague (p. 205). And how do these people reveal their preference for peace of mind? They do so by subscribing to acts and principles that demand complete allegiance, even to the point where such allegiance could result in the death of another. A climate had apparently come to prevail in the world where even those who "were better than the rest could not keep themselves . . . from killing or letting others kill because such is the logic by which they live" (p. 206). Thus the plague manifests itself not in a particularly demonic logic that might have attracted people at a certain point in history. Rather, the very proclivity of humans to subscribe to any logic that might justify the extinction of human life is itself evidence of infection by plague. The plague-stricken exist everywhere because the microbe causing plague occurs plentifully in nature. Everyone carries a latent infection, and everyone possesses the capacity to infect others. The only good people in such a world battle constantly, to the point of a soul-wrenching weariness, to keep from infecting others (p. 207).

There also exist well-meaning people who, although surrounded by plague, hold on jealously to the idea that they possess choices as individuals. They "even contrived to fancy that they were still behaving as free men" (p. 138). Whereas in the early days of infestation and exile, people might still focus solely on the unique ways in which the plague affects their lives, this personalization of the epidemic cannot last. As the plague persists, individual destinies die away to be replaced by collective destiny "made of plague and the emotions shared by all" (p. 138). Consequently, there can be no question of heroism, with its implicit suggestion of personal sacrifice, among those that fight the plague. Fighting a plague merely requires a developed sense of common decency. This common decency could, of course, mean different things to different people. In most people, though, it manifests itself as a desire only to do their jobs (p. 136).

What lessons emerge from Camus's book for those of us who live, work, and study in organizations? First, we understand that "plagues" do not represent transient "crises" (Pauchant & Mitroff, 1992; Shrivastava, 1987; Starbuck, Greve, and Hedberg,

1978) because they emerge from natural causes and are of long duration. Rather, they refer to the pestilence of principles and the absurdity of rules that persistently divorce humans from the experience of their lives. The very values and beliefs that guide humans' conduct as members of families, work organizations, and nations are themselves the microbes that carry disease, for adherence to abstract principle implies a possible willingness, in the name of principle, to participate in the extinction of the one thing that is no abstraction, their humanness.

A second lesson reveals to us the insidious nature of a disease that forces all faced with it to choose between succumbing to it and adopting its own methods to fight against it. We begin to comprehend the futility of appealing to ideas and abstractions to combat the absurdity of lives governed by principle. The commonest way of changing organizational lives, it has been observed, is to replace current ideologies and values with new ones (Gagliardi, 1986). Yet any ideology carries within it seeds of the absurd because it represents a structure of values and beliefs designed to interpret experience and, by the same token, to divorce the interpreting humans *from* experience. Thus the symptoms of the plague lie not in the inappropriateness of a particular set of principles in the governance of individual lives but in the very existence of unquestioned sets of principles.

Finally, fighting against the plague does not denote an act of great bravery or heroism. Organizational members may, for instance, resist edicts that defy reason or resist actions for the good of their organizations that hurt others not from a sense of moral outrage but merely from a desire to display common decency. Thus their roles in organizations are no longer drawn within the narrow confines of organizational objectives but include a sympathy for and a solidarity with all others everywhere. Organizational members could therefore call attention to the potential hazards of their products from a sense of solidarity with those that might use their products, not from a sense of conviction over right and wrong. To prevent a passerby from stepping into the path of a fast-moving car requires no great conviction, merely a sense of common decency.

The Plague at Neighborhood Savings and Loan

The story you have just read draws its inspiration from Camus's *The Plague* in more than one way. At the most obvious level, it points to the sheer absurdity of the crisis that came upon the Neighborhood Savings and Loan Association. Much like death from bubonic plague, the bankrupting of a perfectly healthy institution by the actions of a mentally impaired woman and the confused words of an aspiring college freshman argues against the prevalence of reason in our world. It is not the bankruptcy that represents the plague, however, but the blind adherence of several of the protagonists to their inflexible systems of meaning that is the true sign of infestation.

Jim Bailey's view of the world was probably tinted largely with lenses fashioned in Chicago or New York, lenses that may have only permitted limited views of towns such as Moxahachie in the Florida panhandle. Jim is not a bad man as we understand the term because he had no desire to hurt or defraud anybody. And yet Jim was infected by the plague because he tended to see the town, its citizens, and his job primarily as opportunities for business within the bounds of the law. His adherence to legal principles and the practice of good business put him out of touch with the experiences of those who but for the accident of history were no different from him. Consequently, when mistrust gripped the town and caused its residents to fear for the safety of their wealth, Jim's worldview provided him no assistance in understanding the feelings of the townspeople on whom his livelihood depended. A sense of solidarity with their lives may well have led Jim to address their fears on the morning when they began to emerge. Caught, however, in the trap of his own system of reason, Jim reacted in the only way he knew how, by keeping the doors of the bank closed until it was indeed too late.

The townspeople, unfortunately, were no different from Jim. Their own lenses and heuristics did not permit them to see Jim as anything but a stranger from the North whose intentions could not be trusted or motivations understood. In a purely objective sense, their money was totally safe, a fact that did not affect their actions. Had they extended the same common decency and courtesy to Jim that they would show to one of their own, they might have been prompted to ask Jim just how much at risk their money really was. But their own heuristics probably denied the possibility that any good could come of such an inquiry, for wasn't the man an outsider who could not be trusted?

Of all the protagonists, Stewart Griggs probably came closest to a recognition of the absurd. The night before the run on the bank, as he sat in a bar and heard the fears of the town being bandied about, he could have quelled the people's concern with a few chosen words. He could have explained that the two withdrawals fueling the rumor were perfectly normal and had absolutely no implications for the health of the bank. We cannot be sure that this would have had an impact on events, yet Stewart, for no reason we can understand, did not even try. Whether his silence stemmed from a moment of awareness or a chance aberration, whether his new life represented a quiet determination to do his job without fuss or a fashionable substitution of a bohemian cage for a gilded one remains to be seen.

Conclusion:
The Healthy Organization:
Reuniting the Self,
the Organization,
and the Natural World

Thierry C. Pauchant

It would be very nice to be able to propose in this conclusion a theory and practice of management that address existential issues in a positive way and ensure the health of an organization and its environment. We are, however, still very far away from such praxis; this book is more of an undertaking in progress. It is evident that vanguard managers, scholars, and researchers will need to reflect for a period of time on the critical observations and pragmatic suggestions made in this book and also to reflect on their current daily practice.

In this conclusion, I attempt to answer two pragmatic questions. First, how can one distinguish between an approach that honors existential ideals and one that denies them? This question leads to yet another attempt to define existentialism. Second, how can one assist in a better management of existential issues in one's organization? This leads to suggested diverse avenues for further learning, research, and experimentation.

What Is Existentialism?

We have returned, full circle, to the question raised in the introduction to this book: What is existentialism? This question is not trivial. Its answer would allow us to distinguish between a managerial ethos and management methods that foster existential health and those that can lead to illness.

The difficulty in answering this question precisely resides in the fact that what we have called the *existential tradition* is not an homogeneous tradition. As already pointed out in the preceding pages of this book, Camus and Heidegger refused to be called existentialists; Sartre (1970) defined existentialism as humanism, and others have emphasized that Sartre did not represent the overall thrust of existentialism (Barrett, 1958).

My intent is not to split hairs over a definition that nobody cares about. For example, I am not concerned about knowing whether Kierkegaard is more existentialist than Sartre. However, I am very concerned about defining the meaning of *existential health in organizations*. A better definition of existential health could be instrumental in avoiding another trivialization of existential issues in organizations. The chapters of this book chronicle some of the damage done in and out of organizations as a result of the appropriation of pseudoexistential ideals by people seduced by the search for an organizational and/or individual perfection.

As emphasized by all the authors of this book, the existential tradition urges individuals to determine their choices and take responsibility for them. Furthermore, these authors imply that it is about time that management scholars and managers alike denounce the disastrous approaches and methods currently used in management and act from their personal and political courage to try to stop both the teaching and the practice of such methods. Given this call, it is important to be able to distinguish between approaches that are existentially healthy and those that are not.

Although the authors of this book have properly proposed many different managerial tools and actions for fostering existential health, I do not personally believe that we know enough at the present time on the subject of existentialism in organizations to propose a generic and comprehensive program. Rather, I propose that a set of eight general questions be asked in order to judge whether an approach embraces existential ideals. These questions are derived from the observations made by the authors of this book. (These eight questions appear together, in one list, near the end of this section.)

Question 1. Does the approach address complex issues without trivializing them yet still allow for a democratic dialogue on the concrete reality of individuals and for the development of their fantasies?

Existentialists are first of all concerned about understanding the *concrete* subjective experience of individuals and their *concrete* actions in the world, being attentive to events, experiences, and actions in their day-to-day lives. With this in mind, existentialists should refrain from using mumbo-jumbo jargon and models that are overly sophisticated. As argued by Buber (1958) and Bohm and Edwards (1991), for example, the use of such jargon hinders the possibility of a genuine dialogue between people, negates the possibility of real encounters, and can be used for the protection of the corporatist elite in power, thereby leading to totalitarianism. In addition, existentialists are concerned about sustaining and developing in individuals imagination, dreams, and fantasy that are rich enough to mobilize these individuals into implementing actions.

For me, Sartre is anti-existentialist when he uses unreadable sophisticated jargon in his philosophical books; however, he fully embraces the existential ideals in his novels and plays. In management, authors such as Chanlat and Bédard (1990), Schwartz (1990b), or Zaleznik (1989) have denounced this unfortunate use of language in such areas as corporate finance, strategic management, and all specializations. Other authors have suggested that "researchers may be hurting managers when they prescribe lists and steps that managers should use to improve their thinking" (Weick, 1984, p. 240). In this book, we have attempted to refrain from using jargon and from presenting overly sophisticated models; some of us have also tried to use more artistic modes of exposition, such as stories, to engage the reader's imagination. However, much still needs to be done to make existential material accessible to managers and employees alike so that they can readily use it in their daily practice in organizations.

Question 2. Is the approach grounded in the individual in concrete relation with the world, avoiding an escape into either individualism or collectivism?

It should be clear from this book that existentialism is quite different from individualism. While the existential tradition emphasizes the uniqueness of the individual, grounded in the inescapable experience of loneliness, it also stresses that the individual becomes an individual through encounters and actions with others. This view leads to the paradoxical notion that an individual becomes authentic when he or she can participate actively in a community and that a true community allows individuals to individualize. This aspect of existentialism is emphasized by all the authors in this book, particularly by Robert Kramer in Chapter Seven, where he draws on the work of Otto Rank and Carl Rogers on relationships. This dialectical dance between the self and others avoids the common escape into individualism that is evident in and out of organizations today (Bellah and others, 1985); and it similarly avoids the common escape into so-called team spirit, family spirit, community spirit, and other "holographic" nonsense currently emphasized in many organizations and by many authors of popular books on management.

Question 3. Does the approach encourage the development of an individual source of responsibility and values?

The existential perspective is not only useful for understanding the condition of the individual in relation to the world. As exemplified by the authors of this book, it can also be used for understanding in a different way the experiences and behaviors of individuals in organizations and thus the collective behaviors that are routinized and reinforced (Weick, 1979). The contention that this routinization of problematic behaviors is an escape from the courageous confronting of existential issues is particularly evident in this book in the chapters written by Omar Aktouf (on the current unequal sharing of power and profits) and Nicole Aubert (on the alienating corporate culture of so-called excellent organizations). Yet the existential perspective can also be used as an additional protection against the temptation to sacralize the concept of the organization as if organizations exist on their own, independently of the individuals who compose them. As seen in this book, the existentialist perspective grounds itself in the concrete reality of the individual forming with others a collective system of meaning. Furthermore, existentialists posit that the primary locus of meaning, values, and responsibility is to be found in the existentially healthy individual; it is only secondarily derived from such abstract notions as liberty, community, equality, and efficiency, which are viewed as the fundamental problems of leadership (O'Toole, 1993).

Question 4. Does the approach apprehend the individual and collective subjective realities of individuals in relation to their physiological health?

The existentialist perspective embraced in this book does not lead to an overemphasis on either the psychological or the social realm. While the realm of subjectivity—whether expressed individually or collectively—is particularly important from this perspective, just as important are the concrete physical and biological implications of this subjectivity and their interrelationships. This aspect of existentialism is acknowledged by all the authors in this book and is particularly emphasized by Paul Bracke and James Bugental in Chapter Two, on the relationship between existential addictions and physiological illness, and by myself in Chapter Three, on the negative ecological effects of the current pursuit of excellence. The issue for existentialists is not only that individuals should feel great, as emphasized by most current programs in organizational development, organizational psychology, and corporate culture change in an attempt to gain productivity. Existentialists also believe that individuals should be critical of themselves and of their cultural heritage in order to find a sense of personal meaning *and* to protect the fragile physical health of both individuals and the ecology. As we have argued in this book, the concrete realization of one's fragility and death leads to a realization of both the pain and fragility of the lives of others and of the planet.

From this perspective, a managerial approach that focuses so much on its social implications that it denies its physiological and biological implications is contrary to existential ideals, as further developed below.

Question 5. Are the approach's aims targeted toward an increase in humanistic health and meaning but also compatible with an ecological perspective?

In further developing the previous point, it is important to note that an existential perspective does not lead only to a humanistic perspective; that is, humanist ideals represent only part of the existential quest. The focus of the authors of this book on the relationships between existential issues and physiology or ecology emphasizes the importance of the largest *context* in which individuals live and die. While a traditional humanistic perspective can lead to the sole emphasis that human actions need to better human conditions, the existentialist perspective emphasizes that human beings also have a responsibility toward the larger world. As suggested in the introduction of this book, the original existentialist impulse springs from the pre-Socratic period, and in particular from the philosophy of Heraclitus of Ephesus. Although some authors in existentialism have forgotten this historical heritage, it is fundamental to realize that the spirit of the pre-Socratic period *preceded* that of later times, which increasingly directed the focus of science and philosophy on the achievement of the "good society," meaning the human society. Rather differently, the pre-Socratic spirit emphasized the need for human beings to live in harmony with the entire *cosmos,* of which human beings and society are only a part.

Again, existential ideals stress that we are living not only in a world of organizations but also in a world of organisms. The existential perspective is thus compatible with an ecological view of life and work, including the need for a good society but going beyond this as well. Unlike this perspective, a strictly humanistic perspective can lead to an anthropocentric view, that is, one in which humans are seen as the center of the world and as denying their biological rootedness. In the field of management, a few authors have begun to discuss the desirability of reducing the anthropocentric view and are calling for an ecocentric managerial view (Pauchant and Fortier, 1990; Shrivastava, 1994).

Question 6. Are the approach's aims targeted toward an increase in humanistic health and meaning but also grounded in the transpersonal realm?

This question also springs from the original pre-Socratic ideals. The existentialist tradition has emphasized the need for the sacred, for mythology, for spirituality — understood not as a religious dogma but as a more general way of transcending the concerns of individuals per se, of allowing active commitment. Although not all existentialists honor the pre-Socratic spirit, this basic need is emphasized by many of them, including Campbell, Buber, Frankl, Gide, Heidegger, Kierkegaard, Marcel, Rank, Rogers, Tillich, and Yalom, and it echoes the views developed in other traditions by Dewey, James, Weil, and Whitehead. In this book, this need has been emphasized by many authors, particularly by Frederick Herzberg, who in Chapter Nine proposes that one's motivations be grounded in one's "mystery system" while one remains critical; by Estelle Morin, who argues in Chapter One that the current lack of spiritual grounding leads to a materialistic view of organizational effectiveness; and by Burkard Sievers, who in Chapter Ten emphasizes the needed process of remythologizing organizations. This aspect of existentialism represents yet another potential difference between existential and humanistic ideals.

It is important to remember that one of the founders of the modern humanistic movement in the United States, Abraham Maslow, has warned of the dangers of being stuck in the humanistic phase, a warning not understood by some change agents who wish to develop a strictly humanistic culture in organizations. Not as widely known is the fact that, after he helped found the humanistic movement, Maslow became one of the fathers of another movement in the United States: *transpersonal psychology*. As he explains (1965, pp. iii–iv):

> Humanistic psychology . . . is now quite solidly established as a viable third alternative to . . . behavioristic . . . psychology and to orthodox Freudianism. . . . This Third Psychology is now one facet of a general *weltanschauung,* a new philosophy of life, a new conception of man, the beginning of a new century of work. . . . For any man of good will . . . there is work to be done here, effective, virtuous,

satisfying work which can give rich meaning to one's
own life and to others. . . . I should say also that
I consider Humanistic, Third Force Psychology to
be transitional, a preparation for a still "higher"
Fourth Psychology, transpersonal, transhuman,
centered in the cosmos rather than in human needs
and interest, going beyond humanness, identity,
self-actualization, and the like. . . . Without the
transcendent and the transpersonal, we get sick,
violent, and nihilistic, or else hopeless and apathetic. We need something "bigger than we are" to
be awed by and to commit ourselves to in a new,
naturalistic, empirical, nonchurchly sense, perhaps
as Thoreau and Whitman, William James and John
Dewey did.

Question 7. Does the approach address both the bright and
dark sides of life, focusing on issues such as success and prosperity as well as on losses, despair, and death?

As should be evident by now, existentialists do not focus
only on the bright side of life, on potential or past victories and
successes, on actualization or transcendence. They also emphasize the dark, or tragic, side of life, the moments of despair and
the periods of anguish. Echoing the Scott Peck quotation cited
in the introduction to this book, existentialists also posit that
life is difficult and that an authentic, responsible, and courageous individual needs to address both sides of life in general
and at work. This need has been emphasized by all the authors
of this book, particularly by Howard Schwartz, who in Chapter Eight calls for a better acknowledgment of the dark side,
and by Narayan Pant, who in Chapter Eleven suggests that unauthentic individuals are powerless in preventing crises. This
dialectical view of life is quite different from many approaches
currently used in management, approaches that focus on how-
to methods and solutions for achieving greater success, production, or competitive advantage and place little emphasis on the
dark and destructive side of these activities, including environmental pollution and the pollution of the individual's soul.

Question 8. Does the approach admit the existence of fundamental paradoxes and use a dialectical mode of reasoning? Generalizing even more on the previous point, many existentialists embrace a dialectical perspective. Instead of positing a binary world of life versus death, humans versus nature, material versus spiritual, good versus bad, stability versus change, past versus future, many of them emphasize the necessary dance between life *and* death, humans *and* nature, material *and* spiritual, good *and* bad, stability *and* change, past *and* future. For these existentialists, an individual is, for example, not only determined by his or her past but is also free to create a future. Similarly, a "good" solution always has a problematic side. Moreover, the identity of an individual is not only stable; it is also "becoming," in transformation. This dialectical dance and the challenges it brings to current management principles is emphasized by many of the authors of this book, particularly by Kenwyn Smith in his Chapter Six dialogue between a CEO and an old sage.

The use of the existential perspective does not only challenge many current theories and practices of management. For obvious reasons, it also challenges the emotional robustness of individuals. Quite simply, it is much more difficult to address such anxiety-producing experiences than to deny them, however disastrous the consequences. This lack of existential courage, or the present condition of *bounded emotionality* as we call it in this book, is perhaps, at the emotional level, the strongest reason why the existential tradition has not been widely used in management to date. The dialectical dance I emphasize also carries a challenge at the conceptual level. Most of us, including management scholars, researchers, managers, and other employees, are not used to thinking dialectically. We prefer some variant of binary thinking in which "good" and "bad" really are good and bad.

Perhaps this use of dialectics also explains some of the reasons why the existential tradition is not easy to summarize quickly or classify. To use a rather crude metaphor, existential issues and authors are often like a wet bar of soap that zips away yet is very real in terms of the foam it leaves on the hands as one tries to grasp it from the shower floor.

The eight questions just discussed are listed together below. This list can be used as a "quick and dirty" way to determine whether a managerial approach or method seems to embrace existential ideals or not. As hinted above, *I should warn the reader, however, that this way of proceeding should not be substituted for a real, rich, and personal grounding in the existential tradition for making such a judgment.*

1. Does the approach address complex issues without trivializing them yet still allow for a democratic dialogue on the concrete reality of individuals and for the development of their fantasies?
2. Is the approach grounded in the individual in concrete relation with the world, avoiding an escape into either individualism or collectivism?
3. Does the approach encourage the development of an individual source of responsibility and values?
4. Does the approach apprehend the individual and collective subjective realities of individuals in relation to their physiological health?
5. Are the approach's aims targeted toward an increase in humanistic health and meaning but also compatible with an ecological perspective?
6. Are the approach's aims targeted toward an increase in humanistic health and meaning but also grounded in the transpersonal realm?
7. Does the approach address both the bright and dark sides of life, focusing on issues such as success and prosperity as well as on losses, despair, and death?
8. Does the approach admit the existence of fundamental paradoxes and use a dialectical mode of reasoning?

Obviously, the foregoing questions do not exhaust the existential ideals, and the use of a checklist is rather suspect from an existentialist point of view. Nevertheless, perhaps asking these questions can help managers and employees alike evaluate the corporate policies and other programs currently discussed in their organizations from a more critical perspective — especially the "search for perfection" in organizations, anticipating their dark sides.

Where Do We Go from Here?

We have only scratched the surface of the importance and management of existential issues in organizations. I hope, however, that this book will sensitize managers to the importance of these issues and give researchers the impetus to use this tradition to conduct further inquiries. Use of the existential tradition in management can be a gold mine for courageous individuals who wish to engage themselves in experimentation and research. Five general avenues for pursuing both endeavors are described below.

The Need for Scholarly Research

There is a great need for scholarly works that rediscover and apply the theories of major authors in existentialism to the field of management. Although the field has had the benefit of contributions from economics, sociology, engineering, psychology, political science, and so on, it has not yet profited from the potentially rich integration of the views of existentialists. This lack of integration is particularly disheartening considering that many of the existential authors listed in the introduction include some of the very best minds in human history, among them Hannah Arendt, Martin Buber, Søren Kierkegaard, Paul Tillich, and Simone Weil. While the work of several existentialists — for example, Carl Rogers and R. D. Laing — has already had a modest impact on management thought and practice, additional scholarly work could have an important role in the development and daily practice of management.

As a parallel effort in scholarly research, the rediscovery of classical management authors who have already used existential concepts in their work would also benefit both the theory and practice of management. I have argued elsewhere (Pauchant, in press) that Chester I. Barnard, one of the most illustrious fathers of modern management, strongly embraced existential ideals. Similarly, it would be worthwhile to reexamine Mary Parker Follett's (1949) concept of *dynamic organization* and Abraham Maslow's (1965) notion of *Eupsychian management,* for example.

The rediscovery of classic works and their use by managers are not a new idea, of course. For example, for more than
twenty years, the Aspen Institute has been successfully using
an educational approach based on the reading and discussion
by top executives of classic and challenging authors (O'Toole,
1993). In these seminars, executives read works by Plato, Aristotle, Kant, Locke, Rousseau, and Jefferson, among others. This
grounding in the classics is a healthy counterbalance to the current rush of many academics, consultants, and managers to
popular best-sellers in business; it also reminds us that healthy
management principles are not only to be found in recent articles in the *Harvard Business Review, Fortune,* and *Business Week.*

The Need for the Use of Literary Works for Education

The contribution of existentialism to management thought and
practice should also not be limited to the use of philosophical
and psychological works. Fiction and other literary works are
also relevant to management education (Lapierre, 1992). Such
works not only present complex material in a vivid style and
permit the reader to share in an inner dialogue but also nourish people's imagination, their dreams and fantasies, thereby
allowing them to mobilize themselves for meaningful endeavors (Hillman, 1992). This different function could, in turn, lead
to a less analytical, logical, and dispassionate analysis of problems in business schools and organizations and nourish the
dreams of leaders, be they CEOs or employees at more modest
levels (Bennis, 1989).

A first list of works particularly relevant for managers and
business students would include *Animal Farm* (Orwell), *The
Brothers Karamazov* (Dostoevsky), *The Castle* (Kafka), *Death of a
Salesman* (Miller), *Don Quixote* (Cervantes), *Othello* and *Macbeth*
(Shakespeare), *The Metamorphosis* (Kafka), *Moby Dick* (Melville),
1984 (Orwell), *The Plague* (Camus), and *War and Peace* (Tolstoy).
The reading of books like these often offers the simplest and
deepest introduction to existential concepts. I guarantee that
reading these works of fiction, with an eye on their relationship
to organizational issues, will surprise the reader in terms of their
relevance to the daily and concrete practice of management.

The educational use of existential material, whether philosophical, psychological, or literary, seems particularly important in business schools and organizations alike as an additional way to encourage and stimulate discussion about "big" questions and to nourish the personal dreams of individuals. The relative lack of attention to both issues in formal education has been pointed out by many observers. One of these, the late Fritz Schumacher, recalled:

> The . . . maps which I was supplied at school and university . . . failed to show the large "unorthodox" sections of both theory and practice in medicine, agriculture, psychology, and the social and political sciences. . . . Not surprisingly, the more thoroughly [acquainted] we became with the details of the map, the more we absorbed what it showed and got used to the absence of the things it did not show, the more perplexed, unhappy, and cynical we became. . . . The maps produced by modern materialistic Scientism leave all the questions that really matter unanswered; more than that, they deny the validity of the questions [1977, pp. 3–4].

It seems likely that the use of literary works in management education will increase with the publication of books making more explicit the relationships between the content of these works and managerial practice. The concept of using works of fiction in business education is certainly not utopian. Some of these works are presently being used successfully by senior scholars such as Frederick Herzberg at the University of Utha, Graduate School of Business, and James March at Stanford University's School of Business.

The Need for Research and Experimentation Within Organizations

To address and manage existential issues more effectively in organizations obviously requires much more than reading the existential literature. It also requires research and experimentation within organizations themselves on the effects of these existential issues on individuals and on organizations, their environment, and their potential healthy management. The authors of this book have exemplified the kind of inquiries that can spring from an existential perspective. Some of the questions raised in this book can be used as a beginning list of issues to be further addressed. These issues include the creation of broader criteria for measuring organizational effectiveness (Chapter One), the physiological effects and the potential management of "existential addictions" (Chapter Two), the relationship between the denial of death and industrial pollution (Chapter Three), the challenges of "republicanizing" organizations (Chapter Four), the possibility of relativizing existential creations while remaining competitive (Chapter Five), the development of a more dialectical view of managerial problems (Chapter Six), the existential functions of relationships and the problem they raise for supervision (Chapter Seven), the realization and management of the dark side of organizational life (Chapter Eight), the grounding of motivation in one's cultural and religious backgrounds (Chapter Nine), the challenge of remythologizing organizations (Chapter Ten), and the development of responsibility at work (Chapter Eleven).

Furthermore, internally conducted research needs to document precisely how few managers and CEOs are presently addressing existential issues in their organizations. Again, this type of research is certainly not new, as for example, a 1987 book by Max De Pree, chairman of Herman Miller, Inc., demonstrates, using a number of existential concepts (De Pree, 1987).

The Need to Integrate the Existential Tradition with Other Perspectives

It is important to emphasize that a greater focus on existential issues in organizations should not lead to the creation of an additional independent "school" of management. As exemplified in this book and noted above, existential concepts are relevant to many management domains, including organizational behavior; culture and motivation; managerial decision making;

organizational change, development, crisis, and effectiveness; corporate strategy; and organization theory.

Moreover, it seems that managers could use the richness of the existential tradition for integrating some of the relatively new emphases being developed in management today. As we have seen, the existential tradition is particularly rich: it encompasses the subjective world of the individual and its relationships with behaviors and the cultural world, as well as with the physiological and ecological worlds. Considering this richness, managers could use this perspective for integrating a number of issues in management, including, among others, the trend toward more participative and humanistic management (Lawler, 1990), ethics and managerial integrity (Srivastva and Associates, 1988), value-based management (O'Toole, 1993), organizational learning and the process of collective dialogue (Bohm and Edwards, 1991; Senge, 1990), leadership and vision (Bennis, 1989); crisis management (Pauchant and Mitroff, 1992), the management of dialectical and complex issues (Dupuy, 1982; Morin and Kern, 1993), ecological management (Shrivastava, 1994; Smith, 1993), postmodernism (Bergquist, 1993), and the spiritual basis of work (Cayer, 1993; Hawkins, 1991; Pauchant and Fortier, 1990; Reason, 1993).

The Need for a More Encompassing Mode of Inquiry

It seems likely that the discovery of potential answers to the issues discussed in this book will require much more than traditional efforts in research. Currently, the types of inquiry conducted in organizations and universities for R&D or basic research purposes are often fragmented and cannot address the multiple and transdisciplinary effects of existential issues. The study and the management of these issues require an understanding of the relationships between psychological, social, physical, and biological phenomena. Research based on financial ratio analysis, economics, or even a psychological or cultural model cannot fully address these relationships. To a real extent, the introduction of existential issues in management, with their relationships to the subjective, cultural, physiological, and ecological worlds, triggers in itself a crisis in the fragmented way in which traditional research is conducted.

Although the nature of this challenge is beyond the scope of this book, calling for a discussion in epistemology of science, I would like to suggest a way in which this matter can be addressed. Researchers, with the assistance of practicing managers, will have to invent systemic models that can embrace *transdisciplinary* phenomena. To my knowledge, such practical and working models do not exist at the present time despite advances in systems theory and practice and the search for other inquiry models (see, for example, Reason [1988] or Torbert [1991]). However, it seems that the philosophical framework for developing such an inquiry has already been proposed by such authors as Alfred North Whitehead (1929) and John Dewey (1938). I will close this brief incursion into research methodology with a quotation from Dewey (pp. 487, 492) that emphasizes the necessity of understanding social phenomena from their existential basis, integrating their relationships with the physical and biological worlds:

> The subject-matter of social problems is existential [but] no individual person and no group does anything except in interaction with physical conditions. There are no consequences taking place, there are no social events that can be referred to the human factor exclusively. Let desires, skills, purposes, beliefs be what they will, what happens is the product of the interacting intervention of physical conditions like soil, sea mountain, climate, tools and machines, in all their vast variety, with the human factor. This consideration is fatal to the view that social sciences are exclusively, or even dominantly, psychological. . . . Social phenomena cannot be attacked, qua social, directly. Inquiry into them, with respect both to data that are significant and to their relations or proper ordering, is conditioned upon extensive prior knowledge of physical phenomena and their laws.

These considerations offer a formidable challenge to educators and researchers in management and to the present curricula of business schools and corporate training. Today, an understanding of physiological, biological, and ecological issues in business education is generally viewed as irrelevant. I hope that the current questioning about environmental issues in business will help modify this view, which overemphasizes the importance of the social sciences in business education. I personally believe that the integration of the subjective world with the social and natural worlds, which will require a dialogue between the social and natural sciences, will be one of the greatest challenges of the twenty-first century.

The Courage to Change

The integration of existential issues in management is not a luxury. These issues have direct implications for the mental, physical, social, and economic health of human beings and for the health of the planet. Furthermore, they spring from the concrete suffering of individuals and have been acknowledged since the beginning of science, some twenty-five hundred years ago. Still, existential issues are not readily integrated in management and work activities. The current separation of the world of work from the world of life in general is well captured in the following commentary (quoted in Coles, 1987, pp. 136–137) by a General Motors employee in Framingham, Massachusetts:

> Look, it's no picnic, and I know it every day, and say it every day; it's no picnic going to work there. . . . But I don't go there to have a picnic! I go there to make a living! I don't need anyone feeling sorry for me! . . . Sure, it would be nice if they had better conditions! Sure, it helps to sit and blow off steam — or does it? I don't know! Someone has to do this lousy work, and if it isn't me, it'll be another guy, I guess. . . . These people came through here last year, and they gave us questionnaires, and they sat down with us and asked us more and more ques-

tions, and I know they were trying to do better by us in the long run, but like I told my daughter afterward: to go to work in that factory will never be to sit and study those Shakespeare plays you're reading for your high school English teacher, and that's that!

As stated at the beginning of this book, the field of management is in crisis. Current managerial concepts and tools seem insufficient for addressing the current physiological, subjective, economic, ideological, and ecological crisis. Traditionally, we attempt in management to trigger change by implementing so-called *planned change,* mixing approaches such as education, scientific inquiry, incentive and punishment, psychological and cultural values, and leadership. Much differently, the impetus for change for existentialists is triggered by the experience of a major crisis, leading to a potential renewal (McWhinney, 1992). This positive view of a crisis has been emphasized, for example, by Rollo May (May, Angel, and Ellenberg, 1958, p. 17): "[A] crisis is exactly what is required to shock people out of unaware dependence upon external dogma and to force them to unravel layers of pretense to reveal naked truth about themselves."

In a similar vein, in a beautiful book written on change, McWhinney (1992, p. 224) proposes that "the first and most profound courage is that required to maintain awareness that the world we encounter is of our own choosing. This is the courage to affirm that there is *none among the alternative realities that will assure us of our being."*

I hope that this book will help many people in and out of organizations realize more fully the nature of this crisis and tackle the real problems that confront us today rather than hide themselves behind mumbo jumbo, statistical methods, or fixed logic. To me, the courageous facing of concrete problems is, at bottom, the existential quest: to address critical problems despite one's fears, confusion, dismay, and sense of helplessness. Paul Tillich and Rollo May have written beautiful books on the *courage to be* and the *courage to create.* The authors of this book have demonstrated some of that courage. However, many of today's academics are accused, with perhaps good reason, of being irrelevant to the exercise of business practice. The faith embraced by all the authors of this book is that the introduction, discussion, and use of the existential tradition in business can pragmatically assist courageous men and women in organizations in addressing and managing the multifaceted crisis that confronts us today and in rediscovering meaning for themselves and others.

References

Abraham, K. (1970). *Oeuvres complètes* (Vol. 2). Paris: Payot. (English version: *Selected papers.* New York: Basic Books, 1968.)

Adams, G. B. & Hill Ingersoll, V. (1990). Painting over old works: The culture of organization in an age of technical rationality. In B. A. Turner (Ed.), *Organizational symbolism* (pp. 15–31). Berlin: De Gruyter.

Aktouf, O. (1983). Une approche observation participante et intellectuelle des systèmes de représentation dans les rapports de travail [A participant-observer and an intellectual inquiry into interpretive systems of work relations]. Unpublished doctoral dissertation, École des Hautes Études Commerciales, Montreal.

Aktouf, O. (1986). *Le travail industriel contre l'homme?* [Industrial work against man?] Alger: OPU-SNED.

Aktouf, O. (1989). *Le management entre tradition et renouvellement* [Management between tradition and renewal]. Montreal: Gaëtan Morin.

Aktouf, O. (1990a). Le symbolisme et la culture d'entreprise — Des abus conceptuels aux leçons du terrain [Symbolism and the culture of enterprise — From conceptual abuses to lessons of the field]. In J.-F. Chanlat (Ed.), *L'individu dans l'organisation: Les dimensions oubliées* [The person in the organization: The forgotten dimensions] (pp. 553–588). Quebec: Laval University Press; Paris: Eska.

Aktouf, O. (1990b). *Immortality, managerial taboos, and leadership:*

347

348 References

A theoretical framework and a case study. Working paper, École des Hautes Études Commerciales, Montreal.

Aktouf, O. (1991a), Parole, productivité et travail: Une étude de cas et une perspective comparée [Words, productivity, and work: Case studies and a comparative perspective]. *Minutes of the Third Colloquium on Organizational Communication,* pp. 9–27. Montreal: Department of Communication, University of Montreal.

Aktouf, O. (1991b). Adhésion et pouvoir partagés: Le cas Cascades, Gérer et Comprendre [Shared adherence and shared power: The Cascades case, *Gérer et Comprendre*]. *Annales des Mines, 23,* 44–57.

Aktouf, O. (1992). Management and theories of organizations in the 1990s: Toward a critical radical humanism. *Academy of Management Review, 17*(3), 407–431.

Aktouf, O., Bédard, R., & Chanlat, A. (1992). Management, éthique catholique et esprit du capitalisme: L'exemple québécois [Management, Catholic ethics, and the spirit of capitalism: The example of Quebec]. *Sociologie du Travail, 1,* 83–99.

Allen, D. (1978). *Structure and creativity in religion: Hermeneutics in Mircea Eliade's* Phenomenology and new directions. New York: Norton.

Alvesson, M. (1990). On the popularity of organizational culture. *Acta Sociologica, 33,* 31–49.

American Heart Association (1991). *Heart facts.* Dallas: Author.

American Management Association (1993, April). The pitfalls of poor listening. *Supervisory Sense.*

Anthony, P. D. (1980). Work and the loss of meaning. *International Social Science Journal, 32*(3), 416–426.

Antonovsky, A. (1987). *Unraveling the mystery of health.* San Francisco: Jossey-Bass.

Anzieu, D. (1985). *Le Moi-Peau* [The self-skin]. Paris: Dunod.

Aragon, L. (1944). *Aurélien* [Aurelian]. Paris: Gallimard.

Athos, A., & J. Gabarro. (1978). *Interpersonal behavior: Communication and understanding in relationships.* Englewood Cliffs, NJ: Prentice-Hall.

Aubert, N., & de Gaulejac, V. (1991). *Le coût de l'excellence* [The cost of excellence]. Paris: Seuil.

Aubert, N., & Pagès, M. (1989). *Le stress professionel* [Professional stress]. Paris: Klincksieck.

Auer-Hunzinger, V., & Sievers, B. (1991). Organisatorische Rollenanalyse und -beratung: Ein Beitrag zur Aktionsforschung [Organizational role analysis and consultation: A contribution to action research]. *Gruppendynamik, 22,* 33–46.

Axelos, K. (1962). *Héraclite et la philosophie* [Heraclitus and philosophy]. Paris: Éditions de Minuit.

Bandura, A. (1977). Self-efficacy: Towards a unifying theory of behavioral change. *Psychological Review, 84*(3), 191–215.

Barnard, C. I. (1968). *The functions of the executive.* Cambridge, MA: Harvard University Press. (Original work published 1938)

Barrett, W. (1958). *Irrational man: A study in existential philosophy.* New York: Doubleday.

Barrett, W. (1986). *Death of the soul: From Descartes to the computer.* New York: Doubleday.

Bass, B. M. (1952). Ultimate criteria of organizational worth. *Personnel Psychology, 5,* 157–173.

Bauer, W., Dümotz, I., & Golowin, S. (1980). *Lexikon der Symbole* [Dictionary of Symbols]. Wiesbaden, Germany: Fourier.

Becker, E. (1962). *The birth and death of meaning.* New York: Free Press.

Becker, E. (1973). *The denial of death.* New York: Free Press.

Becker, E. (1975). *Escape from evil.* New York: Free Press.

Bedeian, A. G. (1987). Organization theory: Current controversies, issues, and directions. In C. L. Cooper & I. T. Robertson (Eds.), *International review of industrial and organizational psychology* (pp. 1–33). New York: Wiley.

Bellah, R. N., Madsen, R., Sullivan, W. M., Swidler, A., & Tipton, S. M. (1985). *Habits of the heart: Individualism and commitment in American life.* Berkeley: University of California Press.

Bennis, W. G. (1989). *Why leaders can't lead: The unconscious conspiracy continues.* San Francisco: Jossey-Bass.

Berger, P., & Luckmann, T. (1966). *The social construction of reality.* New York: Doubleday. (French version: *La construction sociale de la réalité.* Paris: Méridiens, Klincksieck, 1986.)

Bergeret, J. (1974). *La personnalité normale et pathologique* [The normal and the pathological personality]. Paris: Dunod.

Bergquist, W. (1993). *The postmodern organization: Mastering the art of irreversible change.* San Francisco: Jossey-Bass.

Berle, A. (1957). *Le capital américain et la conscience du roi: Le néo-capitalisme aux États-Unis.* Paris: Armand Colin. (English version: *The American economic republic* [1st ed.]. Orlando, FL: Harcourt Brace Jovanovich, 1963.)

Bettelheim, B. (1983). *Freud and man's soul.* New York: Knopf.

Beynon, H. (1973). *Working for Ford.* London: Penguin Books.

Biedermann, H. (1989). *Knaurs Lexikon der Symbole* [Knaur's Dictionary of Symbols]. Munich: Droemer Knaur.

Blass-Simmen, B. (1991). *Sankt-Georg. Drachenkampf in der Renaissance. Carpaccio-Raffael-Leonardo* [Saint George: Battles with dragons in the Renaissance—Carpaccio, Raphael, Leonardo]. Berlin: Gebr. Mann.

Bohm, D. (1990). *On dialogue.* (P. Fleming & J. Brodsky, Eds.). Ojai, CA: David Bohm Seminars.

Bohm, D., & Edwards, M. (1991). *Changing consciousness: Exploring the hidden source of the social, political, and environmental crises facing our world.* San Francisco: HarperSanFrancisco.

Bohm, D., & Peat, F. D. (1990). *La conscience et l'univers.* Paris: Éditions du Rocher. (English version: *Science, order, and creativity.* New York: Bantam Books, 1987.)

Boland, R. J., & Hoffman, R. (1983). Humor in a machine shop. In L. R. Pondy, P. Frost, G. Morgan, & T. Dandridge (Eds.), *Organizational symbolism* (pp. 187–188). Greenwich, CT: JAI Press.

Bonnefoy, Y. (1978). Préface à Shakespeare, *Hamlet* et *le Roi Lear* [Preface to Shakespeare, *Hamlet* and *King Lear*]. Paris: Gallimard.

Booth-Kewley, S., & Friedman, H. (1987). Psychological predictors of heart disease: A quantitative review. *Psychological Bulletin, 101,* 343–362.

Borneman, E. (1978), *Lexikon der Liebe: Materialen zur Sexualwissenschaft* [Dictionary of love: Data on sexology]. (Vols. 1–4). Frankfurt: Ullstein.

Borneman, E. (1979). *Das Patriarchat: Ursprung und Zukunft unseres Gesellschaftssystems* [The patriarchy: Origin and future of our social system]. Frankfurt: Fischer-Taschenbuch.

Borrero, I. M., & Rivera, H. A. (1980). Toward a meaning of work. *Journal of Sociology and Social Welfare, 7*(6), 880–894.

Bowles, M. L. (1991). The organization shadow. *Organization Studies, 12*, 387–404.

Bracke, P. E. (1992, March). *An existential-humanistic view of the Type A behavior pattern*. Paper presented at the thirteenth annual scientific session of the Society of Behavioral Medicine, New York.

Braudel, F. (1980). *Civilisation matérielle, économie et capitalisme* (Vols. 1–3). Paris: Armand Colin. (English version: *Civilization and capitalism, 15th–18th century*. New York: Harper-Collins, 1981.)

Braudel, F. (1985). *Dynamique du capitalisme* [The dynamics of capitalism]. Paris: Arthaud.

Braverman, H. (1974). *Labor and monopoly capital*. New York: Monthly Review Press. (French version: *Travail et capitalisme monopolistique*. Paris: François Maspero, 1976.)

Brée, G. (1961). *Camus*. New Brunswick, NJ: Rutgers University Press.

Brée, G. (1985). Prologue. In S. G. Kellman (Ed.), *Approaches to teaching Camus's* The plague (pp. 15–19). New York: Modern Language Association.

Breuk, B. (1966). *Tradition und Neuerung in der christlichen Kunst des ersten Jahrtausends. Studien zur Geschichte des Weltgerichtsbildes* [Tradition and renewal in Christian art from the first millennium. Studies on the history of the portrayal of the Last Judgment]. Vienna: Österreichische Akademie der Wissenschaften.

Brief, A. P., & Nord, W. R. (Eds.). (1990). *Meanings of occupational work*. Toronto: Lexington Books.

Buber, M. (1958). *I and thou* (2nd ed.; R. G. Smith, Trans.) New York: Charles Scribner's Sons.

Buber, M. (1963). *Pointing the way*. New York: Harper Torchbooks.

Bugental, J.F.T. (1965). *The search for authenticity: An existential-analytic approach to psychotherapy*. Troy, MO: Holt, Rinehart & Winston.

Bugental, J.F.T. (1976). *The search for existential identity: Patient-*

therapist dialogues in humanistic psychotherapy. San Francisco: Jossey-Bass.

Bugental, J.F.T., & Bracke, P. E. (1992). The future of existential-humanistic psychotherapy. *Psychotherapy, 29,* 28-33.

Burrell, G. (1984). Sex and organizational analysis. *Organization Studies, 5,* 97-118.

Burrell, G., & Morgan, G. (1979). *Sociological paradigms and organizational analysis: Elements of the sociology of corporate life.* Exeter, NH: Heinemann.

Byrne, J. A. (1992, August 31). Management's new gurus: Business is hungry for fresh approaches to the global marketplace. *Business Week,* pp. 44-52.

Cameron, K. S., & Whetten, D. A. (1983). Organizational effectiveness: One model or several? In K. S. Cameron & D. A. Whetten (Eds.), *Organizational effectiveness: A comparison of multiple models* (pp. 1-26). San Diego, CA: Academic Press.

Campbell, J. (1973). *Myths to live by.* New York: Bantam Books.

Campbell, J. P. (1977). On the nature of organizational effectiveness. In P. S. Goodman & J. M. Pennings (Eds.), *New perspectives on organizational effectiveness* (pp. 13-62). San Francisco: Jossey-Bass.

Camus, A. (1947). *La peste* [*The plague*]. Paris: Gallimard; London: Penguin Books.

Camus, A. (1951). *L'homme révolté.* Paris: Gallimard. (English version: *The rebel: An essay on man in revolt.* New York: Random House, 1991.)

Camus, A. (1967). Three interviews. In P. Thody (Ed.), *Albert Camus: Lyrical and critical* (pp. 259-274). London: Hamish Hamilton.

Carroll, A. B. (1979). A three-dimensional conceptual model of corporate social performance. *Academy of Management Review, 4,* 497-505.

Carroll, D. (1983, November-December). A disappointing search for excellence. *Harvard Business Review,* pp. 78-88.

Cayer, M. (1993). *Bohm's dialogue and action science: Two different approaches.* Working paper. Laval University, Department of Administrative Sciences, Quebec.

Chanlat, A., & Bédard, R. (1990). La gestion: Une affaire de parole [Management: A business of speech]. In J.-F. Chanlat (Ed.), *L'individu dans l'organisation: Les dimensions oubliées* [The person in the organization: The forgotten dimensions] (pp. 79–99). Quebec: Laval University Press; Paris: Eska.

Chanlat, J.-F. (Ed.). (1990). *L'individu dans l'organisation: Les dimensions oubliées.* [The person in the organization: The forgotten dimensions]. Quebec: Laval University Press; Paris: Eska.

Chanlat, J.-F., & Séguin, F. (1987). *L'analyse des organisations: Une anthologie sociologique:* Vol. 2. *Les composantes de l'organisation* [The analysis of organizations: A sociological anthology: Vol. 2. The components of the organization]. Montreal: Gaëtan Morin.

Chasseguet-Smirgel, J. (1985). *The ego ideal: A psychoanalytic essay on the malady of the ideal.* New York: Norton.

Chasseguet-Smirgel, J. (1986). *Sexuality and mind: The role of the father and the mother in the psyche.* New York: New York University Press.

Classics in American business schools. (1993, March 25). *Courrier International,* pp. 36–37.

Coles, R. (1987). *Simone Weil: A modern pilgrimage.* Reading, MA: Addison-Wesley.

Corson, B., Tepper Marlin, A., Schorsch, J., Swaminathan, A., & Will, R. (1989). *Shopping for a better world: A quick and easy guide to socially responsible supermarket shopping.* New York: Council on Economic Priorities.

Crozier, M. (1992). *L'entreprise à l'écoute: Apprendre le management post-industriel* [The listening organization: Learning postindustrial management]. Paris: InterEditions.

Csikszentmihalyi, M. (1990). *Flow: The psychology of optimal experience.* New York: Harper & Row.

Curb, R. K. (1986). Was ist eine lesbische Nonne? [What is a lesbian nun?] In R. Curb and N. Manahan (Eds.), *Die ungehorsamen Bräute Christi: Lesbische Nonnen brechen das Schweigen* [The disobedient brides of Christ: Lesbian nuns break the silence] (pp. 15–27). Munich: Kindler.

Cushman, P. (1990). Why the self is empty. *American Psychologist, 45*(5), 599–611.

Deal, T. E., & Kennedy, A. A. (1982). *Corporate culture: The rites and rituals of corporate life.* Reading, MA: Addison-Wesley.

Dejours, C. (1990). Nouveau regard sur la souffrance humaine dans les organisations [A new look at human suffering in organizations]. In J.-F. Chanlat (Ed.), *L'individu dans l'organisation: Les dimensions oubliées* [The person in the organization: The forgotten dimensions] (pp. 687–708). Quebec: Laval University Press; Paris: Eska.

Deleuze, G. (1969). *Logique du sens.* Paris: Éditions de Minuit. (English version: *The logic of sense.* New York: Columbia University Press, 1990.)

Denhardt, R. B. (1981). *In the shadow of organization.* Lawrence: Regent Press of Kansas.

Denhardt, R. B. (1987). Images of death and slavery in organizational life. *Journal of Management, 13*(3), 529–541.

De Pree, M. (1987). *Leadership is an art.* East Lansing: Michigan State University Press. (French version: *Diriger est un art.* Paris: Rivages/Les Échos.)

Dewey, J. (1938). *Logic: The theory of inquiry.* Troy, MO: Holt, Rinehart & Winston.

Dilthey, W. (1962). *Pattern and meaning in History: Thoughts on history and society.* New York: Harper Torchbooks.

Doise, W. (1985). Les représentations sociales: Définition d'un concept [Social interpretations: Definition of a concept]. *Connexions, 45,* 243–252.

Drewermann, E. (1989). *Kleriker: Psychogramm eines Ideals* [The clergy: Psychogram of an ideal]. Olten, Switzerland: Walter.

Drewermann, E. (1991). *Tiefenpsychologie und Exegese* [Depth psychology and exegesis] (Vol. 2). Olten, Switzerland: Walter.

Drucker, P. F. (1984). The new meaning of corporate social responsibility. *California Management Review, 26,* 53–63.

Dumezil, G. (1987). L'excellence introuvable: Entretien avec *Georges Dumezil* [The elusiveness of excellence: A conversation with Georges Dumezil]. *Autrement, 86.*

Dupuy, J.-P. (1982). *Ordres et désordres: Enquête sur un nouveau para-*

digme [Orders and disorders: Inquiry into a new paradigm]. Paris: Seuil.

Ehrenberg, A. (1987). Héroïsme socialement transmissible [Socially transmittable heroism]. *Autrement, 86.*

Elias, N. (1985). *The loneliness of the dying.* Oxford, England: Basil Blackwell.

Ellmen, E. (1987). *How to invest your money with a clear conscience.* Toronto: James Lorimer.

England, G. E., & Whiteley, W. T. (1990). Cross-national meanings of working. In A. P. Brief & W. R. Nord (Eds.), *Meanings of occupational work* (pp. 65–106). Toronto: Lexington Books.

England, G. W. (1967). Organizational goals and expected behavior of American managers. *Academy of Management Journal, 10,* 107–117.

Enriquez, E. (1983). *De la horde à l'État* [From the mob to the state]. Paris: Gallimard.

Enriquez, E. (1989). L'individu pris au piège de la structure stratégique [The individual caught in the trap of strategic structure]. *Connexions, 54*(2), 145–161.

Enriquez, E. (1990). L'entreprise comme lieu social: Un colosse au pied d'argile [The organization as a social place: A colossus with feet of clay]. In R. Sainsaulieu, *L'entreprise: Une affaire de société* [Business: A social affair] (pp. 203–228). Paris: ENSP.

Erdheim, M. (1986). Das Verenden einer Institution [The death of an institution]. *Psyche, 49,* 1092–1104.

Esambert, B. (1991). *La guerre économique mondiale* [The economic world war]. Paris: Olivier Orban.

Evans, R. (1975). *Carl Rogers: The man and his ideas.* New York: Dutton.

Executive pay: Compensation at the top is out of control. (1992, March 30). *Business Week,* pp. 52–58.

Fassel, D. (1990). *Working ourselves to death.* San Francisco: HarperSanFrancisco.

Firth, R. (1948). Anthropological background to work. *Occupational Psychology, 22,* 94–102.

Flasch, K. (1991). Als Keuschheit Freiheit war. Christentum

vor Augustinus: Elaine Pagels' bemerkenswerte Geschichte des Sünde [When chastity was freedom: Christendom before Augustine — Elaine Pagels's remarkable history of sin]. *Frankfurter Allgemeine Zeitung, 2,* 7.

Follett, M. P. (1949). *Freedom and co-ordination: Lectures in business organisation.* London: Pitman.

Foucault, M. (1976). *Surveiller et punir.* Paris: Gallimard. (English version: *Discipline and punish.* New York: Vintage Press, 1979.)

Foulquié, P. (1989). *L'existentialisme, 253* [Existentialism]. Paris: Presse Universitaire de France.

Fox, W. (1990). *Toward a transpersonal ecology: Developing new foundations for environmentalism.* Boston, MA: Shambhala.

Frankl, V. E. (1963). Man's search for meaning: An introduction to logotherapy. Boston: Beacon Press.

Frankl, V. E. (1966). What is meant by meaning. *Journal of Existentialism, 7,* 21–28.

Frankl, V. E. (1967). *Psychotherapy and existentialism: Selected papers on logotherapy.* New York: Washington Square Press.

French, W., & C. Bell. (1990). *Organization development.* Englewood Cliffs, NJ: Prentice-Hall.

Freud, A. (1968). The widening scope of indications for psychoanalysis. In *The writings of Anna Freud* (Vol. 4, pp. 356–376). New York: International Universities Press. (Original work published 1954)

Freud, S. (1955). *Group psychology and the analysis of the ego:* Vol. 18. J. Strachey (Ed. and Trans.), *The standard edition of the complete psychological works of Sigmund Freud.* London: Hogarth Press. (Original work published 1921)

Freud, S. (1957a). *On narcissism: An introduction:* Vol. 14. J. Strachey (Ed. and Trans.), *The standard edition of the complete psychological works of Sigmund Freud.* London: Hogarth Press. (Original work published 1914)

Freud, S. (1957b). *Civilization and its discontents:* Vol. 21. J. Strachey (Ed. and Trans.), *The standard edition of the complete psychological works of Sigmund Freud.* London: Hogarth Press. (Original work published 1930)

Freud, S. (1958a). The dynamics of the transference. In J. Strachey (Ed. and Trans.), *The standard edition of the complete psychological works of Sigmund Freud.* (Vol. 12, pp. 109–120). London: Hogarth Press. (Original work published 1912)

Freud, S. (1958b). Recommendations to physicians practicing psychoanalysis. In J. Strachey (Ed. and Trans.), *The standard edition of the complete psychological works of Sigmund Freud.* (Vol. 12, pp. 109–120). London: Hogarth Press. (Original work published 1912)

Freud, S. (1958c). Remembering, repeating, and working through. In J. Strachey (Ed. and Trans.), *The standard edition of the complete psychological works of Sigmund Freud* (Vol. 12, pp. 145–156). London: Hogarth Press. (Original work published 1914)

Freud, S. (1958d). *Introductory lectures on psychoanalysis:* Vols. 16, 17. J. Strachey (Ed. and Trans.), *The standard edition of the complete psychological works of Sigmund Freud.* London: Hogarth Press. (Original work published 1916–1917)

Freudenberger, H. (1985). *L'épuisement professionnel, la brûlure interne* [Professional burnout]. Montreal: Gaétan Morin.

Friedlander, F., & Pickle, H. (1968). Components of effectiveness in small organizations. *Administrative Science Quarterly, 13*(2), 289–304.

Friedman, M. (1962). *Capitalism and freedom.* Chicago: University of Chicago Press.

Friedman, M. (Ed.). (1964). *The worlds of existentialism: A critical reader.* New York: Random House.

Friedman, M. (1985). *The healing dialogue in psychotherapy.* Northvale, NJ: Jason Aronson.

Friedman, M., & Rosenman, R. H. (1959). Association of specific overt behavior pattern with blood and cardiovascular findings. *Journal of the American Medical Association, 169,* 1286–1296.

Friedman, M., & Ulmer, D. K. (1984). *Treating Type A behavior and your heart.* New York: Knopf.

Friedman, M. (1994). Reflections on the Buber-Rogers dialogue. *Journal of Humanistic Psychology, 34*(1), 46–65.

Fromm, E. (1947). *Man for himself.* Troy, MO: Holt, Rinehart & Winston.

Fromm, E. (1973). *The anatomy of human destructiveness.* Troy, MO: Holt, Rinehart & Winston.

Fromm, E. (1975). *La passion de détruire: Anatomie de la destructivité humaine.* Paris: Robert Laffont. (English version: *The anatomy of human destructiveness.* Troy, MO: Holt, Rinehart & Winston.)

Fromm, E. (1978). *Avoir ou être? Un choix dont dépend l'avenir de l'homme.* Paris: Robert Laffont. (English version: *To have or to be.* New York: Harper & Row, 1976.)

Frost, P. J., Moore, L. F., Louis, M. R., Lundberg, C. C., & Martin, J. (Eds.). (1985). *Organizational culture.* Newbury Park, CA: Sage.

Fryer, D., & Payne, R. (1984). Working definitions. *Quality of Working Life, 1*(5), 13–15.

Gabriel, Y. (1983). *Freud and society.* London: Routledge and Kegan Paul.

Gabriel, Y. (1986). Unbehagen und Illusion in der psychoanalytischen Kulturtheorie [Discontent and illusion in psychoanalytic theory of (organizational) culture. See also Gabriel, 1991.]. *Psycho, 40,* 21–48.

Gabriel, Y. (1991). Organizations and their discontents: A psychoanalytic contribution to the study of organizational culture. *Journal of Applied Behavioral Science, 27,* 318–336.

Gagliardi, P. (1986). The creation and change of organizational cultures: A conceptual framework. *Organizational Studies, 7*(2), 117–134.

Gagliardi, P. (Ed.). (1990). *Symbols and artifacts: Views of the corporate landscape.* Berlin: De Gruyter.

Gahmberg, H. (1990). Metaphor management: On the semiotics of strategic leadership. In B. A. Turner (Ed.), *Organizational symbolism* (pp. 151–158). Berlin: De Gruyter.

Galbraith, J. R. (1977). *Organization design.* Reading, MA: Addison-Wesley.

Gebara, Y. (1989). Die Mutter Oberin und die geistliche Mutterschaft: Von der Intuition zur Institution [The mother superior and spiritual motherhood: From intuition to institution]. *Concilium, 25,* 483–489.

Gendlin, E. T. (1987). A philosophical critique of the concept of narcissism: The significance of the awareness movement. In D. Levin (Ed.), *Pathologies of the modern self: Postmodern studies on narcissism, schizophrenia, and depression* (pp. 251–304). New York: New York University Press.

Gilmore, J. T. (1986, Summer). A framework for responsible business behavior. *Business and Society Review*, pp. 31–34.

Gini, A. R., & Sullivan, T. (1987). Work: The process and the person. *Journal of Business Ethics, 6*(8), 649–655.

Goffman, E. (1959). *The presentation of self in everyday life.* New York: Doubleday Anchor. (French version: *La mise en scène de la vie quotidienne.* Paris: Éditions de Minuit, 1973.)

Goffman, E. (1973). *Asyle: Über die soziale Situation psychiatrischer Patienten und anderer Insassen* [Asylums: Regarding the social situation of psychiatric patients and other inmates]. Frankfurt: Suhrkamp.

Goodman, P. S., Atkin, R. S., & Schoorman, F. D. (1983). On the demise of organizational effectiveness studies. In K. S. Cameron & D. A. Whetten (Eds.), *Organizational effectiveness: A comparison of multiple models* (pp. 163–183). San Diego, CA: Academic Press.

Gore, A. (1993). *Earth in the balance: Ecology and the human spirit.* New York: Plume Books.

Graves, R., & Patai, R. (1989). *Hebrew myths: The Book of Genesis.* London: Arena.

Green, A. (1985). *Narcissisme de vie, narcissisme de mort* [Narcissism of life, narcissism of death]. Paris: Éditions de Minuit.

Grubel, I. (1990). Lucifer als Seelenfresser: Überlegungen zu einer zentralen Gestalt des mittelalterlichen Jenseitsglaubens [Lucifer as soul-devourer: Reflections on a central figure in medieval belief in the hereafter]. *Zeitschrift für Literaturwissenschaft und Linguistik, 80*, 49–60.

Grunberger, B. (1975). *Le narcissisme* [Narcissism]. Paris: Payot.

Guillaume, M. (1987). L'excellence sacrificielle [Sacrificial excellence]. *Autrement, 86*.

Guillet de Monthoux, P. (1983). *Action and existence: Anarchism of business administration* (D. E. Weston, Trans.). New York: Wiley.

Halper, J. (1988). *Quiet desperation: The truth about successful men.* New York: Warner Books.

Hanna, R. W. (1985). Personal meaning: Its loss and rediscovery. In R. Tannenbaum, N. Margulies, F. Massarik, & Associates (Eds.), *Human systems development* (pp. 42–66). San Francisco: Jossey-Bass.

Hassard, J., & Porter, R. (1990). Cutting down the workforce: Eunuchs and early administrative management. *Organization Studies, 11,* 555–567.

Hawken, P. (1993). *The ecology of commerce: A declaration of sustainability.* New York: HarperBusiness.

Hawkins, P. (1991). The spiritual dimension of the learning organization. *Management Education and Development, 22*(3), 172–187.

Hegel, W. F. (1966). *La phénoménologie de l'esprit* (Vols. 1–2). Paris: Aubier-Montaigne. (English version: *Phenomenology of spirit.* Oxford, England: Clarendon Press, 1977.)

Heidegger, M. (1963). *Being and time* (J. Macquarrie & E. Robison, Trans.). New York: Harper & Row.

Heidegger, M. (1972). *The question concerning technology and other essays* (W. Lovitt, Trans.). New York: Harper & Row.

Heidegger, M., & Fink, E. (1993). *Heraclitus seminar.* Evanston, IL: Northwestern University Press.

Hellinger, B. (1991). Schuld und Unschuld aus systemischer Sicht [Guilt and innocence from a systems perspective]. *Systhema, 5*(1), 19–34.

Herzberg, F. (1959). *Motivation to work.* New York: Wiley.

Herzberg, F. (1966). *Work and the nature of man.* New York: Crowell.

Herzberg, F. (1978, August). Dynamics of caring. *Industry Week.*

Herzberg, F. (1982). *The managerial choice: To be efficient and to be human* (2nd ed.). Homewood, IL: Dow Jones-Irwin.

Herzberg, F. (1984, November–December). Managing egos: East vs. west. *Industry Week.*

Hesse, H. (1951). *Siddharta.* New York: New Directions.

Hillman, J. (1992). *Re-visioning psychology* (2nd ed.). New York: HarperPerennial.

Hills, S. L. (Ed.). (1987). *Corporate violence: Injury and death for profit.* Totowa, NJ: Rowman and Littlefield.

Hitt, M., & Ireland, R. D. (1987). Peters and Waterman revisited: The unended quest for excellence. *Academy of Management Executive, 1*(2), 91–98.

Hoffman, W. (1986). What is necessary for corporate moral excellence? *Journal of Business Ethics, 5,* 233–242.

Horney, K. (1950). *Neurosis and human growth.* New York: Norton.

Ibn Khaldoun. (1978). *Discours sur l'histoire universelle* [Discourse on universal history] (Vols. 1–2). (V. Monteil, Trans.). Paris: Sinbad.

Irigaray, L. (1991). *Die Zeit der Differenz: Für eine friedliche Revolution* [The time of difference: For a peaceful revolution]. Frankfurt: Campus.

Isaacs, W. N. (1993, Autumn). Taking flight: Dialogue, collective thinking, and organizational learning. *Organizational Dynamics,* pp. 24–39.

Jackall, R. (1988). Moral mazes: The world of corporate managers. New York: Oxford University Press.

Janis, I. L. (1972). *Victims of groupthink.* Boston: Houghton Mifflin.

Jankélévitch, V. (1980). *Le Je-ne-sais-quoi et le Presque-rien: Vol. 2. La méconnaissance* [The indefinable something and the almost nothing: Vol. 2. Misreading]. Paris: Seuil.

Jennings, E. E. (1967). *Executive success: Stresses, problems, and adjustments.* New York: Appleton-Century-Crofts.

Johnson, B., Natarajan, A., & Rappaport, A. (1985, Fall). Shareholder returns and corporate excellence. *Journal of Business Strategy,* pp. 52–62.

Jones, E. (1957). *The life and work of Sigmund Freud: The last phase, 1919–1939* (Vols. 1–3). New York: Basic Books.

Jones, J. (1960). Otto Rank: A forgotten heresy. *Commentary, 30.*

Jung, C. G. (1961). *Memories, dreams, reflections.* New York: Vintage Books. (French version: *Ma vie, souvenirs, rêves, et pensées.* Paris: Gallimard, 1966.

Jung, C. G. (1981). *The development of personality.* Princeton, NJ: Princeton University Press.

Kakar, S. (1970). *Frederick Taylor: A study in personality and innovation.* Cambridge, MA: MIT Press.

Kantorowicz, F. (1989). *Les deux corps du roi* [The two bodies of the king]. Paris: Gallimard.

Kaplan, H. R., & Tausky, C. (1974). The meaning of work among the hard-core unemployed. *Pacific Sociological Review, 17*(2), 185–198.

Karpf, F. (1953). *The psychology and psychotherapy of Otto Rank.* New York: Philosophical Library.

Karrh, B. W. (1990). Du Pont and corporate environmentalism. In W. H. Hoffman, R. Frederick, & E. S. Petry, Jr. (Eds.), *The corporation, ethics, and the environment* (pp. 69–76). New York: Quorum Books.

Kaufmann, W. (Ed.). (1956) *Existentialism: From Dostoevsky to Sartre.* New York: Meridian Books.

Kellman, S. G. (1985). Part one: Materials. In S. G. Kellman (Ed.), *Approaches to teaching Camus's* The plague (pp. 3–10). New York: Modern Language Association.

Kernberg, O. (1970). Factors in the psychoanalytic treatment of narcissistic personalities. *Journal of Psychoanalytical Association, 18,* 1.

Kets de Vries, M.F.R., & Miller, D. (1985). *The neurotic organization.* San Francisco: Jossey-Bass. (French version: *L'entreprise névrosée.* Paris: McGraw-Hill.)

Kirk, G. S., Raven, J. E., & Scofield, M. (1990). *The presocratic philosophers: A critical history with a selection of texts.* Cambridge, England: Cambridge University Press.

Kirschenbaum, H. (1979). *On becoming Carl Rogers.* New York: Delacorte Press.

Kirschenbaum, H., & Henderson, V. (Eds.). (1989a). *The Carl Rogers reader.* Boston: Houghton Mifflin.

Kirschenbaum, H., & Henderson, V. (Eds.). (1989b). *Carl Rogers: Dialogues.* Boston: Houghton Mifflin.

Klein, M. (1959). Our adult world and its roots in infancy. *Human Relations, 12,* 291–303.

Klein, S. M., & Ritti, R. R. (1984). *Understanding organizational behavior.* Boston: Kent.

Kobasa, S., & Maddi, S. (1979). Existential personality theory. In R. Corsini (Ed.), *Current personality theory.* Itaska, IL: Peacock Books.

Kobayashi, Y., & Igarashi, H. (1981). An empirical test of the Herzberg theory of job satisfaction. *Tohoku Psychologica Folia, 40,* 74–83.

Kohn-Roelin, J. (1989). Mutter, Tochter, Gott. *Concilium, 25,* 497–502.

Kohut, H. (1985). *Self-psychology and the humanities.* New York: Norton.

Kramer, R. (1989). In the shadow of death: Robert Denhart's theology of organizational life. *Administration and Society, 21*(3), 357–379.

Kübler-Ross, E. (1969). *On death and dying: What the dying have to teach doctors, nurses, clergy, and their own families.* New York: Macmillan.

Laing, R. D. (1970). *Knots.* New York: Vintage Books.

Landier, H. (1988, March). Management: La nouvelle langue de bois [Management: The new frozen paradigm]. *Notes de conjoncture sociale.* Paris.

Lapierre, L. (1992). L'approche clinique: La fiction et la recherche sur le leadership [The clinical approach: Fiction and research on leadership]. In L. Lapierre (Ed.), *Imaginaire et leadership* [Leadership and the imaginary] (pp. 57–88). Montreal: Québec-Amerique et Presses HEC.

Laplanche, J., & Pontalis, J.-B. (1973). *Das Vokabular der Psychoanalyse* [The vocabulary of psychoanalysis]. Frankfurt: Suhrkamp.

Lasch, C. (1978). *The culture of narcissism: American life in an age of diminishing expectations.* New York: Norton. (French version: *Le complexe de narcisse.* Paris: Robert Laffont, 1981.)

Laurin, P. (1973). Remise en question de la participation [Participation reconsidered]. In P. Laurin (Ed.), *Le management, textes et cas* [Management — texts and cases] (pp. 407–417). Montreal: McGraw-Hill.

Lawler, E. E., III (1990). *High-involvement management: Participative strategies for improving organizational performance.* San Francisco: Jossey-Bass.

Lawrence, W. G. (Ed.). (1979). *Exploring individual and organizational boundaries. A Tavistock open systems approach.* Chichester, England: Wiley.

Lawrence, W. G. (1982). *Some psychic and political dimensions of work experiences.* Occasional paper 2, the Tavistock Institute of Human Relations, London.

Legrand, G. (1986). *Vocabulaire de la philosophie* [Vocabulary of philosophy]. Paris: Bordas.

Leherer, J. F., & Hover, L. M. (1989). Fatigue syndrome. *Journal of the American Medical Association, 256,* 842–843.

Le Mouël, J. (1991). *Critique de l'efficacité* [Critique of effectiveness]. Paris: Seuil.

Lesage, P.-B., & Rice, J. (1978). Le sens du travail et le gestionnaire [The manager and the meaning of work]. *Gestion, 3*(4), 6–16.

Lewin, A. Y., & Minton, J. W. (1986). Determining organizational effectiveness: Another look, and an agenda for research. *Management Science, 32,* 514–538.

Lewis, M. (1989). *Liar's poker: Rising through the wreckage on Wall Street.* New York: Norton.

Lieberman, E. (1985). *Acts of will: The life and work of Otto Rank.* New York: Free Press.

Likert, R. (1958). Measuring organizational performance. *Harvard Business Review, 36*(2), 41–50.

Linhart, D. (1991). *Le torticolis de l'autruche* [The ostrich's stiff neck]. Paris: Seuil.

Linhart, R. (1972). *L'établi* [The workbench]. Paris: Seuil.

Lipovetzski, G. (1983). *L'ère du vide* [The age of emptiness]. Paris: Gallimard.

Little, J. P. (1969). Heraclitus and Simone Weil: The harmony of opposites. *Forum for Modern Language Study, 5*(1), 72–79.

Locke, E. A., & Latham, G. P. (1990). *A theory of goal setting and task performance.* Englewood Cliffs, NJ: Prentice-Hall.

Lowith, K. (1991). *Nietzsche: Philosophie de l'éternel retour du même* [Nietzsche: Philosophy of the cycle of eternal repetition]. (A.-S. Astrup, Trans.). (Original work published 1935)

Lydenberg, S. D., Tepper Marlin, A., O'Brien Strub, S., & Council on Economic Priorities. (1986). *Rating America's corporate conscience: A provocative guide to the companies behind the products you buy every day.* Reading, MA: Addison-Wesley.

Maddi, S. (1967). The existential neurosis. *Journal of Abnormal Psychology, 72,* 311–325.

Maddi, S. (1970). The search for meaning. In W. Arnold & M. Page (Eds.), *The Nebraska Symposium on Motivation* (pp. 137–190). Lincoln: University of Nebraska Press.

Mangham, I. L., & Overington, M. (1987). *Organizations as*

theatre: A social psychology of dramatic appearances. Chichester, England: Wiley.

Maquet, A. (1958). *Albert Camus: The invincible summer.* New York: Braziller.

March, J. G., & Olsen, J. P. (1976). *Ambiguity and choice in organizations.* Bergen, Norway: Universitetsforlaget.

Martin, J. (1990). Deconstructing organizational taboos: The suppression of gender conflict in organizations. *Organizational Science, 1,* 339–359.

Marx, K. (1976). *Le capital* [Capital]. Paris: Éditions Sociales.

Maslow, A. (1965). *Eupsychian management: A journal.* Homewood, IL: Richard D. Irwin.

Maslow, A. (1970). *Motivation and personality* (2nd ed.). New York: Harper & Row.

Maslow, A. (1971). *The farther reaches of human nature.* New York: Viking.

Massarik, F. (1984). Searching for essence in executive experience. In S. Srivastva & Associates, *The executive mind* (pp. 243–268). San Francisco: Jossey-Bass.

Massarik, F. (1985). Human experience, phenomenology, and the process of deep sharing. In R. Tannenbaum, N. Margulies, F. Massarik, & Associates (Eds.), *Human systems development* (pp. 26–41). San Francisco: Jossey-Bass.

Maurer, J. (1968). Work as a "central life interest" of industrial supervisors. *Academy of Management Journal, 11*(3), 329–339.

May, R. (1950). *The meaning of anxiety.* New York: Washington Square Press.

May, R. (1960). *Existential psychology.* New York: Random House.

May, R. (1969). *Love and will.* New York: Norton.

May, R. (1973). *Paulus: A personal portrait of Paul Tillich.* New York: Harper & Row.

May, R. (1975). *The courage to create.* New York: Norton.

May, R. (1983). *The discovery of being: Writings in existential psychology.* New York: Norton.

May, R., Angel, E., & Ellenberg, H. F. (Eds.). (1958). *Existence: A new dimension in psychiatry and psychology.* New York: Simon & Schuster.

Mayo, G. E. (1933). *The human problems of an industrial civilization.* New York: Macmillan.

McDannell, C., & Lang, B. (1990). *Heaven: A history.* New Haven, CT: Yale University Press.

McGregor, D. (1960). *The human side of enterprise.* New York: McGraw-Hill. (French version: *La dimension humaine de l'entreprise.* Paris: Gauthier-Villars, 1976.)

McWhinney, W. (1991). *Evil in organizational life: Faustians, professionals, bureaucrats and humanists.* Working paper, the Fielding Institute, Santa Barbara, CA.

McWhinney, W. (1992). Paths of change: Strategic choices for organizations and society. Newbury Park, CA: Sage.

McWhinney, W., & Batista, J. (1988). How remythologizing can revitalize organizations. *Organizational Dynamics, 17*(2), 46–58.

Meeker-Lowry, S. (1988). *Economics as if the earth really mattered: A catalyst guide to socially conscious investing.* Philadelphia: New Society.

Meissner, W. (1991). *What is effective in psychoanalytic therapy: The move from interpretation to relation.* Northvale, NJ: Jason Aronson.

Mentzos, S. (1988). *Interpersonale und institutionalisierte Abwehr* [Interpersonal and institutionalized defense]. Frankfurt: Suhrkamp.

Merleau-Ponty, M. (1942). *La structure du comportement.* Paris: Presse Universitaire de France. (English version: *Structure of behavior.* Boston: Beacon Press, 1963.)

Messine, P. (1987). *Les saturniens* [The Saturnians]. Paris: Découverte.

Miller, D. (1992). *Le paradoxe d'Icare.* Quebec: Laval University Press. (English version: *The Icarus paradox.* New York: Harper Business, 1990.)

Miller, T., Turner, C., Tindale, R., Posavac, E., & Dugoni, B. (1991). Reasons for the trend toward null findings in research on Type A behavior. *Psychological Bulletin, 110,* 469–485.

Mills, A. J., & Tancred, P. (Eds.). (1992). *Gendering organizational analysis.* Newbury Park, CA: Sage.

Mintzberg, H. (1984). *Le manager au quotidien.* Montréal: Agence d'Arc. (English version: *The nature of managerial work.* New York: Harper & Row, 1973.)

Mintzberg, H. (1987). Les organisations ont-elles besoin de stratégies? [Do organizations need strategies?] *Revue Internationale de Gestion, 12*(4), 5–9.

Mintzberg, H. (1989). *On management: Inside our strange world of organizations.* New York: Free Press.

Mitroff, I. I. (1983). *Stakeholders of the organizational mind: Toward a new view of organizational policy making.* San Francisco: Jossey-Bass.

Mitroff, I. I. (1987). *Business NOT as usual.* San Francisco: Jossey-Bass.

Mitroff, I. I., Mason, R., & Barabba, V. (1983). Policy as argument: A logic for ill-structured decision problems. *Management Science, 28,* 1391–1404.

Mitroff, I. I., & Pauchant, T. C. (1990). *We're so big and powerful nothing bad can happen to us.* New York: Caroll Publishing.

Mitroff, I. I., Pauchant, T. C., & Shrivastava, P. (1988). Conceptual and empirical issues in the development of a general theory of crisis management. *Technological Forecasting and Social Change, 33,* 83–107.

Morgan, G. (1986). *Images of organization.* Newbury Park, CA: Sage. (French version: *Images de l'organisation.* Québec: Laval University Press; Paris: Eska, 1989.)

Morin, E. (1990, September 22). L'ère Damocléenne [The age of Damocles]. *Le Monde,* pp. 1–2.

Morin, E., & Kern, A. B. (1993). *Terre-patrie* [Motherland]. Paris: Seuil.

Morin, E. M. (1989). *Vers une mesure de l'efficacité organisationnelle: Exploration conceptuelle et empirique des représentations* [Toward measuring organizational effectiveness: Conceptual and empirical exploration of the social interpretations]. Unpublished doctoral dissertation, University of Montreal.

Morin, E. M. (1993). Enantiodromia and crisis management: A Jungian perspective. *Industrial and Environmental Crisis Quarterly, 7*(2), 91–114.

Morin, E. M., Savoie, A., & Beaudin, G. (1994). *L'efficacité des organisations: Théorie, représentations et mesures* [The effectiveness of organizations: Theory, interpretations, and measurement]. Boucherville, Quebec: Gaëtan Morin.

Morse, N. C., & Weiss, R. C. (1955). The function and meaning of work and the job. *American Sociological Review, 20*(2), 191–198.

Moser, T. (1976). *Gottesvergiftung* [God-Poisoning]. Frankfurt: Suhrkamp.

Moser, T. (1990). Die eine Zukunft und die zwei Vergangenheiten: Psychoanalytische Erwägungen zum deutschen Einigungsprozess [The one future and the two pasts: Psychoanalytical reflections on the process of German reunification]. *Das Plateau, 1,* 2, 4–15.

Moss, G. E., Dielman, J. (1986). Demographic correlates of SI assessments of Type A behavior. *Psychosomatic Medicine, 48,* 564–574.

MOW International Research Team. (1987). *The meaning of working.* San Diego, CA: Academic Press.

Multiple Risk Factor Intervention Trial Group. (1979). The MRFIT behavior pattern study 1: Study design, procedures, and reproducibility of behavior pattern judgment. *Journal of Chronic Disease, 32,* 293–305.

Nietzsche, F. (1972). *Ainsi parlait Zarathoustra: Un livre pour tous et pour personne* [Thus spake Zarathustra. A book for everyone and for no one]. Paris: Le Livre de Poche.

Olivier, C. (1989). *Jokastes Kinder: Die Psyche der Frau im Schatten der Mutter* [Jocasta's children: Woman's psyche in the mother's shadow]. Munich: Deutscher Taschenbuch.

Olivier, C. (1991). *F wie Frau: Psychoanalyse und Sexualität* [F as in Female [Woman]: Psychoanalysis and sexuality]. Dusseldorf: Econ.

Orzack, L. (1959). Work as "central life interest" of professionals. *Social Problems, 7*(2), 125–132.

O'Toole, J. (1993). *The executive compass: Business and the good society.* New York: Oxford University Press.

Pagels, E. (1991). *Adam, Eva und die Schlange: Eine Theologie der Sünde* [Adam, Eve, and the snake: A theology of sin]. Hamburg: Rowohlt.

Pagès, M. (1984). *La vie affective des groupes: Esquisse d'une théorie de la relation humaine* [The affective life of groups: Sketch of a theory of human relations]. Paris: Dunod.

Pagès, M., Bonetti, M., de Gaulejac, V., & Descendre, D. (1979). *L'emprise de l'organisation* [The ascendancy of the organization]. Paris: Presse Universitaire de France.

Palmade, J. (1988). Le management post moderne ou la technocratisation des Sciences de l'homme [Postmodern management or the technocratization of the humanities]. In J. Palmade (Ed.), *Organisation et management en question* [Organization and management in question]. Paris: L'Harmattan.

Pascale, R. T., & Athos, A. G. (1981). *The art of Japanese management.* New York: Simon & Schuster. (French version: *Le management est-il un art Japonais?* Paris: Éditions d'Organisation, 1984.)

Pascarella, P. (1980). Herzberg the humanist takes on scientific management. *Industry Week, 206*(6), 45–50; *206*(7), 69–72.

Patch, A. R. (1984). Reflections on perfection. *American Psychologist, 39*(4), 386–390.

Pauchant, T. C. (1991). Transferential leadership: Towards a more complex understanding of charisma in organizations. *Organization Studies, 12*(4), 507–527.

Pauchant, T. C. (1993). In search of existence: On the use of the existential tradition in management and organization development. In F. Massarik (Ed.). *Advances in organization development* (pp. 2, 103–127). Norwood, NJ: Ablex.

Pauchant, T. C. (in press). Chester I. Barnard and the guardians of the managerial state. *Academy of Management Review.*

Pauchant, T. C. & Cotard, N. (in press). Votre enterprise est-elle "apprenante" ou "porte-crise": La gestion des crises et de la contre-production au Canada [Is your organization "learning" or "crisis-prone": Crisis management and the management of "counterproduction" in Canada]. *Revue Internationale de Gestion.*

Pauchant, T. C., & Fortier, I. (1990). Anthropocentric ethics in organizations: Strategic management and the environment. In P. Shrivastava and R. Lamb (Eds.), *Advances in strategic management* (pp. 99–114). Greenwich, CT: JAI Press.

Pauchant, T. C., & Mitroff, I. I. (1992). *Transforming the crisis-prone organization: Preventing individual, organizational, and environmental tragedies.* San Francisco: Jossey-Bass.

Pauchant, T. C., & Morin, E. M. (1994). Preventing crises and learning from them: The existential courage to manage complexity. In *The emergency planning college: Crises in a complex society* (pp. 59–74). Easing Wold, York, England: The Emergency Planning College.

Pauck, W., & Pauck, M. (1989). *Paul Tillich: His life and thought.* New York: Harper & Row.

Peck, M. S. (1978). *The road less traveled: A new psychology of love, traditional values, and spiritual growth.* New York: Simon & Schuster.

Perls, F., Hefferline, R., & Goodman, P. (1951). *Gestalt therapy.* New York: Delta Books.

Perrenoud, P. (1987). Sociologie de l'excellence ordinaire [Sociology of ordinary excellence]. *Autrement, 86.*

Perrow, C. (1979, May). *Organizational theory in a society of organizations.* International Conference on Public Administration. Quebec City, Quebec.

Peters, T. J. (1986). In search of arrogance. In R. Nadler & W. Taylor (Eds.), *The big boys: Power and position in American business* (pp. ix–xv). New York: Pantheon Books.

Peters, T. J. (1988). *Thriving on chaos: Handbook for a management revolution.* New York: Knopf.

Peters, T. J. (1992). *Liberation management: Necessary disorganization for the nanosecond nineties.* New York: Knopf.

Peters, T. J., & Austin, N. (1985). *A passion for excellence: The leadership difference.* New York: Random House.

Peters, T. J., & Waterman, R. H., Jr. (1982). *In search of excellence: Lessons from America's best-run companies.* New York: Harper & Row. (French version: *Le prix de l'excellence.* Paris: Inter-Éditions, 1983.)

Pondy, L. R., Frost, P., Morgan, G., & Dandridge, T. (Eds.). (1983). *Organizational symbolism.* Greenwich, CT: JAI Press.

Post, J. (1986a). Hostility, conformity, fraternity: The group dynamics of terrorist behavior. *International Journal of Group Psychotherapy, 36,* 211–224.

Post, J. (1986b). It's us against them: The group dynamics of political terrorism. *Terrorism, 10,* 23–36.

Preston, L. E. (1978). Analyzing corporate social performance: Methods and results. *Journal of Contemporary Business, 7,* 135–150.

Price, V. A. (1988). Research and clinical issues in treating Type A behavior. In B. K. Houston & C. R. Snyder (Eds.), *Type A behavior pattern: Research, theory, and intervention* (pp. 275–311). New York: Wiley.

Quinn, R. E. (1977). Coping with Cupid: The formation, impact, and management of romantic relationships in organizations. *Administrative Science Quarterly, 22,* 30–45.

Quinn, R. E. (1988). *Beyond rational management: Mastering the paradoxes and competing demands of high performance.* San Francisco: Jossey-Bass.

Quinn, R. E., & Rohrbaugh, J. (1981). A competing values approach to organizational effectiveness. *Public Productivity Review, 5*(2), 122–139.

Quinn, R. E., & Rohrbaugh, J. (1983). A spatial model of effectiveness criteria: Toward a competing values approach to organizational analysis. *Management Science, 29*(3), 363–377.

Rank, O. (1945). *Will therapy and truth and reality.* New York: Knopf.

Rank, O. (1958). *Beyond psychology.* New York: Dover Books. (Original work published 1941)

Rank, O. (1961). *Psychology and the soul.* New York: A. S. Barnes. (Original work published 1930)

Rank, O. (1973). *The trauma of birth.* New York: Harper & Row. (Original work published 1924)

Rank, O. (1978a). *Will therapy: An analysis of the therapeutic process in terms of relationship* (J. Taft, Trans.). New York: Norton. (Original work published 1936)

Rank, O. (1978b). *Truth and reality: A life history of the human will* (J. Taft, Trans.). New York: Norton. (Original work published 1936)

Rank, O. (1989). *Art and artist: Creative urge and personality development* (C. Atkinson, Trans.). New York: Norton. (Original work published 1932)

Rank, O. (in press). *Otto Rank: Selected American lectures* (R. Kramer, Ed.). Princeton, N.J.: Princeton University Press.

Reason, P. (Ed.). (1988). *Human inquiry in action: Developments in new paradigm research.* Newbury Park, CA: Sage.

Reason, P. (1993). Reflections on sacred experience and sacred science. *Journal of Management Inquiry, 2*(3), 273–283.

Reed, B. (1976). Organizational role analysis. In I. L. Cooper (Ed.), *Developing social skills in managers* (pp. 89–102). London: Macmillan.

Regis, P. F. (1932). *Der Klosterobere: Sein Amt und seine Persönlichkeit. Aszetisch-praktische Grundsätze für Vorsteher und Vorsteherinnen klösterlicher Niederlassungen* [The convent head — Office and personality: Ascetic/practical principles for father and mother superiors in convent settings]. Wiesbaden, Germany: Matthias-Grünewald.

Reich, R. B. (1992, January 9). Is Japan really out to get us? *New York Times Book Review,* pp. 1, 24–25.

Reinke, E. (1987). Über frühzeitige Ichentwicklung und weibliche Selbstentwertung: Eine moderne Variante weiblicher Emanzipation [Regarding early ego development and low self-esteem in women: A modern variation on women's emancipation]. In K. Brede & others. (Eds.), *Befreiung zum Widerstand. Aufsätze zu Feminismus, Psychoanalyse, und Politik* [Freedom for resistance: Essays on feminism, psychoanalysis, and politics] (pp. 204–212). Frankfurt: Fischer.

Rice, J. H. (1960). Existentialism for the businessman. *Harvard Business Review, 38*(2), 135–143.

Riley, P. F. (1990). Michel Foucault, lust, women, and sin in Louis XIV's Paris. *Church History, 59,* 35–50.

Roethlisberger, F. (1977). *The elusive phenomena: An autobiographical account of my work in organizational behavior at the Harvard Business School.* Boston: Harvard Business School, Division of Research.

Rogers, C. (1951). *Client-centered therapy: Its current practice, implication, theory.* Boston: Houghton Mifflin.

Rogers, C. (1959). A theory of therapy, personality, and interpersonal relationships as developed in the client-centered framework. In S. Koch (Ed.), *Psychology: A study of a science* (pp. 184–256). New York: McGraw-Hill.

Rogers, C. (1961a). *On becoming a person.* Boston: Houghton Mifflin.

Rogers, C. (1961b). Two divergent trends. In R. May (Ed.), *Existential psychology* (pp. 85–93). New York: Random House.

Rogers, C. (1980). *A way of being.* Boston: Houghton Mifflin.

Rogers, C. (1983). *Freedom to learn for the 80s.* Columbus, OH: Merrill.

Rogers, C., & Roethlisberger, F. (1952, July-August). Barriers and gateways to communication. *Harvard Business Review, 30*(4), 46–52.

Roman, J. (1987). Excellence, individualisme, et légitimité [Excellence, individualism, and legitimacy]. *Autrement, 86.*

Rondeau, A., & Boulard, F. (1992, February). Gérer des employés qui font problème, une habileté à développer [Managing problem employees, a skill to develop]. *Gestion,* pp. 32–42.

Rosenman, R. H., Brand, R. J., Scholtz, R. I., & Friedman, M. (1966). Coronary heart disease in the Western Collaborative Group Study: A follow-up experience of two years. *Journal of the American Medical Association, 195,* 130–136.

Rosenman, R. H., Brand, R. J., Scholtz, R. I., & Friedman, M. (1976). Multivariate prediction of coronary heart disease during 8.5 year follow-up in the Western Collaborative Group Study. *American Journal of Cardiology, 37,* 903–910.

Rosenman, R. H., Swan, G. E., & Carmelli, D. (1988). Definition, assessment, and evolution of the Type A behavior pattern. In B. K. Houston & C. R. Snyder (Eds.), *Type A behavior pattern: Research, theory, and intervention* (pp. 8–31). New York: Wiley.

Rosset, C. (1976). *Le réel et son double* [The real and its double]. Paris: Gallimard.

Rowan, J. (1988). *Ordinary ecstasy: Humanistic psychology in action.* London: Routledge.

Ruffin, J. E. (1984). The anxiety of meaninglessness. *Journal of Counseling and Development, 63*(1), 40–42.

Russell, P., & Evans, R. (1992). *The creative manager: Finding inner vision and wisdom in uncertain times.* San Francisco: Jossey-Bass.

Sarason, S. B. (1972). *The creation of settings and the future societies.* San Francisco: Jossey-Bass.

Sartre, J.-P. (1945). *Les chemins de la liberté:* Vol 2. *Le sursis.* Paris: Gallimard. (English version: *The age of reason.* London: Penguin Books, 1961.)

Sartre, J.-P. (1966). *Being and nothingness.* New York: Washington Square Press.

Sartre, J.-P. (1970). *L'existentialisme est un humanisme*. Paris: Nagel. (English version: *Existentialism and humanism*. Brooklyn, NY: M.S.G. Haskell House, 1977.)

Sayers, J. (1991). *Mothers of psychoanalysis: Helen Deutsch, Karen Horney, Anna Freud, Melanie Klein*. New York: McGraw-Hill.

Schaberg, J. (1989). Die Stammütter und die Mutter Jesu [The ancestress and the mother of Christ]. *Concilium, 25,* 528–533.

Schaef, A. W., & Fassel, D. (1988). *The addictive organization*. San Francisco: HarperSanFrancisco.

Schein, E. H. (1985). *Organizational culture and leadership*. San Francisco: Jossey-Bass.

Schein, E. H. (1987). The clinical perspective in fieldwork. *Qualitative Research Method, 5.* Newbury Park, CA: Sage.

Schmidbauer, W. (1991). Ich wollte doch nur helfen . . . [But I only wanted to help . . .]. *Psychologie Heute, 18,* 8, 50–53.

Schmidt, H., & Schmidt, M. (1982). *Die vergessene Bildersprache christlicher Kunst: Ein Führer zum Verständnis der Tier-, Engel- und Mariensymbolik* [The forgotten pictorial language of Christian art: A guide to understanding the symbolism of animals, angels, and Mary]. Munich: C. H. Beck.

Schumacher, E. F. (1977). *A guide for the perplexed*. New York: HarperCollins.

Schumacher, E. F. (1979). *Good work*. New York: HarperCollins.

Schwartz, H. (1983). Maslow and the hierarchical enactment of organizational reality. *Human Relations, 36*(10), 933–956.

Schwartz, H. (1985). The usefulness of myth and the myth of usefulness: A dilemma for the applied organization scientist. *Journal of Management, 11*(1), 31–42.

Schwartz, H. S. (1987a). Anti-social actions of committed organizational participants: An existential psychoanalytic perspective. *Organization Studies, 8*(4), 327–340.

Schwartz, H. S. (1987b). On the psychodynamics of organizations' totalitarianism. *Journal of Management, 13*(1), 42–54.

Schwartz, H. S. (1990a). The symbol of the space shuttle and the degeneration of the American dream. In P. Gagliardi (Ed.), *Symbols and artifacts: Views of the corporate landscape*. (pp. 303–322). Berlin: De Gruyter.

Schwartz, H. S. (1990b). *Narcissistic process and corporate decay:*

The theory of the organization ideal. New York: New York University Press.

Scott, W. R. (1987). *Organizations: Rational, natural, and open systems*. Englewood Cliffs, NJ: Prentice-Hall.

Seashore, S. E., & Yutchman, E. (1967). Factorial analysis of organizational performance. *Administrative Science Quarterly, 12*(3), 377–395.

Segal, H. (1972). A delusional system as a defence against the re-emergence of a catastrophic situation. *International Journal of Psycho-Analysis, 53,* 393–401.

Senge, P. M. (1990). *The fifth discipline: The art and practice of the learning organization*. New York: Doubleday.

Sennett, R. (1979). *Les tyrannies de l'intimité* [The tyrannies of intimacy]. Paris: Seuil.

Sennett, R., & Cobb, J. (1972). *The hidden injuries of class*. New York: Vintage Books.

Serres, M. (1990). *Le contrat naturel* [The natural contract]. Paris: Éditions François Bourin.

Shepherdson, K. V. (1984). The meaning of work and employment: Psychological research and psychologists' values. *Australian Psychologist, 19*(3), 311–320.

Shorris, E. (1981). *The oppressed middle: Politics of middle management, scenes from corporate life*. New York: Doubleday Anchor.

Shrivastava, P. (1987). *Bhopal: Anatomy of a crisis*. New York: Ballinger.

Shrivastava, P. (1993). Crisis theory/practice: Towards a sustainable future. *Industrial and Environmental Crisis Quarterly, 7*(1), 23–42.

Shrivastava, P. (1994). *Greening business: Toward sustainable corporations*. Unpublished manuscript. Bucknell University, Lewisburg, PA.

Sievers, B. (1986a). Participation as a collusive quarrel over immortality. *Dragon 1*(1), 72–82.

Sievers, B. (1986b). Beyond the surrogate of motivation. *Organization Studies, 7*(4), 335–351.

Sievers, B. (1989). "I will not let thee go, except thou bless me!" Some considerations about the constitution of authority, inheritance, and succession. In F. Gabelnick, & A. W. Carr

(Eds.), *Contributions to social and political science: Proceedings of the First International Symposium on Group Relations* (pp. 155–173). Washington, DC: A. K. Rice Institute.

Sievers, B. (1990a). Curing the monster: Some images and considerations about the dragon. In P. Gagliardi (Ed.), *Symbols and artifacts: Views of the corporate landscape.* (pp. 207–231). Berlin: De Gruyter.

Sievers, B. (1990b). Thoughts on the relatedness of work, death, and life itself. *European Management Journal, 8*(3), 321–324.

Sievers, B. (1990c). The diabolization of death: Some thoughts on the obsolescence of mortality in organization theory and practice. In J. Hassard and D. Pym (Eds.), *The theory and philosophy of organizations: Critical issues and new perspectives* (pp. 125–136). London: Routledge.

Sievers, B. (1990d). La motivation: Un ersatz de significations [Motivation: A substitute for meaning]. In J.-F. Chanlat (Ed.), *L'individu dans l'organisation: Les dimensions oubliées* [The person in the organization: The forgotten dimensions] (pp. 337–361). Quebec: Laval University Press; Paris: Eska.

Sievers, B. (1992, June 30–July 3). *Characters in search of a theatre: Organization as theatre for the drama of childhood and the drama of work.* Paper presented at the tenth anniversary Standing Conference on Organizational Symbolism, Lancaster University.

Sievers, B. (1993). *Love in the time of AIDS.* Working papers from the economic studies subject area of the Bergische University, Wuppertal, Germany.

Sievers, B. (1994). *Work, death, and life itself: Essays on management and organization.* Berlin: De Gruyter.

Simon, H. A. (1947). *Administrative behavior: A study of the decision-making process in administrative organization.* New York: Free Press. (French version: *Administration et processus de décisions.* Paris: Economica, 1983.)

Simon, H. A. (1973a). Applying information technology to organization design. *Public Administration Review, 33*(3), 268–279.

Simon, H. A. (1973b). Organization man: Rational and self-actualizing. *Public Administration Review, 33*(4), 354–358.

Slipp, S. (Ed.). (1982). *Curative factors in dynamic psychotherapy.* New York: McGraw-Hill.

Smircich, L. (1983). Concepts of culture and organizational analysis. *Administrative Science Quarterly, 28,* 339–358.

Smith, D. (Ed.). (1993). *Business and the environment: Implications of the new environmentalism.* London: Paul Chapman.

Smith, K. K. (1982). Philosophical problems in thinking about organizational change. In P. S. Goodman & Associates, *Change in organizations.* San Francisco: Jossey-Bass.

Smith, K. K., & Berg, D. N. (1987). *Paradoxes of group life: Understanding conflict, paralysis, and movement in group dynamics.* San Francisco: Jossey-Bass.

Spiegel, der. (1990). Bei Triebschub beten: Juristen, Theologen und Mediziner streiten über Sexualität [To pray under the press of inner drives: Lawyers, theologians, and doctors argue about sexuality]. *Psychiatrie und Behinderten-Heimen, 2,* 100–110.

Srivastva, S., & Associates. (1988). *Executive integrity: The search for high human values in organizational life.* San Francisco: Jossey-Bass.

Starbuck, W. H., Greve, A., & Hedberg, B.L.T. (1978). Responding to crises. *Journal of Business Administration, 9,* 111–137.

Steers, R. M. (1977). *Organizational effectiveness: A behavioral view.* Santa Monica, CA: Goodyear.

Steiner, J. (1990). Die Wechselwirkungen zwischen pathologischen Organisationen und der paranoid-schizoiden und depressiven Situation [The reciprocal effects between pathological organizations and the paranoid-schizoid and depressed situation]. In Elisabeth Bott Spilius (Ed.), *Melanie Klein Heute: Entwicklungen in Theorie und Praxis* [Melanie Klein today: Developments in theory and practice] (pp. 408–431). Munich: Internationale Analyse.

Strati, A. (1992). Aesthetic understanding of organizational life. *Academy of Management Review, 17,* 568–581.

Sutherland, J. E., Pershy, V. W., & Brody, J. (1990). Proportionate mortality trends: 1950 through 1986. *Journal of the American Medical Association, 264,* 3178–3184.

Taft, J. (1968). *Otto Rank: A biographical study based on notebooks, letters, collected writings, therapeutic achievements, and personal associations.* New York: Julian Press.

Tannenbaum, R., & Hanna, B. W. (1985). Holding on, letting

go, and moving on: Understanding a neglected perspective on change. In R. Tannenbaum, N. Margulies, F. Massarik, & Associates (Eds.), *Human systems development* (pp. 95–121). San Francisco: Jossey-Bass.

Tausky, C. (1969). Meaning of work among blue-collar men. *Pacific Sociological Review, 12*(1), 49–55.

Taylor, F. W. (1911). *The principles of scientific management.* New York: Harper & Row. (French version: *La direction scientifique des entreprises.* Paris: Dunod, 1965.)

Terkel, S. (1972). *Working.* New York: Pantheon. (French version: *Gagner sa croûte.* Paris: Fayard, 1976.)

Theobald, M. (1990). Heilige Hochzeit: Motive des Mythos im Horizont von Eph. 5:21–33 [Holy matrimony: Mythical motifs in the light of Eph. 5:2–33]. In K. Kartelge (Ed.), *Metaphorik und Mythos im Neuen Testament* [Metaphor and myth in the New Testament] (pp. 220–254). Freiburg, Germany: Herder.

Thoresen, C. E., & Bracke, P. E. (1993). Reducing coronary recurrences and coronary prone behavior: A structural group approach. In J. Spira (Ed.), *Group therapy for the medically ill.* New York: Guilford Publications.

Thorne, B. (1992). *Carl Rogers.* Newbury Park, CA: Sage.

Tillich, P. (1948). *The shaking of the foundations.* New York: Scribner's.

Tillich, P. (1952). *The courage to be.* New Haven, CT: Yale University Press.

Tillich, P. (1966). *On the boundary.* New York: Scribner's.

Torbert, W. R. (1991). *The power of balance: Transforming self, society, and scientific inquiry.* Newbury Park, CA: Sage.

Toulmin, S. (1958). *The uses of argument.* Cambridge, England: Cambridge University Press.

Treiber, H. (1990). Der Fabrikherr des 19. Jahrhunderts als Moral-Unternehmer: Über die Fabrikation von "Berufsmenchen" in einer entzauberten Welt [The nineteenth-century factory owner as a morale-entrepreneur: Regarding the production of "career people" in a world deprived of magic]. In H. König, B. von Grieff, & H. S. Mauer (Eds.), *Sozialphilosophie der industriellen Arbeit* [Social philosophy of industrial work] (pp. 149–177). Opladen, Germany: Westdeutscher.

Trost, C. (1990, May 2). Women managers quit not for family but to advance their corporate climb. *Wall Street Journal,* pp. B1, B2.

Türk, K. (1976). *Grundlagen einer Pathologie der Organisation* [Rudiments of a pathology of the organization]. Stuttgart: Ferdinand Enke.

Türk, K. (1980). Pathologie der Organisation [Pathology of the organization]. In E. Grochla (Ed.), *Handwörterbuch der Organisation, 1855–1864* [A pocket dictionary of the organization]. Stuttgart: Poeschel.

Turner, A., & Lombard, G. (1969). *Interpersonal behavior and administration.* New York: Free Press.

Turner, B. A. (Ed.). (1990). *Organizational symbolism.* Berlin: De Gruyter.

Turner, B. A. (1992). The symbolic understanding of organizations. In M. Reed & M. Hughes (Eds.), *Rethinking organization: New directions in organization theory and analysis* (pp. 46–66). Newbury Park, CA: Sage.

Vaill, P. (1985). Integrating the diverse directions of the behavioral sciences. In R. Tannebaum, N. Margulies, F. Massarik, & Associates, *Human systems development* (pp. 547–577). San Francisco: Jossey-Bass.

Vaill, P. (1989). *Managing as a performing art: New ideas for a world of chaotic change.* San Francisco: Jossey-Bass.

Van Der Meersch, E. (1987). Résistance au temps ou vitesse de notoriété [Resistance to time or speed of notoriety]. *Autrement, 86.*

Van de Ven, A. H. (1980). A process for organization assessment. In E. E. Lawler, D. A. Nadler, & C. Cammann (Eds.), *Organization assessment: Perspectives on the measurement of organizational behavior and the quality of work life* (pp. 548–568). New York: Wiley.

Van de Ven, A. H., & Delbecq, A. L. (1974). The effectiveness of nominal, Delphi, and interacting group decision making processes. *Academy of Management Journal, 17*(4), 605–621.

Van Egeren, L. F. (1991). *A "success trap" theory of Type A behavior.* Corte Madera, CA: Select Press.

Vecchio, R. (1980). The function and meaning of work and

the job: Morse and Weiss, 1955. *Academy of Management Journal, 23*(2), 361–367.

Vedder, J. N. (1992). How much can we learn from success? *Academy of Management Executive, 6*(1), 56–66.

Vogel, D. (1986). The study of social issues in management: A critical appraisal. *California Management Review, 28*(2), 142–151.

Weber, M. (1964). *L'éthique protestante et l'esprit du capitalisme.* Paris: Plon. (English version: *The Protestant ethic and the spirit of capitalism.* New York: Scribner's, 1958.)

Weick, K. E. (1979). *The social psychology of organizing.* New York: Random House.

Weick, K. E. (1984). Managerial thought in the context of action. In S. Srivastva and Associates, *The executive mind: New insights on managerial thought and action* (pp. 221–242). San Francisco: Jossey-Bass.

Weigand, W., & Sievers, B. (1985). Rolle und Beratung in Organisationen [Role and consultation in organizations]. *Supervision, 7,* 41–61.

Weil, S. (1949). *L'enracinement: Prélude à une déclaration des devoirs envers l'être humain* [Rootedness: Prelude to a declaration of duties toward the human being]. Paris: Gallimard.

Weil, S. (1964). *La condition ouvrière* [The condition of workers]. Paris: Gallimard.

Weil, S. (1970). *First and last notebooks.* Oxford, England: Oxford University Press.

Weil, S. (1988a). A propos de la condition humaine [Regarding the human condition]. In P. Devaux & F. De Lussy (Eds.), *Simone Weil: Oeuvres Complètes: Vol. 2. Écrits historiques et politiques* [S.W. Complete works: Vol. 2. Historical and political writings]. Paris: Gallimard. (Original work published 1933)

Weil, S. (1988b). *Simone Weil: Écrits historiques et politiques* [Simone Weil: Historical and political writings]. (G. Leroy, Ed.). Paris: Gallimard.

Weisbord, M. (1987). *Productive workplaces: Organizing and managing for dignity, meaning, and community.* San Francisco: Jossey-Bass.

Weisskopf-Joelson, E. (1967). Meaning as an integrating factor. In C. Bühler & F. Massarik (Eds.), *The course of human life: A study of goals in the humanistic perspective.* New York: Springer.

Wells, L. (1980). The group-as-a-whole: A systemic socioanalytic perspective on interpersonal and group relations. In C. P. Alderfer and C. L. Cooper (Eds.), *Advances in experiential social processes.* New York: Wiley.

Wells, S., & Taylor, G. (Eds.). (1987). *The complete Oxford Shakespeare: Vol. 1. Histories.* Oxford, England: Oxford University Press. (Original work published 1597 and 1600)

Westerlund, G., & Sjöstrand, S.-V. (1981). *Organisationsmythen* [Organizational myths]. Stuttgart: Klett-Cotta.

White, K. (1987). Residential care of adolescents: Residents, carers and sexual issues. In G. Horobin (Ed.), *Sex, Gender and Care Work* (pp. 52–65). London: Jessica Kingsley.

White, R. W. (1959). Motivation reconsidered: The concept of competence. *Psychological Review, 66*(4), 297–323.

Whitehead, A. N. (1929). *Process and reality: An essay in cosmology.* New York: Free Press.

Whitehead, A. N. (1961). *Adventures of ideas.* New York: Free Press. (Original work published 1933)

Who's excellent now? (1984, November 5). *Business Week,* pp. 76–88.

Wilden, A. (1972). *System and structure.* London: Tavistock. (French version: *Système et structure.* Montreal: Boréal Express, 1983.)

Winnicott, D. W. (1950). Some thoughts on the meaning of the word democracy. *Human Relations, 3,* 175–186.

Wolf, W. B. (1974). *The basic Barnard: An introduction to Chester I. Barnard and his theories of organization and management.* Ithaca, NY: Cornell University, Industrial and Labor Relations Press.

Yalom, I. D. (1970). *Theory and practice of group psychotherapy.* New York: Basic Books.

Yalom, I. D. (1980a). *Existential psychotherapy.* New York: Basic Books.

Yalom, I. D. (1980b). The mental health care revolution: Will psychology survive? *American Psychologist, 44,* 703–708.

Yalom, I. D. (1989). *Love's executioner and other tales of psychotherapy.* New York: Basic Books.

Yalom, I. D. (1992). *When Nietzsche wept.* New York: Basic Books.

Yates, R. (1988, November 13). Japanese live and die for their work. *Chicago Tribune.*

Zahra, S. A., & Latour, M. S. (1987). Corporate social responsibility and organizational effectiveness: A multivariate approach. *Journal of Business Ethics, 6,* 459–467.

Zaleznik, A. (1989). *The managerial mystique: Restoring leadership in business.* New York: Harper & Row.

Zeri, F. (1987). *Behind the image: The art of reading paintings.* London: Heinemann.

Zimmerman, M. E. (1983). Toward a Heideggerian ethos for radical environmentalism. *Environmental Ethics, 5,* 99–131.

Name Index

Subject Index